Praise for

THE COMPLETE BOOK OF
VINYASA YOGA

"Srivatsa Ramaswami's book is nothing less than a treasure for yoga students at every level of ability. Its informative introduction to practice, combined with clear descriptions of literally hundreds of yoga postures, have brought Krishnamacharya's vision of *asana* teaching to life. Each pose is skillfully embedded within a classical family of movements—a *vinyasa* sequence—and these are illustrated by well-chosen photographs. Equally valuable, the text grounds each reader in the fundamental idea of vinyasa—the integration of movement, breath, and mindfulness that is so vital to a rewarding yoga practice. Aided by its simple and agreeable style of writing, this book will undoubtedly become a standard reference for those seeking to understand the spirit of yoga."

—ROLF SOVIK, PsyD., Spiritual Director, Himalayan International Institute, coauthor of *Yoga: Mastering the Basics*

"This book is a precious contribution to yoga; ancient knowledge brought forth by Professor T. Krishnamacharya and faithfully presented to us by his dear student Ramaswami. You can place these vital principles into the yoga that you already know and love to make your practice powerful, safe, and efficient. This is the full spectrum of yoga from the "teacher of our teachers." With no agenda except to accurately represent yoga, Ramaswami duplicates his teacher's knowledge gathered over thirty-three years of private lessons with him. Study this book. It is straight from the source."

—MARK WHITWELL, author of *Yoga of the Heart*

"*The Complete Book of Vinyasa Yoga* is truly comprehensive as it incorporates proper breathing guidance coordinated with an incredible variety of yoga vinyasas. Techniques for stretching and strengthening the thoracic muscles associated with breathing and increasing the length of inhale and exhale makes this book useful even in therapeutic settings. In teaching yoga to cancer patients at the USC (University of Southern California) cancer hospital, breath awareness and control (pranayama) is the most important ingredient for decreasing pain. Additionally, bandhas are essential for restoring strength to the inner core of pelvic muscles in prostate cancer patients. Ramaswami has included all. This book supplies me with a complete array of tools to help my students."

—VIVIAN RICHMAN, yoga therapist, USC/Norris Cancer Center

"Beautiful. Masterful. Complete. The full spectrum of Krishnamacharya's asana teaching methods. Instructions are clear, concise, accurate, fully illustrated, and given in exquisite detail. Here for the first time are all eleven sequences including the Visesha (special) sequences and a chapter on the proper way to end a practice. Ardent students and serious teachers of the yoga of Krishnamacharya will rejoice."

—DAVID HURWITZ, yoga instructor

THE
COMPLETE BOOK OF
VINYASA
YOGA

SRIVATSA RAMASWAMI

THE
COMPLETE BOOK OF
VINYASA
YOGA

AN AUTHORITATIVE PRESENTATION—BASED ON 30 YEARS
OF DIRECT STUDY UNDER THE LEGENDARY YOGA
TEACHER KRISHNAMACHARYA

MARLOWE & COMPANY
NEW YORK

THE COMPLETE BOOK OF VINYASA YOGA
An Authoritative Presentation—Based on 30 Years of Direct Study
Under the Legendary Yoga Teacher Krishnamacharya
Copyright © 2005 by Srivatsa Ramaswami
Photographs copyright © 2004 by Srivatsa Ramaswami

Published by
Marlowe & Company
An Imprint of Avalon Publishing Group Incorporated
245 West 17th Street • 11th Floor
New York, NY 10011-5300

AVALON
publishing group incorporated

Library of Congress Cataloging-in-Publication Data
Ramaswami, Srivatsa.
The complete book of vinyasa yoga: an authoritative presentation, based on 30 years of direct study under the legendary yoga teatcher Krishnamacharya / Srivatsa Ramaswami.
p. cm.
Includes bibliographical references and index.
ISBN 1-56924-402-2 (pbk.: alk. paper)
1. Yoga. I. Krishnamacharya, T., b. 1888. II. Title.

RA781.7.R32 2005
613.7'046—dc22
2005000398

9 8 7 6 5 4 3 2 1

Designed by Pauline Neuwirth, Neuwirth & Associates

Printed in Italy

DEDICATED TO

My Lord, My Pal

Who Creates All

Who Sustains All

Who Survives All

CONTENTS

ACKNOWLEDGMENTS

MY SINCERE THANKS to three people who had a very positive influence on my life, my mother, my father, and my guru, Sri. Krishnamacharya. They were always willing to give affection, resources, and knowledge, desiring only happiness for me and nothing for themselves in return.

My wife, Uma, has been very supportive all along. With her medical background, she helped me to look at yoga more dispassionately, which has been very helpful. My sons, Prasanna and Badri, continue to help me with mature advice. My daughters-in-law, Tina and Audrey, always chipped in with genuine interest.

I am beholden to all my young friends/students, Tatyana Popova, Girija, Ranjit Babu, Dr. Mahendran, Kirti, Klaus Koenig, and Thiruchelvan, for willingly giving the time and expertise to help landscape the book with their exquisite yoga pictures. My sincere thanks are due to Sri. P. N. Srinivasan of Krishna Photo Stores in Chennai India, for shooting, scanning, and editing all the pictures. He has been our family photographer for more than fifty years now.

Dr. Jaime Schmitt, herself the author of a beautiful book, *Every Woman's Yoga,* read the first few chapters of my manuscript and gave many useful suggestions, and I am thankful to her. Others including Yogi Dave, John Coon, Badri, Mini Shastri and Prasanna have also given useful input; thank you all.

I am thankful to many yoga stalwarts, especially Dr. Rolf Sovik, Shiva Rea, Dr. Chris Chapple, Suddha Weixler, and Nishit Patel for their support. The yoga world is now saturated with several branded systems. Still, many schools were willing to afford me opportunities to present this vinyasa krama method. I am thankful to

Kalakshetra (where I taught for more than twenty years), Public Health Center, Sri. Ramachandra Medical University, and Yoga Brotherhood in Chennai, India; Loyola Marymount University, Esalen Institute (Big Sur), Yoga Works, Yoga Garden Studios and Heartofyoga in California; Sonic Yoga, Beyoga, Yoga Tree, Breathing Project, and Yogaforwellbeing, in New York State; Himalayan Institute of Yoga in Honesdale, PA, Buffalo, NY, Chicago, and New York City, NY; Yoga Center in Houston; Yoga Mind in Chicago; Yogavita, Teaneck, NJ; Yogagarage in Cincinnati; and others. Many individual students and teachers have studied vinyasa yoga in depth with me. Many of them have also incorporated essentials of vinyasa krama into their teaching and practice, even from Day 1, and have given me useful feedback that was helpful in shaping this book. In this regard, I must thank C. S. Sampath, Prof. Janardhanan, Dr. Rangaswamy, Pam Hoxsey, John Coon, Yogi Dave, Mark Whitwell, Vivian Richman, Pam Johnson, Hilary Nixon, Shawn White, Fran Ubertini, Sri. Ramanathan, Debbie Mills, Rita Varghese, Sarah Mata, Sherie Scheer, Lisa Leeman, Chris Bannister, Cristhal Bennett, Linda Chausee, Ampro Denney, Arun Deva, Crystal Fu, Mike Gandolfi, Merrilee Gilson, Tonya Riley, Karen Goldsmith, Rebecca Greenbaum, Jessica Harper, Barry Liss, Cathy Mah, Michael Manoogian, Robyn Marin, Suheila Mouammar, Jessica Russel, Ross Smith, Christine Sugiyama, Kathaleen Shraddha Sweeney, Trampas Thompson, Deborah Woody, Yukiko Amaya, Charlotte Holtzerman, Chris Arns, Kit Barile, Linda Dynek, Leah Finch, Cheeko Lal, Herbert Lube, Beth Marik, Barbra Noh, Melissa Noble, and Jake Quealy.

My experience with my agent, Bob Silverstein of Quicksilver books, has been wholesome. I have made another good friend in Matthew Lore of Marlowe & Company, the publisher of the book. I am also beholden to Kylie Foxx, senior editor of Marlowe & Company for her energy, guidance, and expert editorial input to my book.

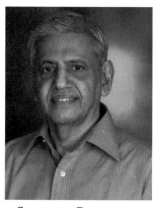

SRIVATSA RAMASWAMI

PREFACE

MY STUDY OF yoga and related subjects under my guru, Sri. T. Krishnamacharya, spanned over three decades. I first met him when I was about fifteen years old, when he, at the request of my father, came to my house to teach yoga to my somewhat handicapped brother. Soon all the members of our family were his students. With my guru I studied hatha yoga, Vedic chanting, and important yoga and related texts, such as the *Yoga Sutras*, the *Upanishads*, the *Bhagavat Gita*, *Samkhya*, elements of *Tarka,* and others. I started teaching only after more than fifteen years of rather intense study with him. I taught hatha yoga to students of Kalakshetra, which is recognized as an institution of national importance by the government of India. I taught for more than twenty years. Since the students were young and artists and dancers, their interest and quality of practice were of a high order. My guru taught me vinyasa krama over three decades, in a comprehensive manner, with all the beautiful flowing sequences linked closely to smooth, deliberate breaths—the unique yoking of body and mind that vinyasa krama provides. I also observed Krishnamacharya teach other students and give demonstrations, which all helped me to slowly understand the unfolding of yoga practice as a consummate art. I have attempted to present this gift from my guru in this book.

My guru, T. Krishnamacharya, was born in 1888. He died in 1989. I can divide his one hundred years into three stages. Sri. Krishnamacharya spent the first forty years meeting with sages in different parts of India, studying and acquiring deep spiritual knowledge and practices, and earning an array of impressive diplomas and titles in subjects ranging from Sanskrit and yoga to Vedic studies. Under the benevolence of the then Maharaja of Mysore. Krishnamacharya settled down in the region and took charge of the Yoga School set up at the Mysore Palace, where he trained a number of students, including members of the royal family, in yoga. He did this until the early 1950s.

During this earlier period, two of Sri. Krishnamacharya's students went off to work independently. One was Mr. B. K. S. Iyengar, Sri. Krishnamacharya's student and brother-in-law. Being young and an early student of my guru, Iyengar developed a very physical style of yoga that was an aggressive form of the method he'd learned from Krishnamacharya. Iyengar's tremendous control over his body and incredible ability to do difficult postures with considerable ease made him an instant success in the West. Iyengar yoga became very popular, and stalwart practitioners like J. Krishnamurti, Yehudi Menuhin, and others helped make Iyengar a celebrity. Iyengar's book, *Light on Yoga*,

> "Sri. Krishnamacharya spent the first forty years meeting with sages in different parts of India, studying and acquiring deep spiritual knowledge and practices, and earning an array of impressive diplomas and titles . . ."

with its breathtaking poses, became immensely popular throughout the world, especially in the West. However, Iyengar's method omitted several important ingredients of Krishnamacharya's teaching, such as progression or sequencing of asanas, use of counterposes, and the complete synchronization of breath. Nevertheless, Iyengar's system caught the imagination of millions of yoga enthusiasts and made him more famous than his teacher. While Iyengar globetrotted and ran a prestigious school in India, Krishnamacharya continued to teach in a low-key, mostly one-on-one basis. He never went abroad—nor did he wish to—but did have a few Western students, like Indira Devi, who came to him.

The other student of Krishnamacharya from the Mysore days was Pattabhi Jois, who also became tremendously popular. He based his method on Krishnamacharya's small book from the early 1930s, *Yoga Makaranda,* and christened it Ashtanga yoga after the eight-limbed classical yoga (although the two were not really related). Ashtanga followed a system of rapid movements strung together in a sequence, although it lacked the slow, deliberate, smooth, and coordinated breathing central to Krishnamacharya's method. Further, Ashtanga practice mainly adopted sequences mentioned in *Yoga Makaranda* as well as a few Jois learned from his guru during their relationship—a bulk of sequences Krishnamacharya would later teach to his students was therefore left out. Still, the Pattabhi Jois system of Ashtanga yoga, which looks like gymnastic floor exercises and requires tremendous skill and power, has become very popular throughout America and the West. Jois's yoga is now practiced by millions of people and is almost as popular as the Iyengar system.

The third student of Krishnamacharya who came into prominence in the 1970s was Krishnamacharya's own son, T. K. V. Desikachar. He excelled in adapting asanas to individual needs and in the therapeutic application of Krishnamacharya's yoga. His *asana vinyasas* were generally milder than others, and as such many people who were intimidated by the blatantly aggressive styles of Iyengar and Pattabhi Jois found Desikachar's asanas more accessible. His was perhaps the closest to the system that Sri. Krishnamacharya taught in the third part of his life.

But, I believe that each of these methods represents only a portion of the vinyasa krama that Sri. Krishnamacharya taught me during our three decades of study together. The system I teach includes several hundred variations and provides a comprehensive treatment of vinyasa krama. Here every movement is done slowly and with complete synchronization of the breath. I teach not only asanas but also breathing exercises, Vedic chanting, and textual studies. My method is beneficial to both beginners and experts alike, and is the most comprehensive rep-

> "Whatever Krishnamacharya taught had a stamp of authority, sincerity, and profundity."

resentation of Krishnamacharya's teachings of *yogasana* practice.

It is not surprising that no individual or volume has been able to encompass the entirety of Krishnamacharya's teachings. No one student of Krishnamacharya can claim to represent his teachings completely because he was like a university, teaching different subjects to different people differently at different times. Like a diamond he had many facets, each brilliant in its own way. Whatever Krishnamacharya taught had a stamp of authority, sincerity, and profundity. From memory he would teach and chant passage after passage of mantras from the Vedas, without missing a note (swara) or mispronouncing a syllable. He covered various subjects, like the Vedas, Sanskrit grammar, the *Upanishads,* the *Bhagavad-Gita*, and hatha yoga texts. He was an expert in religious studies as well; students with that interest came to him to study epics like the *Ramayana* and several Vaishnava texts. Others came to him for counseling: his background in astrology helped him suggest astrological remedies, while his Ayurveda knowledge helped him offer a holistic approach. Whether he was teaching a long-standing student or a novice, he gave the same total attention. Krishnamacharya never withheld any knowledge; the only problem was his students, like me—there was only so much one could understand.

It was a great opportunity to study under such a rare soul—he had a hard exterior, but like the South Indian tender coconut, was all sweetness and nourishment inside. At the end of each of almost all the several hundreds of hours of learning under him, I would come out with a sense of fulfillment at having learned something new, something insightful.

Chanting alongside him was always joyful and uplifting.

It is from this that my desire arises to present the full set of Krishnamacharya's ASANA teachings in a single volume. I hope this book will give you a similar feeling.

"It was a great opportunity to study under such a rare soul—he had a hard exterior, but like the South Indian tender coconut, was all sweetness and nourishment inside."

INTRODUCTION

WHAT IS VINYASA KRAMA YOGA?

VINYASA KRAMA YOGA is an ancient practice of physical and spiritual development. It is a systematic method to study, practice, teach, and adapt yoga. This vinyasa krama (movement and sequence methodology) approach to *yogasana* (yoga posture) practice is unique in all of yoga. By integrating the functions of mind, body, and breath in the same time frame, a practitioner will experience the real joy of yoga practice. Each of the important postures (asanas) is practiced with many elaborate *vinyasas* (variations and movements). Each variation is linked to the next one by a succession of specific transitional movements, synchronized with the breath. The mind closely follows the slow, smooth, deliberate *ujjayi* yogic breathing; and the yoking of mind and body takes place with the breath acting as the harness.

The legendary yogi Sri. T. Krishnamacharya, my guru of thirty years, brought this method of yoga back to use and prominence. As I mentioned earlier, in the 1930s he wrote a small book titled *Yoga Makaranda* (Honey of Yoga), in which he explained with considerable fluidity the system of vinyasa krama. He chose a few sequences using about one hundred vinyasas in all, and presently some schools teach those very sequences under the umbrella of vinyasa krama. But in his book my guru also mentioned that he had learned about seven hundred asanas from his teacher, indicating that what was included in *Yoga Makaranda* was just a small sample. For example, in *Yoga Makaranda*, asanas like the headstand and shoulder stand were shown without any vinyasas. In contrast, I personally studied exhaustive vinyasa sequences with Krishnamacharya in these asana groups. *The Complete Book of Vinyasa Yoga* is therefore my attempt to offer as broad a picture as possible of vinyasa krama yoga, based on my studies, observations, and experiences with my wonderful mentor.

Vinyasa krama yoga strictly follows the most complete definition of classical yoga. Yoga is typically defined in two ways: In one definition it is defined as union, or *yukti* in Sanskrit; in the other, it is mental peace, or *samadhana (samadhi)*. By using the breath as a harness, vinyasa krama yoga integrates body and mind and so is the yoga of union. And because the mind follows the breath, the mind is made part of the whole process and achieves an elevated level of mental peace (samadhana). Thus the undercurrent of peace and joy is established permanently.

THE PARAMETERS OF VINYASA YOGA

The Sanskrit word *vinyasa* comes from a prefix *vi*, which means variation, and a suffix *nyasa*, which means "within prescribed parameters." The parameters prescribed in classical yoga with respect to yogasanas, as contained in *Yoga Sutra of Patanjali*, are:

STEADINESS (STHIRA). For a posture to qualify as a yogasana, it should afford the practitioner the ability to remain steady in that posture, be it standing on his or her feet (*tadasana*) or standing on his or her head (*sirsasana*).

COMFORT (SUKHA). Use of breath and the close attention of the mind to the breath, which are the hallmarks of yoga, ensure that there are considerable joy and relaxation for the practitioner.

SMOOTH AND LONG BREATHING (PRAYATNA SITHILA). This is the method prescribed by Patanjali to facilitate yoga practice. *Prayatna* (effort) here refers to *jivana prayatna*, or effort of life, which, as you can guess, is breathing. This condition stipulates that while practicing asanas, the breath should be smooth and long. So, while doing yoga correctly, one should not pant heavily. In contrast to aerobic exercise (which itself has benefits), neither the breathing rate nor heart rate should increase while practicing yoga. Our normal breathing rate is about fifteen to twenty breaths per minute. Since the movements are slow in vinyasa yoga, one has to slow one's breathing rate as well. A good guideline to follow is taking no more than six breaths per minute. One should inhale for five seconds during an expansive movement (such as stretching the arms or legs or bending backward) and exhale smoothly when folding forward, turning, twisting, bending the knees, or doing similar body contractions.

The smooth inhalation accompanying expansive movement is known as *brahmana kriya*, or expansive (breathing) action; the exhalation during contraction of the body is *langhana kriya,* or reducing or contracting (breathing) action. When you inhale while making an expansive movement and correspondingly exhale during contraction, this is known as *anuloma,* or "with the grain" movement/breathing. Anuloma exercise creates harmony between the tissues of the breathing organs and the body.

Though anuloma is the general rule, there are situations in which one might or should exhale during an expansive movement. (The converse, however, is never the case because contractive movements cannot be performed while inhaling.) This might be recommended when the practitioner is tense, obese, old, or stiff. Take the example of the cobra pose. From the lying-down position, moving into cobra pose is an expansive movement should be done on inhalation. But some especially tense people find this extremely uncomfortable because they tend to stiffen their muscles and virtually prevent their back from bending. A similar situation may arise with obese people because the belly tends to add pressure while inhaling. So, people with these conditions may breathe out while doing expansive movements. It is for the student and/or teacher to determine what type of breathing is appropriate for a particular vinyasa. One general rule is, "When in doubt, do the movement while exhaling."

BREATH RATE IN VINYASA PRACTICE

During the practice of vinyasa yoga one should perform ujjayi, or throat, breathing, because ujjayi facilitates the unaided control of breathing, which is necessary. If, while doing several vinyasas in a sequence, one feels overworked or out of breath, one should take a rest of one or two minutes to regain one's breath. People who practice these vinyasas often find that their breath rate gradually decreases over a period of time, both during practice and also habitually; the mind becomes more calm and joyful as well. There are yogis who can do yoga at the consistent rate of about four breaths per minute, even during an hour of practice. Some adepts maintain a rate of just two breaths per minute, without feeling choked or hurried. Such people demonstrate extreme relaxation while remaining in a complex pose, such as the shoulder stand, headstand, posterior stretch, or mahamudra.

FOCUSING THE MIND ON THE BREATH (ANANTA SAMAPATTI)

The Sanskrit word *ana* means breath (ana the equivalent of *swasa,* a well-known Sanskrit word that also means breath). *Samapatti* is total mental concentration. One should focus mentally on the breath during vinyasa practice. Every time one's mind wanders, one should gently coax it back to concentrating on the breath. By and large, most people find it easy to maintain mental attention on their breath and thus enjoy the process.

Vinyasa krama in yoga asana practice was the mainstay of my guru's asana teaching. For thirty years I studied this method with him, watched him teach others, and participated in his lecture-demonstrations. Never once did I see him teach asana practice without vinyasas and/or coordinated breathing to accompany the movements. This is the key to teaching vinyasa krama properly. One must maintain the practice of slow, smooth breathing, and also know the full range of asanas. It is only through full knowledge of and careful selection from the entire range of asanas that teachers and therapists can adequately design programs for students with a variety of needs.

HOW TO USE THIS BOOK

It is always difficult to write a book that meets the requirements of all readers. I wanted to write a book on vinyasa that would not intimidate beginning and intermediate students, but would still serve as a useful and comprehensive resource for experts. This book, representing the system of vinyasa krama, contains a progression of vinyasas. In each sequence and subroutine, the flow progresses from simple movements to those that may appear impossible at first glance. The purpose of vinyasa krama is to train the body and mind so that the practitioner can make sure and steady progress. Without vinyasa krama, the possibility of making any great strides is not great. So, even though the book contains several challenging vinyasas, one should remember that, with the help of slow breathing and total attention, one will be able to make considerable progress.

To facilitate better use of the book by both beginners and experts, I have, on the basis of my assessment, assigned each vinyasa a ranking of one to five diamonds (◆) to indicate the degree of difficulty, with five diamonds (◆◆◆◆◆) being the most difficult. With this general guidance the beginner may attempt 1◆ and some 2◆ vinyasas. The intermediate student may do 2◆ or 3◆ vinyasas, and the advanced student may attempt up to 4◆. The gifted student may be able to do a few of the 5◆ vinyasas. To use the book, choose one vinyasa sequence and attempt to practice all the asanas within your ability within that sequence. There may be vinyasas that you are not able to do; please make your best attempt, even if you are unable to reach the ultimate position of the vinyasas. If you prefer, you may even skip a particularly difficult vinyasa and proceed to another vinyasa.

It is always necessary to have a plan before you start your daily yoga practice. Depending upon the time available, you should apportion time to various requirements. My guru used to ask me to do asanas for about forty minutes and then allot the following twenty minutes for pranayama, meditation, or chanting.

You should find a good deal of satisfaction in the progress you make day by day. When working through the book, go from the possible to the difficult. When the difficult poses become possible to do, then the impossible ones will appear to be just difficult ones—possible with effort. If you are an absolute beginner, however, I do strongly recommend that you take some classes with a competent teacher (*gurumukha*).

My guru believed that the correct vinyasa method is essential in order to receive the full benefits from yoga practice. The following quote, which I translated from *Yoga Makaranda*, perfectly captures this sentiment.

IMPORTANT ANNOUNCEMENT

From time immemorial the Vedic syllables ... are chanted with the correct (high, low, and level) notes. Likewise, sruti (pitch) and laya (rhythm) govern Indian classical music. Classical Sanskrit poetry follows strict rules of chandas (meter), yati (caesura), and prasa (assemblage). Further, in mantra worship, nyasas (usually the assignment of different parts of the body to various deities, with mantras and gestures)—such as Kala nyasa, Jiva nyasa, Matruka nyasa, Tatwa nyasa—are integral parts. Likewise yogasana (yogic poses), pranayama (yogic breathing exercises), and mudras (seals, locks, gestures) have been practiced with vinyasas from time immemorial.

However, these days, in many places, many great souls who teach yoga do so without the vinyasas. They merely stretch or contract the limbs and proclaim that they are practicing yoga.

. . .

That any activity done without the proper procedures (niyama) will not produce the intended results is well known to everyone. That being the case, one can hardly stress that this would be the case with such lofty practices like yoga, Vedic chants, or mantra meditations. Because of wrong association, people who are merely interested in material benefits practice the perennial yoga and other disciplines, but do not derive any tangible benefits.

I would say that there are two main reasons for that.

1. They do not follow the disciplines of vinyasas and others mentioned in the texts.
2. Their teachers do not bring out the nuances of the system when they teach to their students. . . .

Just as music without proper pitch (*sruti*) and rhythm (*laya*) will not give happiness, yogasana practice without the observance of vinyasas will not give health. That being the case what can I say about long life, strength, and other benefits?

The significance of this quote was illustrated to me a few years ago, when I did a workshop in the United States. An Indian student came to me at the end of the program and mentioned that she was an ardent yoga student who had observed closely the systems of Sri. Krishnamacharya's well-known students. She had noticed that they all teach differently, and that the way I teach is still another cup of tea. How could there be so much difference?

It was then that I realized that a large portion of Krishnamacharya's teachings was being neglected. Except for asanas, none of his other yogic teachings—such as textual studies, his focus on therapeutic applications, and his vast Vedic chanting experiences—was adequately taught. So, I prepared a manuscript detailing the yoga philosophy along with several asana sequences and many therapeutic applications. I used

 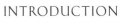

the manuscript for my lessons, and even christened it *Yoga: An Art, a Therapy, a Philosophy*. It was this manuscript, considerably modified, that was published as *Yoga for the Three Stages of Life* (Inner Traditions) in 2001. I followed the thought process of Patanjali to incorporate what I had learned about yoga from my guru. In the book, I explained that yoga's overarching goal is "freedom," and I covered chants, yoga philosophy, yogic breathing exercises, and meditation, as well as many important therapeutic applications of yoga. I also included a few representative asana vinyasa sequences, but because the book was already bulky, covering many topics, I could not cover the entire range. Thus, I have provided the full spectrum of asanas in *The Complete Book of Vinyasa Yoga*.

By using it over time, with mindfulness of the breath, you can learn to practice vinyasa yoga as T. Krishnamacharya taught it to me. Good luck with your vinyasa yoga practice.

ABOUT THE AUDIO CD

THIS BOOK IS accompanied by a compact disc audio recording of some useful and important Sanskrit chants.

First, it contains a hymn for Lord Ganesa, the remover of impediments. This is followed by the recitation of the *Yoga Sutras of Patanjali*, which, as I learned from my guru, Sri. Krishnamacharya, is the yoga bible. (My teacher would say that any practice unacceptable to *Yoga Sutras* should be rejected in toto by a serious yoga student.) It is included for serious students and practitioners of yoga so that they can read the Sanskrit text correctly and learn how to chant it. Or, they may listen to the CD while simultaneously reading the text.

The CD also contains chanting of a very famous Vedic hymn of Lord Shiva. This is followed by fervent prayer to Shiva for wealth, health, and, above all, spiritual knowledge and abiding mental peace. This may be chanted or listened to at the end of a yoga class or individual practice. One can study the meaning of the text and then listen to the chanting as a form of meditative practice.

There is also chanting of the famous Gayatri Mantra, followed by ten peace chants, again drawn from the Vedas. All or some of the chants can be used at the beginning and/or end of a yoga session as a means of meditative practice. Most of the chants on the CD were taught to me by Sri. T. Krishnamacharya.

ON
YOUR FEET
YOGASANAS

T HE FIRST ASANA sequence in the vinyasa method of doing yogasana practice is the standing sequence known as the hill pose. The hill pose, or what is known in Sanskrit as *tadasana*, is a posture that lends itself to a variety of vinyasa sequences, which are exceptionally useful in exercising the entire body. The progression of vinyasas proceeds from the fingers to the knuckles, wrists, elbows, and shoulders, then the neck, thorax, thoracic spine, and lumbar spine. The *krama* (order of postures) then sequentially involves the hip joint and the pelvis, the knees, ankles, and dorsum of your feet. Thus the entire body is involved. And tadasana is the centerpiece of this sequence, which contains several important poses such as the forward bend (*uttanasana*) and the squat (*utkatasana*).

THE BALANCE

One of the parameters that defines asana is steadiness, or good balance. Whether you are on your feet or standing on your head, steadiness is a vital ingredient of asana practice. Tadasana and its various vinyasas help to improve your sense of balance considerably. When you are agitated you cannot stand steadily and tend to lose your balance. Tadasana, when practiced regularly, will instill a good sense of balance and produce a sense of mental calm, which manifests as steadiness at the physical level.

Stand erect with both feet together, ankle bones touching (you may also keep your thighs touching). The muscles in the lower extremities—the thighs, calves, and gluteal muscles—should all be kept relaxed. Your knees in particular should be kept relaxed, but not bent. Do not pull your kneecaps up, nor push your knees back or your hamstrings will be kept taut. Now, nudge your pelvis slightly forward, so that your legs are straight without being rigid. You should lift your chest slightly, and bring your shoulder blades toward each other, so that your upper body also is straight. Keep your head steady. *(See figure 1-1.)*

Figure 1-2 gives the frontal view.

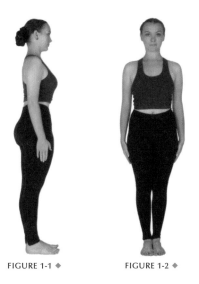

FIGURE 1-1 ◆   FIGURE 1-2 ◆

This position is called *tadasana-samasthiti*. *Samasthiti* means a state of balance. *Sama* in Sanskrit is the cognate for the word "same" in English. When there is the same amount of bodyweight distributed on both the feet it is called samasthiti. In this position, the weight of your body is transmitted through your legs without any of your leg muscles being tightened. This is the starting point of this entire sequence of tadasana vinyasas.

Now, press your chin to the sternoclavicular notch or, if possible, against the sternum itself, still keeping your back straight *(see figure 1-3)*. This is called *jalandhara bandha*.

Closely observe your balance. Your body

may sway a little to either side, but the amplitude of the swinging will gradually diminish as you observe your "balancing act." Stay in this position for at least one minute, observing your balance.

Before we proceed, please permit me to digress a little and look at some less common samasthiti positions, which require a better sense of balance. Tadasana, or the hill pose—some call it the tree pose (*vrikshasana*)—is another form of samasthiti. In this form, you raise your arms and interlock your fingers as you raise your heels (keeping your ankles together). Stay in this position for five seconds, holding your breath, or stay in this position for a few breaths. Closely watch how you balance *(see figure 1-4)*.

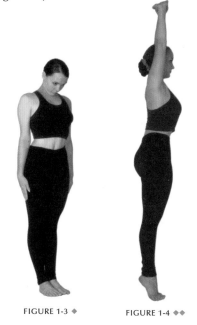

FIGURE 1-3 ◆   FIGURE 1-4 ◆◆

Over time, try to increase how long you can remain in this state.

Another standing vinyasa of samasthiti is to turn your feet out laterally by 90 degrees, with your heels touching. Keep your hands alongside your body, or keep your palms together in the gesture of respect (*anjali mudra*) *(see figure 1-5)*. This posture and gesture can be seen in some icons in Indian temples. A rear view of this variation, which is called the penguin pose, is shown in figure 1-6.

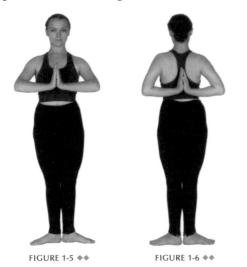

FIGURE 1-5 ◆◆   FIGURE 1-6 ◆◆

THE CHECKS

Now that we have discussed balance, let us check a few parameters, starting with the first samasthiti we have discussed. As explained in the introduction, one of the important ingredients of vinyasa krama yogasana practice is the use of breath to connect or harness the mind and body when movements are performed. A popular definition of yoga is the integration of the mind and body. Breath is the means by which this is achieved, according to Patanjali (*Yoga Sutra* chapter II sutra 46) and the experts in vinyasa krama such as my revered guru, Sri. T. Krishnamacharya. Hence the next step will be to initiate the process of integrating your mind and breath before you initiate the

movements. So, stand erect but relaxed in samasthiti, keeping your head down, and direct your attention to the center of your thoracic cavity (inside your chest). Next, we will attend to the second aspect of vinyasa practice, which is awareness of breath. Keeping your eyes closed, turn your attention to the inside of your chest. Locate the place where you feel your breathing is centered: a point from which inhalation appears to start and into which exhalation converges. It is not the air you breathe that you want to watch, but the slow outward and inward movement of prana. This position is also called *pranasthana*, or "the place of breath." Watch your breath at this point for at least a minute and in this way connect your mind to the breath.

Continue to pay attention to your breath for three to six long, smooth inhalations and exhalations that create a rubbing sensation in your throat. My teacher used to say that the smooth hissing sound produced should resemble that of a cobra. This is called ujjayi breathing. Smooth inhalation and slow exhalation through a partially closed glottis produce ujjayi's characteristic hissing sound.

The next goal is to connect your breath to your movements with the total involvement of your mind. Let us further investigate this important aspect of vinyasa krama yoga.

Our normal breathing rate is about fifteen breaths per minute. In the vinyasa krama, we reduce the rate of breathing considerably. Beginners may breathe at the rate of about six breaths per minute while practicing vinyasa krama. With diligent practice, it is possible for experts to reduce their breathing rate to about two breaths per minute for almost the entire duration of their yoga asana practice, with rest pauses.

Having connected with the center of breathing (pranasthana), now perform ujjayi breathing a few times, keeping your head down. Remember to breathe with a hissing sound and a rubbing sensation in your throat, from the partial closure of the glottis. Both inhalation and exhalation should be smooth and uniform. In fact, some of the yoga texts, such as the ancient *Yoga Upanishads*, specify that the inhalation should be like drinking water through the stem of a blue water lily (*nilotpala nala*). That is, the inhalation should be at a uniform rate, unbroken as when you drink water through a straw. In the same way, exhalation is likened to the flow of oil (*taila dharaavat*), meaning that the exhalation should be smooth and uniform as when you pour oil from a ladle.

Now, you are ready to start the vinyasa krama in tadasana. The first set of movements (vinyasas) will involve basically the movements of the arms. These vinyasas are called *hasta vinyasas*, vinyasas or movements pertaining to the arms. Please keep in mind that the default position of the head is a chin-down position (*see figure 1-3*),

except when the head should be turned to either side as required in most of the twisting movements, bending back, or similar situations. The chin-down (or preferably chin-lock) position helps you to maintain good balance, maintain control ujjayi breathing, and keep your spine stretched. (Not all the figures in this book show the chin-down position because in some cases it was necessary to keep the head upright for clarity in the picture.)

MOVEMENTS OF THE ARMS (HASTA VINYASAS)

The Lateral Side (Parsva Bhaga) Movement

Start from samasthiti. The first vinyasa involves stretching the arms overhead when you slowly inhale the ujjayi way. As you complete the inhalation, the arm movement is also to be completed, ending with the fingers interlaced and the palms turned out. The sequences of arm positions as you "shoulder the arms" is shown in figures 1-7 through 1-10.

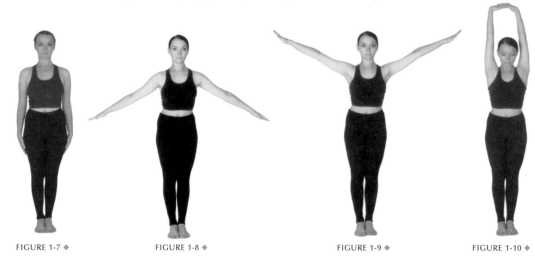

FIGURE 1-7 ◆   FIGURE 1-8 ◆   FIGURE 1-9 ◆   FIGURE 1-10 ◆

When you turn your interlocked palms out, pull your arms up so that both sides (*parsva bhaga*) of your body are well stretched (*see figure 1-11*).

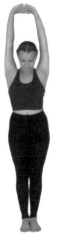

FIGURE 1-11 ◆

This is a complete side stretch, and the slow synchronous inhalation helps to expand the chest muscles from inside. Remain in the stretched position for a second or so, and then while exhaling, slowly lower your arms to samasthiti, the initial position. The duration of inhalation and exhalation can be equal—though should be a minimum of five seconds—and you can increase the duration slowly as your control over the movements improves. While performing the movements, please make sure that you closely watch and follow your breath. Repeat the movements three times, stretching a bit more on each successive attempt.

The Frontal (Purva Bhaga) Stretch

The second movement in the sequence stretches the front portion of the body by moving the arms upward in front (*purva bhaga*). Turn your palms inward (*see figure 1-12*).

As you are slowly inhaling, raise your arms all the way up in front of you, taking a minimum of five seconds. Keep your palms facing forward. As you raise your arms and inhale, expand your chest and make sure that the front of your body is also stretched (*see figure 1-13*). Hold the breath for a second. On the following exhalation, slowly lower your arms, completing the movement as you finish the exhalation.

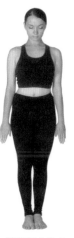

FIGURE 1-12 ◆

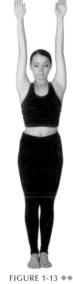

FIGURE 1-13 ◆◆

FIGURE 1-14 ◆◆

You may also stretch your abdominal muscles, as shown in the side view of the pose (see figure 1-14).

This gives a good stretch to the front portion of the body, all the way up the arms to the fingertips. Repeat the movements three times, stretching more intensely on each successive movement. These two movements are invigorating because of the robust inhalation and full stretching of the torso, inside and outside. (Just as when we are tired, we reach our arms up and stretch, and feel refreshed.) These two vinyasas kick-start the asana practice.

The Sweeping Movement (Prasarana)

Keep your arms crossed in front of you, placing each palm on the opposite thigh (see figure 1-15).

when you do the movement with deep inhalation. Follow your breath closely during these movements. Spend at least five seconds on the inhalation and exhalation.

The Elbow Movement

As you inhale slowly, raise your arms and interlock your fingers. As you exhale slowly, lower your arms, bending your elbows and keeping your hands interlaced. Keep your hands behind your neck, further opening your chest in the process (see figure 1-17).

When you reach the final position of the vinyasa, your shoulder blades will be close together. Persons with stiffness in the neck should not force the movement beyond the point where they feel some strain. Repeat the movement three times. The rear view of this vinyasa is shown in figure 1-18.

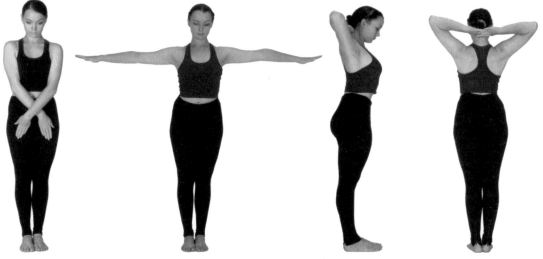

FIGURE 1-15 ◆   FIGURE 1-16 ◆   FIGURE 1-17 ◆◆   FIGURE 1-18 ◆◆

As you inhale slowly, swing your arms outward up to shoulder level (see figure 1-16).

Stay that way for a second. During the next exhalation lower your arms. You may repeat the movement three times. This is a nice way to open up the chest—especially

Hands-on-Shoulder-Blades Vinyasas

There are several more movements leading to different hand positions (hasta vinyasas) that are helpful in strengthening the arms, shoulders, neck, and torso as well. Inhale and raise your arms overhead, and as you slowly exhale bend your elbows, lower your hands toward your back, and place your palms on the respective shoulder blades (*see figure 1-19*).

A close-up view is shown in figure 1-20.

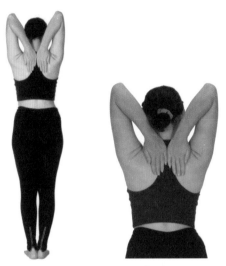

FIGURE 1-19 ◆◆   FIGURE 1-20 ◆◆

Hold this position for three to six long inhalations and exhalations, expanding your chest nicely on each slow inhalation. Then,

finally, inhale and raise your arms to the tadasana position. As you are exhaling slowly, lower your arms to your sides to return to the tadasana-samasthiti position (the starting position of the sequence).

The next vinyasa is the same, except that you place your palms on the opposite shoulder blades (*see figure 1-21*).

A close-up view is shown in figure 1-22.

Hold this position for three to six smooth inhalations and exhalations—at least five seconds—expanding your chest during every inhalation. Return to samasthiti, as you exhale slowly (*see figure 1-23*).

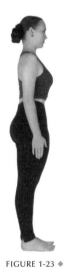

FIGURE 1-23 ◆

These movements help to open the chest, especially the pectoral and supraclavicular region of the chest. The apical region of the lungs also comes into play.

Hands-Locked-Behind Vinyasas

The next few hand or hasta vinyasas can be practiced independently; they can also be used in other more involved asanas for balance and to enhance the effectiveness of some of the postures. Standing in tadasana, while inhaling, raise your arms

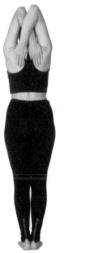
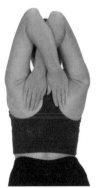

FIGURE 1-21 ◆◆   FIGURE 1-22 ◆◆

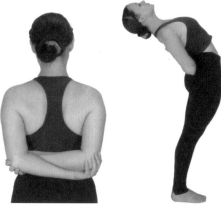
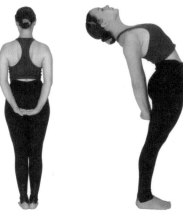

FIGURE 1-24 ◆◆   FIGURE 1-25 ◆◆   FIGURE 1-26 ◆◆   FIGURE 1-27 ◆◆

overhead. Then as you slowly exhale, swing your arms behind and around your back and hold your elbows (see figure 1-24).

Open your chest. This hand position, which effectively locks the hands in forward movement, is used for several forward-bending poses as in uttanasana. This arm position also facilitates bending backward very effectively. On the next deep inhalation, slowly bend backward, lifting your chest up, dropping your shoulders, and bringing your shoulder blades closer together in the process (see figure 1-25).

Hold your breath for one or two seconds and on exhalation return to asana sthiti. Repeat the movement three to six times.

Now on exhalation in tadasana, slowly drop your arms behind your back, interlace them, and turn them outward (see figure 1-26).

Stay in this position for a few breaths. As in the earlier vinyasas, inhale slowly as you stretch your arms, bend back, and lift your chest up. You may press your shoulders down so that your shoulder blades touch each other (see figure 1-27).

Stay in this posture for three to six breaths, and then return to tadasana sthiti while exhaling slowly. These vinyasas, in which you keep your arms locked behind your back, help to open your chest and also facilitate the backward bending movement of your torso.

The Back-Salute (Prishtanjali)

Another hasta vinyasa is the back salute position (prishtanjali; prishta = back; anjali = salutation). Begin the movement from samasthiti. While inhaling slowly, raise your arms overhead. Stay that way for a second. Now as you are exhaling, lower your arms. As you continue to exhale, join your hands palm to palm at the bottom of your spine, turn them upward, and gently slide them along your spine until they reach a position near your shoulders (see figure 1-28).

Your hands will be on your back with your palms together and fingertips pointing up in a gesture of salutation (anjali mudra). Stay that way for a few breaths. You may also do some back bending (while inhaling of course) with your hands in the back salute (see figure 1-29).

Return to samasthiti while you smoothly exhale. This variation of the hand position completely locks the hands so that all further movement of the torso will require

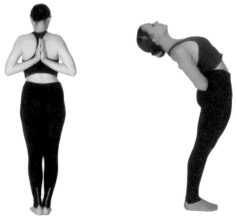

FIGURE 1-28 ◆◆◆   FIGURE 1-29 ◆◆◆   FIGURE 1-30 ◆◆   FIGURE 1-31 ◆

mobility of the spine; hence, this position of the hands is very effective for thoracic expansion, while doing deep inhalation. People with stiff neck and shoulders may find it difficult to do the movement to its completion. With slow exhalation and perseverance, it will be possible to do the movement successfully. One should move cautiously, however.

The Shoulder Rotation Vinyasas

The shoulder joint is a ball-and-socket joint providing the ability to rotate the shoulder and arm. Shoulder stiffness is a common malady, and because of disuse people slowly lose the full range of rotation over time. The two vinyasas described next will help you to maintain the flexibility of this robust, but complex, joint.

The first movement begins with the arms overhead with fingers interlaced. Now, while inhaling slowly, bend back (*see figure 1-30*).

Then on the following exhalation, rotate your shoulders in an outward arc and bring your arms forward to about shoulder level; at the same time, with your hands facing upward, straighten your back (*see figure 1-31*).

Take care that you do the movement as close to your body as possible. Hold this position for a second. Now as you inhale, retrace the movement and bring your arms back to the starting position. You don't have to bend back on the return movement. Those who cannot bend their back much can do the entire downward movement on exhalation in one go.

The second part of this shoulder movement sequence is as follows: Beginning from the arms-raised position (*see figure 1-32*), slowly and smoothly exhale while lowering your arms in front of you to shoulder level (*see figure 1-33*).

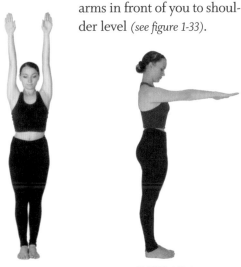

FIGURE 1-32 ◆   FIGURE 1-33 ◆

Spread your arms sideways, keeping them at shoulder height (*see figure 1-34*).

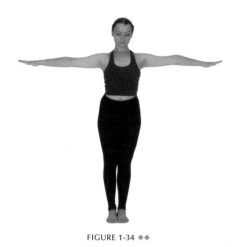

FIGURE 1-34 ◆◆

Do this all in one continuous movement. Stay in the position for a second. Then during the subsequent slow inhalation, bring your arms forward and up. Next, as you exhale, slowly lower your arms to samasthiti. You can see that between the earlier vinyasas and this one, you get a complete rotation for the shoulder joints. Since the whole movement is done slowly and deliberately, the stretch is very effective. Do the movement three times to get the full benefit. The movements are to be done slowly and carefully, with your mind closely following your breath.

SIDE POSES (PARSVA BHANGI)

The previous vinyasas were for the arms, shoulders, and thoracic spine. The next two subgroups are called side poses and use side-bending and -twisting movements that are aided by the spine. Please note, however, that there should absolutely be no twisting of the spine in these vinyasas.

Side-Bending Pose of the Torso (Parsva Bhangi I)

From samasthiti, as you slowly inhale, raise both arms overhead and interlock your fingers (*see figure 1-35*).

Then as you slowly exhale, pressing through your feet, nudge your pelvis gently to the left, and bend your torso to the right (*see figure 1-36*).

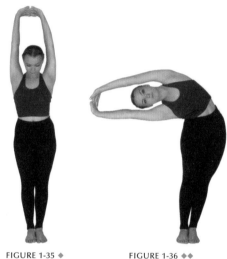

FIGURE 1-35 ◆   FIGURE 1-36 ◆◆

Be sure to anchor your feet well so that you can maintain good balance. Upon inhalation, return to the starting position slowly and deliberately. (Many practitioners spring back quickly to the erect body position, but I recommend taking at least five seconds to effect the movement, synchronizing the movement with the inhalation.) Repeat the movement three to six times. After some practice, you may want to remain in the posture for some length of time, say about six breaths. During that period, on every slow, smooth exhalation, you should try to bend a little more. This posture is called *dakshina-parsva bhangi* (right-side pose). Make sure that you do not twist your spine by looking down at the floor or turning your neck and looking up. The entire movement should be confined to the vertical plane, neither looking down nor up, but rather straight ahead. This will ensure that your bending is correct and optimum.

After returning to the starting position, repeat the same movement on the left side—this is known as left-side pose (*vama-parsva bhangi*) (*see figure 1-37*).

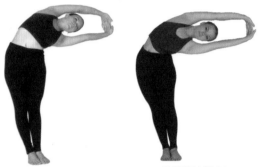

FIGURE 1-37 ◆◆   FIGURE 1-38 ◆◆

Another view of the same vinyasa (*see figure 1-38*).

These two exercises improve the flexibility of the spine and also stretch the thoracic muscles.

Side Twist of the Torso (Parva Bhangi II)

Now we can look at the turning or twisting movement of the torso and thoracic spine. It is difficult for many to maintain good balance while performing the twisting movement. So, this is done step by step in three different hand vinyasa positions.

First, begin in samasthiti; while inhaling, raise your arms laterally to shoulder level, keeping your chin down (*see figure 1-39*).

Then while slowly exhaling, firmly anchor your feet and gradually turn to the right side. As you complete the movement,

turn your head to look over your right shoulder (*see figure 1-40*).

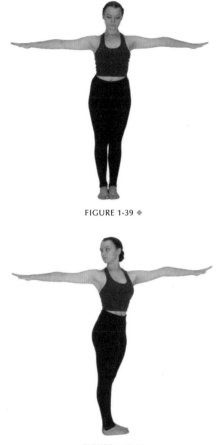

FIGURE 1-39 ◆

FIGURE 1-40 ◆◆

Remain in this position for a second and then, while slowly inhaling, return to the starting position. Repeat the movement three to six times, turning a little more each time. You may also opt to stay in the final position and repeat three slow, smooth inhalations and exhalations, turning a bit more each time as you squeeze air out of your lungs. (Note that due to the bending of the body in this movement, you may feel the urge to lift the side of the foot that is opposite the side on which movement occurs. Refrain from doing so by watching the position of your feet—there should be no movement of the feet, because you are in tadasana sthiti right through to the end.)

In a similar fashion, repeat the movements on the left side (see figure 1-41).

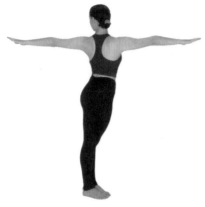

FIGURE 1-41 ◆◆

Twisting Different Hand Position (Parsva Bhangi Vinyasa)

The same twisting movement can be done with a different arm position, which will help in improving the quality of the turn. Here, instead of keeping your arms at shoulder level which will, to some extent, help you balance a little better, you bring your arms overhead and interlock your fingers (see figure 1-42).

Now try the same turning movement during a slow ujjayi (see page 4). In this exercise, the spine is pulled further up and the twist is better, with less distortion. As you exhale slowly turn to the right side (see figure 1-43).

Stay in this position for one or two breaths. For a further extension of the posture, as you slowly inhale, bend back with your spine still twisted to the right side (see figure 1-44).

(If bending back is difficult, you may try to bend back a little bit at the end of the previous movement itself when you turn.)

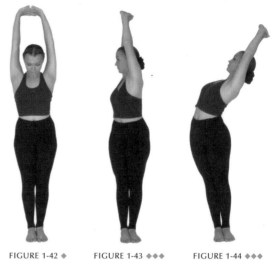

FIGURE 1-42 ◆   FIGURE 1-43 ◆◆◆   FIGURE 1-44 ◆◆◆

From the bending-back position, in which you are slowly exhaling, return to the previous position; then on the next inhalation, return to the asana sthiti. During your next slow exhalation, lower your arms to return to samasthiti. Repeat the movement three to six times. This, if done with slow breathing and unhurriedly, is very invigorating.

Now do this movement on the left side, following the same procedure. The three positions are shown in figures 1-45 through 1-47.

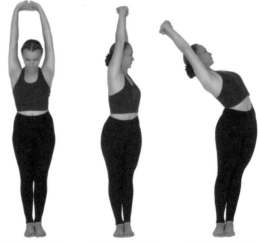

FIGURE 1-45 ◆   FIGURE 1-46 ◆◆◆   FIGURE 1-47 ◆◆◆

Twisting Arms in Back Salute
(Parsva Bhangi-Prishtanjali)

In the next vinyasas, the arms are completely locked so that you have to perform the vinyasas with correct balance and movement of only the torso and thoracic spine. From tadasana (arms-raised position), while you slowly exhale, swing your arms behind your back and do the back salute (prishtanjali, see page 8) (see figure 1-48).

Stay in that position for three long inhalations and exhalations. Then as you exhale long and smoothly, slowly turn your body and head to the right side; look over your right shoulder. Stay in that position for three to six breaths, twisting a little bit more on each of the exhalations (see figure 1-49).

Then as you are inhaling, return to the starting position, keeping your hands in prishtanjali. The same movement should be practiced on the left side (see figure 1-50).

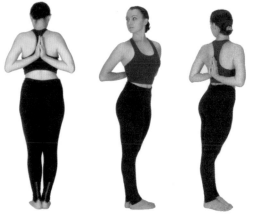

FIGURE 1-48 ◆◆◆   FIGURE 1-49 ◆◆◆   FIGURE 1-50 ◆◆◆

With this we have completed the different vinyasas for the torso in a comprehensive manner. You can see that the various vinyasas will ensure that all auxiliary muscles associated with the breathing apparatus are exercised. Further, because all the movements are done with deep, slow inhalations and exhalations, the efficacy of the stretching movements is enhanced by the stretching of the inside of the chest. The synchronized breathing ensures a complete stretch, both inside and out. In fact, the combination of internal and external stretching helps stretch the spine—especially the thoracic portion—which is very difficult to stretch. The vital capacity is increased. Asthmatics get a good workout by using the muscles of the torso, which they seldom use. (In fact, people with breathing deficiencies may selectively use several of the vinyasas; those who are ill and cannot do some of the vinyasas while standing can do them seated in a yoga posture or even a chair; some of the movements can be done even while lying down.)

THE FORWARD BEND
(Uttanasana)

In this section, we focus on other portions of the body: the lumbar spine, hips, legs, and feet. Uttanasana is a classical yoga posture and helps to stretch the posterior portion of the body (and also the anterior portion) very well. The intense stretch improves the circulation of all the muscles concerned and thus increases the strength and tone of the posterior muscle groups—the thigh, calf, gluteal muscles, and back. These rear muscles are relatively massive and difficult to access and exercise. Hence, the forward stretch sequence is very important. Furthermore, these sequences enhance your sense of balance considerably, because you have to do all the variations with your feet together. Your breathing also should be kept smooth and long. If however, your breath gets short at any time, stay in samasthiti for a short while until your breath normalizes.

The Half-Forward-Stretch Pose (Ardha-Uttanasana)

This sequence involves forward bending, essentially stretching the posterior portion of the body, and should be done before the full forward stretch (*purna uttanasana*). From tadasana, with your arms raised (*see figure 1-51*), slowly exhale while nudging your buttocks back.

Lower your upper body, keeping it straight, until your upper body is horizontal. The thigh, calf, gluteal muscles, and the hamstrings are stretched considerably (*see figure 1-52*), and your spine, especially the lumbar portion, is stretched as well.

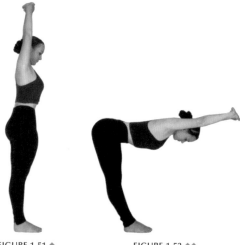

FIGURE 1-51 ◆   FIGURE 1-52 ◆◆

The posture, as my guru used to say, should look like the numeral 7. Stay in this position with your chin down for three long inhalations and exhalations. (Prior to that, you can practice the movement by bending halfway forward while exhaling, and return-

ing to samasthiti upon inhalation.) This posture is good for stretching the spine and preparing for the full forward stretch.

There are some beneficial variations on this half-forward stretch. One is a vinyasa of ardha-uttanasana known as *khagasana*, or bird posture (a bird flying with wings outstretched). To do it, start from the arms-stretched position explained in the half-forward stretch pose. While exhaling deeply, bring your arms to shoulder level (*see figure 1-53*).

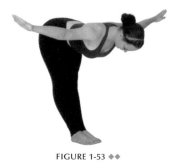

FIGURE 1-53 ◆◆

Then during the following inhalation, stretch your arms overhead, and in the process lengthen your spine and stretch your thigh and gluteal muscles. (There are a number of vinyasas done in this posture with arms in different hasta vinyasas, such as the back salute, hands held behind, and others.)

The Complete Forward Stretch (Purna-Uttanasana)

The complete forward stretch, or purna uttanasana, an important asana of uttanasana. Here it is along with its different variations.

Begin again in samasthiti, raising your arms while inhaling (*see figure 1-54*). Exhale, then while inhaling again slowly bend back (*see figure 1-55*).

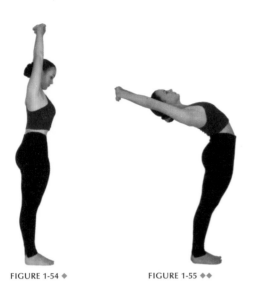

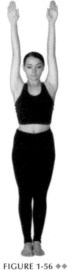

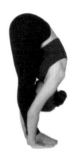

FIGURE 1-54 ◆   FIGURE 1-55 ◆◆   FIGURE 1-56 ◆◆   FIGURE 1-57 ◆◆◆

Now release the finger lock and keep the hands free (*see figure 1-56*).

Then, while slowly exhaling, stretch your upper body up and over, pressing down through your feet, especially the balls of your feet. Still exhaling and firmly anchoring your feet, slowly bend all the way down and place your palms on the floor beside your feet (*see figure 1-57*).

Tilt your pelvis down as much as possible in the process. While you are exhaling, draw in your rectal muscles and gradually tuck in your abdomen. Hold this position for a second. Then as you inhale, return to tadasana with your arms still raised. Repeat these movements very slowly three to six times, concentrating on your exhalations and the bending forward movement.

After some practice, you may be able to remain in this posture for a longer period, working on increasing the duration of your exhalation. For example, while in the forward bending position (uttanasana), keep your inhalations short—about three seconds or so—but concentrate on making your exhalations very long and smooth. In addition, it is helpful to practice both abdominal and rectal locks (*uddiyana* and *mula bandhas*) after exhalation and while holding your breath after exhaling. (*Mula bandha* means to pull up the rectum and keep it drawn inward for a short period, say about five seconds. *Uddiyana bandha* means to keep the rectum drawn in while continuously pulling the pelvic floor up and the rectus abdominis inward.) The locks are released after holding them for about five seconds and before beginning the next inhalation.

This posture helps to stretch the hamstrings and the calf, thigh, and gluteal muscles as well as the whole back. It is a beneficial posture that is a favorite among yogis. It lends itself to many different arm positions, some of which are described on the following pages.

THE FORWARD BEND—FURTHER VINYASAS

Hand-Feet Posture (Pada Hastasana)

Start in tadasana (the arms raised position) (*see figure 1-58*).

During a long smooth exhalation, complete the full forward bend described earlier and place the palms of your hands beneath your feet (*see figure 1-59*).

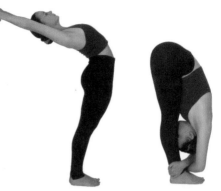

FIGURE 1-60 ◆◆   FIGURE 1-61 ◆◆◆

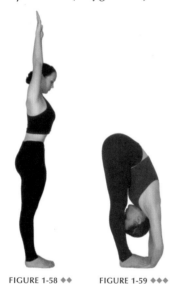

FIGURE 1-58 ◆◆   FIGURE 1-59 ◆◆◆

Hold this position for three to six breaths. Then on the next inhalation, slowly raise your arms and then your head and trunk to return to tadasana.

The next vinyasa involves holding your legs with crossed hands (*parivritta*). Again begin in tadasana. With your arms raised, slowly inhale and bend back (*see figure 1-60*).

While you are exhaling, bend forward and grasp your right ankle with your left hand and your left ankle with your right hand (*see figure 1-61*).

On every exhalation, move your elbows out to the side and try to stretch your torso forward and down. Remain in this position

for three to six breaths, maintaining very long exhalations. The inhalations can be short. Return to the tadasana position while inhaling slowly and smoothly. If you are unable to bend forward completely and can't reach your ankles, try holding part of your legs, knees, or shins. Rest in that position for a few breaths, until you feel a good stretch. Try to stretch a little more on each exhalation. Exhalation tends to relax the muscles and will help you proceed slowly.

Forward-Stretch Pose, without Support (Niralamba Uttanasana)

The forward bending vinyasas we have seen so far are *salamba*, or with support. You hold some part of the body—the feet, ankles, shins—or the floor itself in order to anchor yourself for a good stretch. But with practice, it should be possible to do forward bending without holding onto your body or any external props.

There are several hand positions (hasta vinyasas) in which you can do the unsupported forward-bending exercises. For the first, begin in the tadasana position and put your hands in the back salute (prishtanjali) (*see figure 1-62*).

To do this, raise your arms on inhalation, and during the following smooth

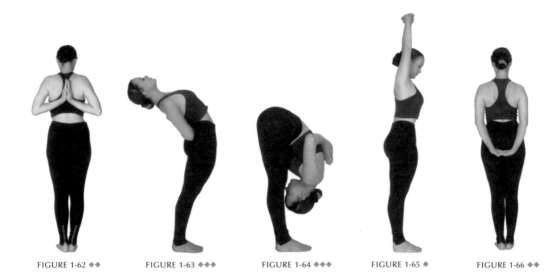

FIGURE 1-62 ◆◆   FIGURE 1-63 ◆◆◆   FIGURE 1-64 ◆◆◆   FIGURE 1-65 ◆   FIGURE 1-66 ◆◆

exhalation, swing your hands behind your back and into the salutation gesture (anjali mudra). Remain in this position for three breaths; on the next inhalation, bend backward *(see figure 1-63)*.

Slowly breathe out and fold your body forward, placing your forehead on your knees or shins *(see figure 1-64)*.

Remain in this position for three to six breaths. Return to tadasana with a slow, smooth inhalation, arching your back as you move upward. As you exhale, return to samasthiti by lowering your arms.

Now from samasthiti, raise your arms overhead while inhaling; keep your chin down *(see figure 1-65)*.

During the next exhalation, lower your arms and bring them behind your back, interlocking your fingers and turning your palms out *(see figure 1-66)*.

On the next inhalation, slowly bend back to open up your chest. (Many people do this vinyasa without turning their palms out, in which case their shoulders tend to slide inward and they tend to crouch. If you turn your palms out, your arms and shoulders will also open out, with your shoulder blades touching each other.) *(See figure 1-67)*.

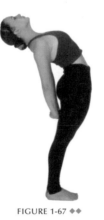

FIGURE 1-67 ◆◆

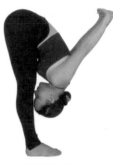

FIGURE 1-68 ◆◆◆

Then while you do smooth long ujjayi exhalation, bend forward, pulling your arms away from your body behind your back. Place your face on your knees or shins. *(See figures 1-68 and 1-69)*.

Stay in this position for three to six

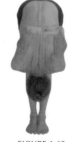

FIGURE 1-69
(BACK VIEW) ◆◆◆

breaths. Finally as you are inhaling, raise your head and return to tadasana sthiti.

The next variation is also *niralamba uttanasana*. From tadasana, as you inhale, raise both arms laterally to shoulder level (*see figure 1-70*).

Then while you are doing smooth, long ujjayi exhalation, stretch your back and bend forward, placing your head on your knees or shins (*see figure 1-71*).

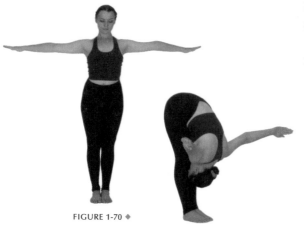

FIGURE 1-70 ◆

FIGURE 1-71 ◆◆◆

Stay in this position for three to six breaths. While you are inhaling, slowly come up. On the next exhalation, lower your arms to return to samasthiti.

Sideward-Forward Stretch (Parsva Bhaga Uttanasana)

The next *niralamba*, or unsupported forward bend uses a different arm position. If your forward bending is good and you feel you can stretch a little more, this may help you do just that. The two movements in the sideward-foreward stretch make the hip joint and the sides of the lower extremities supple. The vinyasa requires you not only to bend forward, but also to turn to one side to give your hip joint a forward movement and

sideward twist. (These are difficult vinyasas that should be attempted only when your usual forward bending (uttanasana) is very good. Persons with hip problems or lumbago should avoid this pose.)

In right-side forward-stretching pose (*dakshina-parsva bhaga uttanasana*), you turn to the right side, bend forward, and place your hands beside your right foot. To do this, begin in tadasana, and while inhaling raise your arms and interlock your fingers (*see figure 1-72*).

Then as you exhale slowly, turn to the right (*see figure 1-73*).

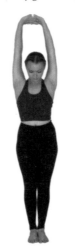

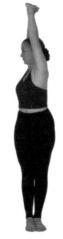

FIGURE 1-72 ◆◆

FIGURE 1-73 ◆◆

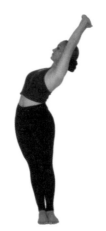

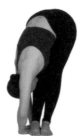

FIGURE 1-74 ◆◆

FIGURE 1-75 ◆◆◆

While inhaling, arch your back to the left side *(see figure 1-74)*.

During the next exhalation, very slowly bend forward to the right side of your body; place your interlocked hands on the outside of your right foot with your hands parallel to your feet. Touch the outside of your right leg with your face *(see figure 1-75)*.

Hold this position for three to six breaths. Concentrate on an extended exhalation. Return to samasthiti afterward.

Repeat these movements on the left side *(vama-parsva bhaga uttanasana)*: Raise your arms overhead while inhaling; turn to the left side on a slow exhalation *(see figure 1-76)*.

Then bend back upon inhalation *(see figure 1-77)*.

As you exhale, bend forward and place your hands by the side of your left foot; place your face against the side of your left leg *(see figure 1-78)*.

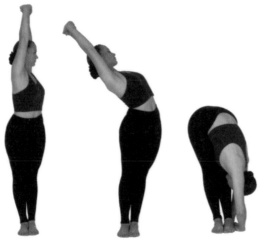

FIGURE 1-76 ♦♦   FIGURE 1-77 ♦♦   FIGURE 1-78 ♦♦♦

Hold this pose for as long as you held it on the right. Return to samasthiti on a slow smooth ujjayi inhalation.

Standing Turtle Pose Variation (Kurmasana Vinyasa)

A purist might frown upon the next vinyasa, which involves complicated forward bending, because it may require the feet to be spread apart (typically, the tadasana sequence requires you to keep the feet together). But it is necessary to spread the legs about a foot apart in order to accommodate the torso when the pelvis is folded.

Start from samasthiti. While inhaling, raise your arms overhead *(see figure 1-79)*.

During the next exhalation, spread your legs apart by about one foot. Inhale again, and in the following, long exhalation bend forward and insert your torso between your legs *(see figure 1-80)*.

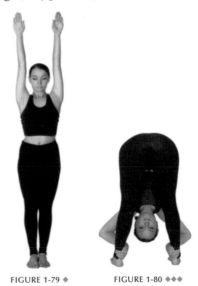

FIGURE 1-79 ♦   FIGURE 1-80 ♦♦♦

Hold this position for a few breaths; inhale as you return to your starting position.

Alternately, you can round your back as in turtle pose *(kurmasana)* and bring your head further beyond your legs: While you exhale, bend forward to bring your shoulders inside your thighs; bring your arms around your legs, and hold them together *(see figures 1-81 through 1-83)*.

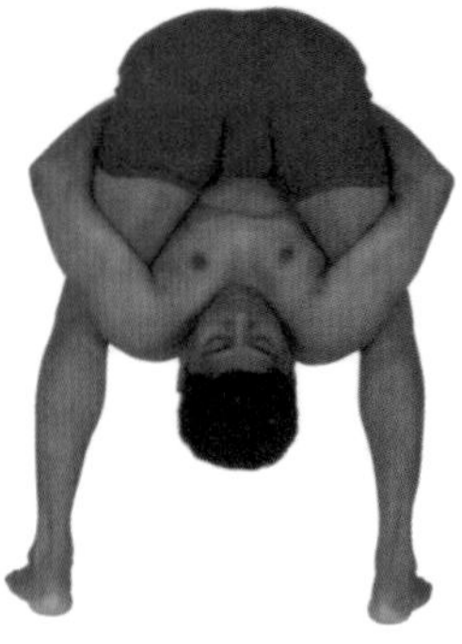

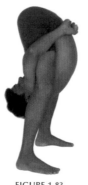

FIGURE 1-81
(FRONT VIEW) ◆◆◆◆

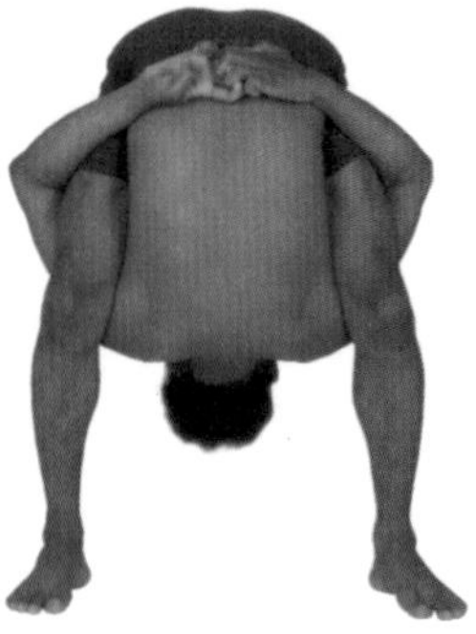

FIGURE 1-82
(BACK VIEW) ◆◆◆◆

FIGURE 1-83
(SIDE VIEW) ◆◆◆◆

Hold this position for three to six inhalations and exhalations, and then return to the standing position. Then as you are inhaling, bring your feet together for tadasana-samasthiti. This posture is considered a very difficult variation of turtle pose (kurmasana), but it is beneficial in that the hip joint and pelvic tilt reach maximum flexion.

Standing Complete Back Stretch Pose (Tiryang-Mukha-Uttanasana)

The next posture in uttanasana takes a slightly different direction from that of the movements we have seen so far. It is called the full circle posture (*purna chakrasana*), but is more correctly known as the back-ward-facing stretching posture (tiryang-mukha-uttanasana). Stand in tadasana-samasthiti, and while inhaling raise both arms overhead *(see figure 1-84)*.

Exhale deeply and on the next inhalation, slowly bend back and place your palms on the floor close to and behind your feet *(see figure 1-85)*.

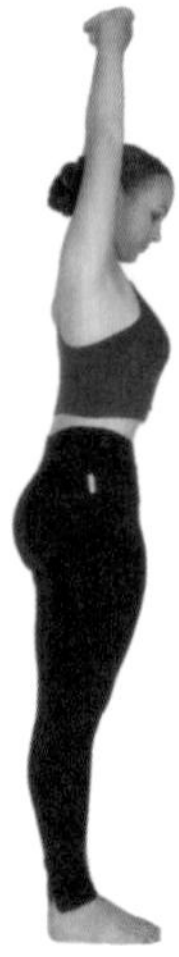

FIGURE 1-84 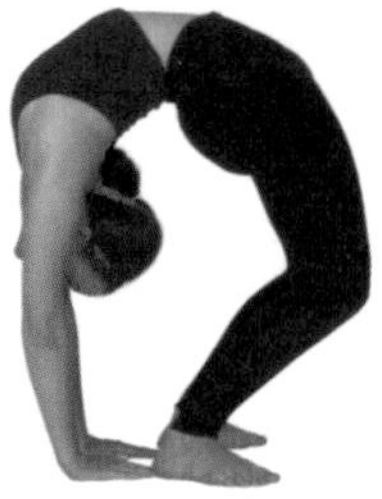 ◆   FIGURE 1-85 ◆◆◆◆

Stay in this position for three to six breaths. During the exhalation, move back slowly to tadasana.

With this we come to the conclusion of a variety of standing forward (and backward) stretching sequences.

THE HIP-STRETCH OR HIP SQUAT POSE (UTKATASANA)

The next set of vinyasas centers around another important pose known as the hip stretch posture (utkatasana). It is preceded by half-squat pose (*ardha-utkatasana*), which will be explained momentarily. These two are very effective and helpful for the knee joints.

The Half-Squat or Chair Pose (Ardha-Utkatasana)

The half-squat pose, which resembles a chair and so is also known as the chair pose, is a very effective posture for stretching the hip joint and knees. There are several arm positions used; the easiest of these is the arms-forward position, which follows.

From tadasana, slowly raise your arms in front of your body up to shoulder level (*see figure 1-86*).

Stay in this position for a few breaths. Then as you slowly exhale, keeping your feet, ankles, and thighs together, bend your knees and lower your trunk to the half-squat pose (*see figure 1-87*).

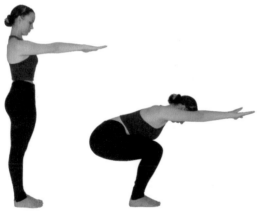

FIGURE 1-86 ◆   FIGURE 1-87 ◆◆

(Be sure to keep your thighs horizontal, with your knees bent at a 90-degree angle—they should not feel any strain.) While inhaling, slowly return to a standing position with your mind following your breath. You may stand in tadasana for a few breaths and then repeat the movement two more times, taking a break in between if necessary. After some practice, you may attempt to stay in the pose for three to six breaths.

When first attempting this pose you may feel the urge to lean forward, but with practice you will achieve the correct posture (*see figure 1-88*).

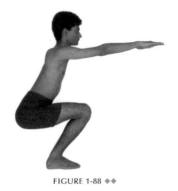

FIGURE 1-88 ◆◆

Many people tend to bend only about one-fourth of the way, attempt to hold the position, and strain their knees in the process. In addition, some people experience a quickening of the breath because the stomach is compressed. It may be helpful to slowly draw in the rectum and tummy along with the downward movement of the body. Those who practice these locks may attempt to do them while remaining in the posture after exhalation is complete and only while holding the breath out. Let us look at this posture from a different angle. Stand in tadasana. Now inhale and raise your arms frontward up to shoulder level (*see figure 1-89*).

Stay in this position for three breaths. Very slowly exhaling, do a half-squat, keeping your chin down and also doing the abdominal and rectal locks (*see figure 1-90*).

In the next hand position, you keep your arms stretched to the sides. From the tadasana position, slowly inhale and raise your arms out to the sides to shoulder level (*see figure 1-91*).

Stay in the position for one long inhalation and exhalation. As you are slowly exhaling, flex your knees and lower your

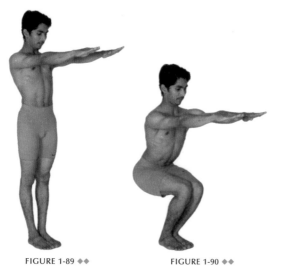

FIGURE 1-89 ◆◆   FIGURE 1-90 ◆◆

buttocks to a half-squat position, with your arms still stretched outward (*see figure 1-92*).

You may try to keep your chin down for better balance and better control over your

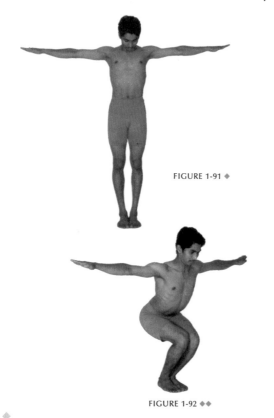

FIGURE 1-91 ◆

FIGURE 1-92 ◆◆

breathing. Stay in this position for three breaths, and as you are slowly inhaling return to tadasana-samasthiti.

The next version is a bit more difficult because the arms are not used for balance. Begin again from samasthiti. As you inhale, slowly raise both arms overhead, interlock your fingers, and turn your hands outward (with the palms pointing toward the ceiling). (*See figure 1-93.*)

Stay in this position for three long inhalations and exhalations. Now, keeping your chin down and exhaling very slowly, flex your knees; lower your body until you get to the half-squat position (*see figure 1-94*).

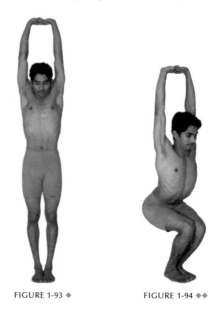

FIGURE 1-93 ◆   FIGURE 1-94 ◆◆

Keep your back nicely arched. You may do both rectal and abdominal locks (see above). Stay in this position for three breaths before raising your trunk back to samasthiti, while inhaling slowly.

The following half-squat vinyasas are increasingly difficult and require the arching of the spine in order to maintain proper balance.

Again start from samasthiti. Inhaling, raise both arms overhead. While exhaling, bend your elbows and place your palms on your shoulder blades. Your elbows should be pointing upward *(see figure 1-95)*.

Stay in this position for three long inhalations and exhalations, and then as you breathe out, holding your chin down in jalandhara bandha, ease your torso into the chair pose *(see figure 1-96)*.

and move your hands back, placing them on the opposite shoulder blades *(see figure 1-97)*.

Stay in this position for three long inhalations and exhalations, expanding the chest well during every inhalation. Then while you are exhaling smoothly, keep your chin down and lower your trunk, bending your knees carefully until you are in a half-squat pose *(see figure 1-98)*.

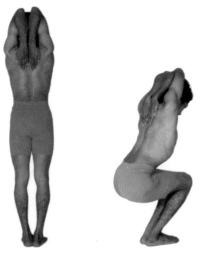

FIGURE 1-95 ◆◆   FIGURE 1-96 ◆◆◆

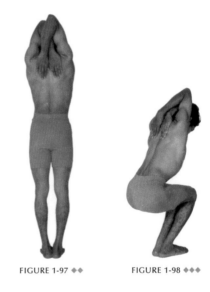

FIGURE 1-97 ◆◆   FIGURE 1-98 ◆◆◆

You can effectively draw in your rectum and lower abdomen as you move into the posture. Stay in this position for a few breaths, starting both the rectal and abdominal locks during exhalation and holding the locks as you hold the breath out for a few seconds. The inhalations also will be very effective in improving your vital capacity because the chest is nicely opened out when the hands are held behind the back. After a few breaths, while slowly inhaling return to samasthiti.

From samasthiti, once again inhale slowly, raising your arms overhead. As you start exhaling slowly, start bending your elbows

It is good to draw in your rectal and abdominal muscles as you are breathing out and moving your body downward. Stay in the pose for a few breaths, maintaining the rectal and abdominal locks when you hold your breath after exhalation. Return to samasthiti.

Once again from samasthiti, raise your arms overhead. Stay in this position for a few breaths and, on the next exhalation, slowly lower your arms, but swing them behind your back and join your hands at the bottom of your spine. In a continuous motion, join your palms, turn your hands upward, and move them along the canal of your back. This position, as we have seen already is the back salute (prishtanjali) *(see figure 1-99)*.

Stay in this position for a few breaths, expanding your chest during every smooth, long inhalation. Now, as you smoothly exhale through a constricted throat, facilitated by the chin lock, lower your trunk, bending your knees *(see figure 1-100)*.

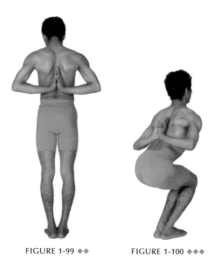

FIGURE 1-99 ◆◆   FIGURE 1-100 ◆◆◆

Once you lower your body to the half-squat position, stay in this position for a few breaths, doing the abdominal and rectal locks during the pause in breath after exhalation and before starting your inhalation. Stay in this position for a few breaths and then, while inhaling, return to samasthiti, with your hands still in back salute position. Another variation is to keep your arms folded behind you *(see figure 1-101)*.

While you exhale, bend your knees and lower your body to the chair pose *(see figure 1-102)*.

Then on the following exhalation, lower your arms to samasthiti *(see figure 1-103)*.

THE FULL HIP-STRETCH POSE (PURNA UTKATASANA)

The complete squat pose is an important pose in this sequence of vinyasas. The Sanskrit name of the pose indicates that it is the full hip-stretch pose *(purna utkatasana)*. It is also considered the counterpose *(pratikriya)* for the involved forward stretch pose (uttanasana) discussed earlier.

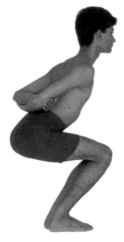

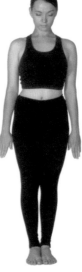

FIGURE 1-101 ◆◆   FIGURE 1-102 ◆◆◆   FIGURE 1-103 ◆

Now we will examine all the important vinyasas pertaining to the full hip stretch pose, purna utkatasana. First, as you inhale, raise your arms in front of you, up to shoulder level (see figure 1-104).

Stay in this position for three breaths. Then as you slowly exhale, bend your knees; lower your trunk so that you are sitting on your haunches (see figure 1-105).

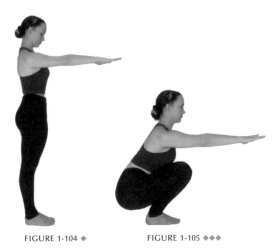

FIGURE 1-104 ◆   FIGURE 1-105 ◆◆◆

You may stay in the posture for a considerable amount of time, concentrating on your exhalation and the bandhas, or locks. You may also include the chin lock (jalandhara bandha), which will help you to maintain good control over your breathing. Since your arms are stretched in front of you, you will be able to maintain a good balance as you move down into the pose. This posture is popular when doing religious ablutions in India as part of the sun worship at dawn and at dusk. You can see hundreds of villagers sitting in this position while doing seated household work or agricultural work in the fields. It stretches and pulls up the pelvis from the hip joints. The thighs, gluteal muscles, and lower back are also pleasantly stretched. It is a nice pose in which to do

the three locks, the rectal, the abdominal, and the chin. It is very good exercise, and is beneficial for the lower abdomen and improves the functioning of *apana*, or the downward-flowing force, which is said to control many of the pelvic organs or organs close to the lower abdomen, such as the uterus, prostate, bladder, and colon.

We shall presently look at other vinyasas pertaining to this wonderful pose, utkatasana. In this vinyasa pertaining to utkatasana, or the hip stretch pose, the arms are raised overhead and the movement performed. While raising your arms overhead for this vinyasa, you will have to bend back a little more to maintain balance. As you inhale, very slowly raise both arms overhead and interlock your fingers (see figure 1-106).

Stay in this position for three long inhalations and exhalations. Now as you slowly exhale, maintain the chin lock (jalandhara bandha), and smoothly lower your trunk by bending your knees until you are sitting on your haunches (see figure 1-107).

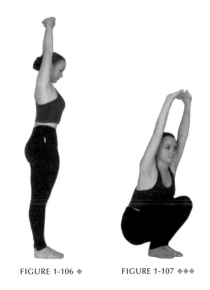

FIGURE 1-106 ◆   FIGURE 1-107 ◆◆◆

Stay in this position for a few breaths. All three locks can be practiced with appropriate breathing in this vinyasa.

The third vinyasa will involve keeping the arms stretched to the sides at shoulder level. This makes it a little more difficult and requires more attention from the practitioner to maintain balance. As you inhale, raise your arms to shoulder level laterally *(see figure 1-108)*.

Stay in this position for three long inhalations and exhalations. Then slowly, as you are exhaling (ujjayi), bend your knees and sit on your haunches, still keeping your arms spread out *(see figure 1-109)*.

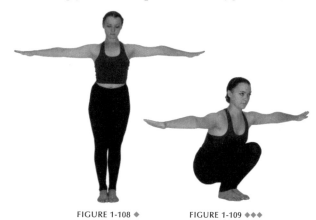

FIGURE 1-108 ◆   FIGURE 1-109 ◆◆◆

Stay in this position for three to six breaths. This posture is also a vinyasa of the bird pose (khagasana). It looks like a bird about to fly off or one that has just landed and is about to lower its wings.

The fourth vinyasa will require you to swing your hands behind your back. Inhaling for at least five seconds, raise both arms overhead, and as you slowly exhale, bend your elbows and place your palms on your shoulder blades *(see figure 1-110)*.

Stay in this position for a few breaths, then as you slowly exhale, bend your knees

and slowly sit down on your haunches *(see figure 1-111)*.

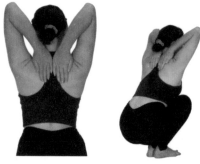

FIGURE 1-110 ◆◆   FIGURE 1-111 ◆◆◆

This will be more intricate than the previous vinyasas. Stay in the position for at least three breaths. You may practice all the three bandhas during the breath holding after exhalation. You can see that your chest opens perceptibly in this vinyasa, and you will feel the stretch in your upper chest as well.

In the fifth vinyasa, the hands are placed on the opposite shoulder blades. Inhaling, raise your arms overhead. While you are exhaling, bend your elbows and place your right palm on the left shoulder blade and your left palm on your right shoulder blade *(see figure 1-112)*.

Stay in this position for three breaths. Then while you smoothly do ujjayi exhalation, bend your knees and squat on your haunches *(see figure 1-113)*.

Stay in this position for a long time, concentrating on very smooth, long exhalation. You may also do all of the bandhas after the exhalation is over.

The sixth vinyasa brings out the best of this full squat pose. By opening the chest completely and requiring you to maintain perfect balance, this vinyasa necessitates your concentrating completely. Let us look

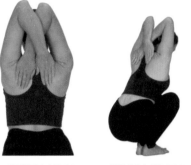

FIGURE 1-112 ◆◆   FIGURE 1-113 ◆◆◆

at the procedure. Raise your arms as you smoothly inhale. Then as you are breathing out, lower your arms, swing them behind your back, join them at the bottom of your spine, and turn your palms upward. Gently slide them along your spine up close to your shoulder blades in the back salute (prishtanjali) *(see figure 1-114)*.

Stay in this position for a few breaths. Now as you do slow, smooth ujjayi breathing, bend your knees and slowly ease into the hip stretch position (utkatasana). *(See figure 1-115.)*

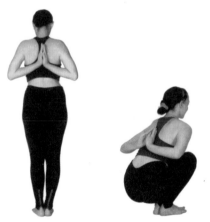

FIGURE 1-114 ◆◆   FIGURE 1-115 ◆◆◆◆

This is one more vinyasa of utkatasana, and perhaps the most involved. Stay in the position for a few breaths. As you inhale, you may return to tadasana.

You can see that the last three vinyasas are very good hip stretches, working on the knees as the knees are fully flexed, and equally important, they help to open up the thorax tremendously. If you stay in this pose, concentrating on both inhalation and exhalation, your vital capacity will improve.

Breathing in utkatasana tends to speed up until you are able to achieve perfection in the different vinyasas. This is so mainly because the posture compresses the abdomen, which can affect your breathing. So, many people, especially those with a large belly, breathe heavily while practicing utkatasana variations. With practice you will be able to breathe more smoothly in this posture. You should, however, not continue with the exercise when your breathing becomes heavy. You should rest between movements in the samasthiti position, regaining your smooth breathing before continuing. In vinyasa krama yoga practice, you should not compromise the quality of your breathing just to achieve a postural advantage. Further, in utkatasana, many people tend to lift their heels, which again is not correct. Rather you may use a windowsill, a chair, or a helping hand to do the posture without raising the heels. And your feet should be kept together.

THE TURTLE SQUAT POSE (KURMASANA)

The next vinyasa is similar to the previous group, but while you go down into the posture, you may open your hips, thereby spreading your knees (still keeping your feet together). Start the sequence of movements from tadasana. As you inhale, raise your arms. Then as you slowly exhale, open the hips and bend your knees, and start to squat while spreading your knees. As you sit on your haunches with your knees spread, insert your torso between your legs. You can grasp your heels with your hands from behind, by swinging your arms around your bent legs (*see figure 1-116*).

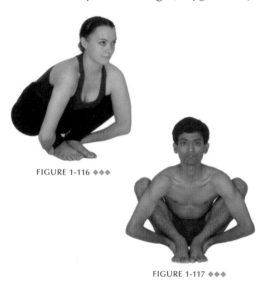

FIGURE 1-116 ◆◆◆

FIGURE 1-117 ◆◆◆

This posture is called kurmasana and is another variation of the turtle pose. The back is nicely curved like the shell of a turtle. Curving the back is an important exercise for the spine. Normally, we give considerable importance to arching the spine backward, but curving or rounding the spine is also necessary to maintain the flexibility of the entire spine. Free forward and backward movement of the spine is very useful when practicing postures requiring fine control of the spine, as in the headstand. This posture is mentioned as a practice for daily ablutions in many Indian books written more than 1,000 years ago. Stay in this position for three to six breaths. The front view is shown in figure 1-117.

THE GOLDEN BELT POSE
(KANCHYASANA)

The next vinyasa is an extension of the kurmasana we have already seen (the side view is shown in figure 1-118).

Some people call it the garland pose, or *malasana*. Staying in kurmasana, as you slowly exhale, take your hands from your feet, and then hold your hands behind your back like a belt. Inhale, then bend forward and place your head on the floor. Since you are still on your feet (on haunches), your buttocks do not touch the floor (*see figure 1-119*).

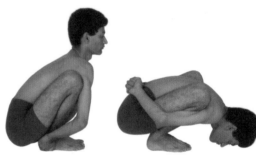

FIGURE 1-118 ◆◆◆   FIGURE 1-119 ◆◆◆

A front view of the same pose is seen in figure 1-120.

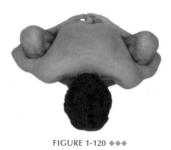

FIGURE 1-120 ◆◆◆

This pose is considered a part of the tadasana sequence. It is known as the golden belt pose (*kanchyasana*). Stay in this position for three to six breaths and on the next inhalation, stretch your arms overhead to get back to utkatasana, and then rise to tadasana.

The next vinyasa is a variant of the turtle pose (kurmasana). Remaining in malasana, do three long inhalations and exhalations. Then as you are slowly exhaling, round your back as much as you can, draw your head very close to your feet, and place the crown of your head in front of your feet (*see figure 1-121*).

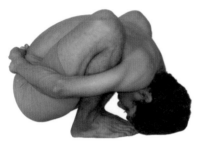

FIGURE 1-121 ◆◆◆◆

Your feet should still be planted firmly on the floor in utkatasana position. Stay in this position for three breaths, concentrating on making your exhalation as long as possible. The curving of the backbone is very pronounced in this exercise, and this is an important exercise, like back bending for the back.

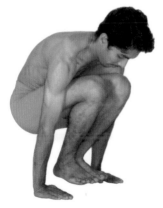

FIGURE 1-122 ◆◆◆◆

The next vinyasa is as follows. As you are exhaling, lower your arms while you are positioned in utkatasana. Exhale completely and holding the breath out, press through your palms and pump your body up, keeping the integrity of the utkatasana pose intact. Stay in the position for a few seconds, and then lower your body back into the squatting position. Repeat the movements a few times. This is *utkatasana utpluti* (*see figure 1-122*).

THE NOOSE POSE (PASASANA)

The next posture in this vinyasa sequence is known as the noose pose (*pasasana*). In a way it is similar to utkatasana except that you are turning sideways rather than looking straight ahead as in utkatasana. It is a "twist" in this group. Start the sequence from tadasana. As you inhale, slowly raise your arms overhead, interlock your fingers, and turn your palms outward. Stay in the position for a few slow ujjayi breaths. Then as you smoothly exhale, turn your torso to the right, still keeping your feet together and your toes pointing forward (*see figure 1-123*).

Inhale, and again when you are exhaling, bend your knees and squat, still keeping your torso turned to the right. It may be easygoing up to a point as you lower your body, but after you reach the halfway stage your body will tend to unwind. With very deep continuous exhalation, firmly anchor your feet and also tuck in your stomach as in the mula and uddiyana bandhas. Sit on your haunches, looking sideways. Stay in this position for one or two breaths. Then as you exhale, bend down slightly, place your left underarm around your right knee, and then swing your left arm around both the knees. Now swing your right arm around your back, and clasp your hands. The arms encircle or embrace the legs around the knees like a noose, hence the name of this pose (*see figure 1-124*).

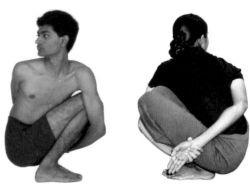

FIGURE 1-125 ◆◆◆◆   FIGURE 1-126 ◆◆◆◆

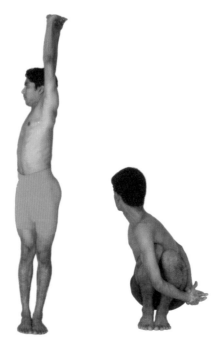

FIGURE 1-123 ◆◆   FIGURE 1-124 ◆◆◆◆

This is a very effective twisting pose. Hatha yogis interested in kundalini yoga practice it regularly. According to Nathamuni, an ancient yogi, this is one of the poses recommended for contraception, because it produces considerable pressure and torsion on the pelvic organs, especially the uterus. The side view is shown in figure 1-125.

Another view is shown in figure 1-126.

The side twist is very powerful and complete, in this case because the whole upper body will have to be taken outside of the range of the legs. You may stay in this position for a few breaths, concentrating on a very smooth, long exhalation, while the inhalation will be short. While inhaling, return to tadasana sthiti. Lower your arms while exhaling to return to samasthiti. You may also repeat the movements a few times to get the posture correct.

Repeat the movement on the left side as well. The view shown in figure 1-127 is the turning position before you start the descent.

Pasasana on the left side twist is shown in figure 1-128, and the front view is shown in figure 1-129.

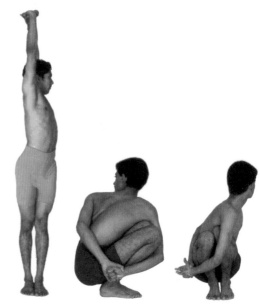

FIGURE 1-127 ◆◆   FIGURE 1-128 ◆◆◆◆   FIGURE 1-129 ◆◆◆◆

AIDED SQUATS
(Utkatasana-Sahaya Sahita)

As we conclude the utkatasana variations, I'd like to mention that keeping the feet together is an essential element of this entire sequence. Many people who are quite supple but do not normally squat on the floor find it difficult to practice this sequence. Many yoga experts who can do very difficult bends, handstands, and other postures balk at this very versatile, useful, and artistic asana sequence, perhaps because the fear of falling down makes them tight. So, in the initial stages you can hold a stable chair, table, or window frame for support. Sometimes a teacher will help a student through these poses by holding his or her hands and sitting down and rising up along with the student. See the figures, which indicate the starting utkatasana (*figure 1-130*), half-utkatasana (*figure 1-131*), and full utkatasana (*figure 1-132*) aided by a teacher.

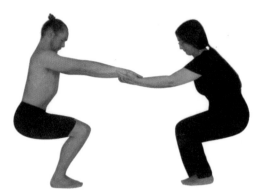

FIGURE 1-131 ◆◆

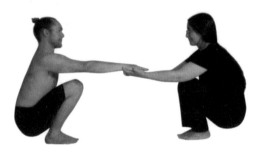

FIGURE 1-132 ◆◆

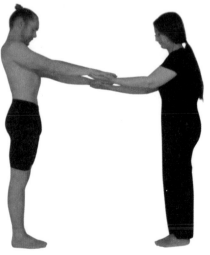

FIGURE 1-130 ◆

A large number of physical therapists and some professionals do not think going all the way down as described in the utkatasana variations is beneficial or even possible for many except perhaps the adepts. According to conventional wisdom among yogis, any part of the body, especially the joints, if left disused could become the breeding ground for ailments. My guru used to exhort many of his older students to keep moving their limbs (*vyayama*) by doing vinyasas. Since it is possible for many people (except those who have some organic, structural problems of the knees) to squat with some help, as shown earlier in this section, it is good to perform the squats regularly in yoga practice. In most cases, practitioners tend to stiffen the knees while trying to do the squat for fear of falling down, but with help they are able to

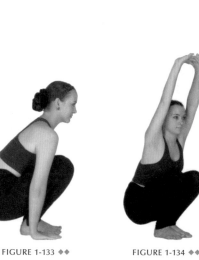

FIGURE 1-133 ◆◆

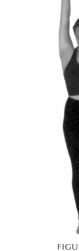

FIGURE 1-134 ◆◆

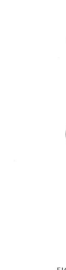

FIGURE 1-135 ◆

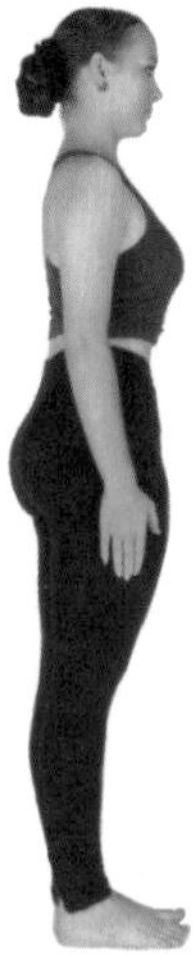

FIGURE 1-136 ◆

do the movement rather easily. Since the knee joints need to be flexed periodically, utkatasana may be included on a regular basis. The massaging stretch to the knees, and the stretching of the hips, thighs, and gluteal muscles are beneficial aspects of this pose and its vinyasas.

Now let us look at the return to samasthiti. You are now in full squat with both the palms on the floor (see figure 1-133).

Remaining in full squat (utkatasana), inhale, raise both your arms, interlock your fingers, and turn your hands outward (see figure 1-134).

Stay in this position for a couple of breaths and then, while inhaling, raise your trunk back to tadasana with your arms still raised (see figure 1-135).

During the next exhalation, slowly lower your arms to return to samasthiti (see figure 1-136).

Another way to return to samasthiti is to go through uttanasana, especially if you have been working with the vinyasas of

squats (utkatasana). Start from utkatasana sthiti with your palms firmly pressing on the floor (see figure 1-137).

While inhaling, straighten your knees for the forward stretch (uttanasana). See figure 1-138.

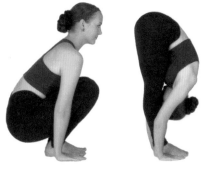

FIGURE 1-137 ◆◆◆

FIGURE 1-138 ◆◆◆

This will help stretch your knees, hamstrings, thighs, and calf muscles. It could be considered a counterpose (pratikriya) to the sequence of squat poses. Stay in the position for three breaths before returning to samasthiti (see figures 1-139 and 1-140).

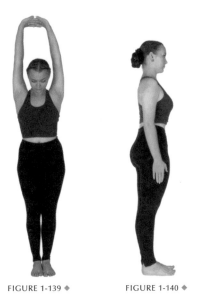

FIGURE 1-139 ◆   FIGURE 1-140 ◆

of your feet are stretched fully in this pose. Look at the "balancing" practice here.

THE CORPSE POSE (SAVASANA)

It is a good practice to have rest pauses during the vinyasa sequences. At the end of the session, it will be advisable to take rest in the corpse pose (*savasana*) *(see figure 1-142)*.

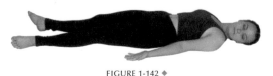

FIGURE 1-142 ◆

THE COMPLETE HILL POSE (TADASANA)

The last part of the sequence is tadasana. Here the movement is done is two stages. As you inhale, raise your arms overhead. Stay in the position for three breaths. Then while you are exhaling, raise your heels so that you are balancing on the balls of your feet *(see figure 1-141)*.

In the process you will be stretching the torsa of your feet as well. Try to stay in the position for three to six breaths. Then during the next inhalation, lower your heels. During the next exhalation, lower your arms to samasthiti. This movement helps to stretch your whole body. The ankles and dorsa

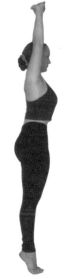

FIGURE 1-141 ◆◆◆

Lie down on your back. Keep your feet slightly apart and your feet turned slightly outward. Keep all your joints loose. Turn your head slightly to one side. Relax all your big joints deliberately. Relax your toes and your feet. Watch your heels relax and your calf muscles. Then relax your hamstrings and your knees. Direct your attention to your thighs and relax them next. Relax your buttocks, hip joints, and lower back. Next, relax your spine and neck. Then slowly move your attention to your shoulders and relax those joints. Relax your arms, elbows, and wrists. Then the knuckles and fingers should be relaxed. Wait for a moment, and then slowly move your attention to inside of your chest and watch your breath slow down, and allow it to slowly become nice and smooth. If your mind wanders, coax it back to your breath. Take about two to three minutes to relax in the corpse pose, and then proceed to the next item of practice on your agenda.

This completes the tadasana, or hill pose, sequence per the vinyasa method of yoga posture practice. This is the sequence of choice to start the vinyasa krama yoga. With this sequence, you can comprehensively exercise your whole body, and according to hatha yogis, it aligns the centers of the body (the chakras) nicely. Balance (*sthiratwa*) is an essential ingredient of yoga posture practice. This group instills a very fine sense of balance. The sequence is logically built, covering first movements of the arms, then the upper body, then the lumbar region, then the back, and finally the lower extremities.

Those not able to do all the vinyasas may attempt only those movements that they can do well unaided. Then they may attempt to do poses with aid or support, but should endeavor to dispense with supports and props as soon as possible.

The upper body exercises are very good for persons with breathing problems, especially those with bronchial asthma. The arm and thoracic movements exercise the entire breathing apparatus. The constant ujjayi breathing employed simulates asthmatic breathing and thus stimulates the sympathetic nervous system, which will help in opening the bronchial tubes for easier breathing. Normally, these exercises can be taught during periods when the attacks are minimal, and the patient learns to breathe with a constricted airway and hence develops some degree of self-confidence. Further, all the thoracic muscles that are disused in the asthmatic are also toned up, enabling a freer movement of the chest muscles. People who have breathing problems and also older people may be taught to do some of the upper body exercises while seated or even lying down.

The versatile tadasana sequence lends itself to some innovative and abbreviated subsequences. Repeated forward bend/pelvic tilt movement and the squat sequence will tone the muscles of the lower extremities. The well-known sun salutation sequence is an extension of the tadasana cycle. The bird posture sequence and salutations to the directions (*diknamaskara*) are some of the other classical sequences culled out of this major vinyasa krama. These special sequences are explained in chapter eleven.

2

ASYMMETRICAL SEATED VINYASA SEQUENCE

THE NEXT VINYASA group consists of seated postures that are asymmetrical. In the previous sequence, tadasana, basic alignment of the entire body was taken up and the all major muscles and joints were considered. Since it is basically seated sequence that is important for pranayama and other meditative efforts (*sadhanas*), it is imperative to master the basics for seated poses. The asymmetrical seated poses help to correct any imbalance by working both sides of the body separately, especially the lower extremities. Though many Westerners are eager to practice yoga, some are not particularly enthusiastic about doing seated postures, such as the lotus pose, hero pose, and others, which involve the hip joints, knees, and ankles. My guru used to say that the yogi should guard against an expanding waist and bludgeoning thighs, and this sequence is ideally suited in this regard. The vinyasas of varying difficulties help a practitioner attain *asana siddhi* (perfection in seated poses).

THE LEAD SEQUENCE

In vinyasa krama, it is customary to start all sequences from samasthiti. For seated poses, the beginning or hub pose is *dandasana*, or the staff pose. So in this sequence, we will start from samasthiti and go through a small sequence of vinyasas to reach the staff pose.

Please note that this sequence involves a few jump-throughs, which may be difficult for people who are older, new to yoga, or overweight. If you feel that you might have difficulty with a particular vinyasa, do not force yourself to do it. Pushing yourself to do every vinyasa in a group can result in injury, so please be cautious and do what you can. One shortened sequence would be to do samasthiti through utkanasana (see page 25) and then to sit down stretching your legs to dandasana. Or, you could begin in dandasana itself and proceed from there, skipping the preliminaries.

Samasthiti

Begin in samasthiti (see figure 2-1), and pay attention to your balance for one minute.

Then for one more minute, keep your eyes closed, your chin down, and your attention turned to the breath inside your chest.

As you inhale slowly (take five to ten seconds or more), raise both your arms, stretch, and interlace your fingers (see figure 2-2).

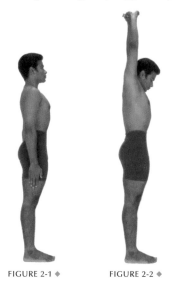

FIGURE 2-1 ◆   FIGURE 2-2 ◆

Stay like this for three long inhalations and exhalations. (This is a tadasana variation.) This gives a nice stretch to one's sides, and the upward movement of the arms also facilitates a nice inhalation and internal expansion of the chest.

The Forward Bend (Uttanasana)

Stretch thoroughly as you exhale. Bend forward and place your palms on the floor next to your feet (see figure 2-3).

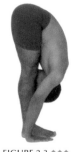

FIGURE 2-3 ◆◆◆

Try to place your face on your knees or a little bit lower, on your shins. (See page 15 for more on uttanasana.) This posture gives a nice forward tilt to the pelvis and also helps to tone the muscles of the posterior portions of the lower extremities, back, and neck.

THE FULL SQUAT OR SITTING-ON-YOUR-HAUNCHES POSE (UTKATASANA)

Slowly inhale. As you slowly and smoothly exhale, sit on your haunches. As you go down, you may slowly draw in your rectum and lower abdomen in coordination with your exhalation (see figure 2-4).

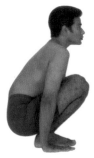

FIGURE 2-4 ◆◆◆

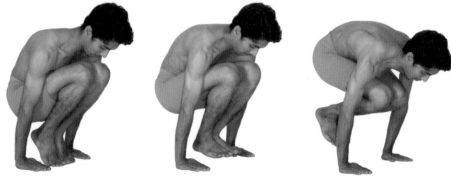

FIGURE 2-5 ◆◆◆◆   FIGURE 2-6 ◆◆◆◆   FIGURE 2-7 ◆◆◆◆

(This posture is a variation of utkatasana [the hip stretch] and is also known as *utkatakasana*, or the sitting-on-your-haunches pose.) Again hold this position for three breaths, concentrating on maintaining a very long exhalation.

Utpluti (Lifting Up)

This vinyasa is good preparation for jumping (*plavana*) backward into the next pose. Breathe out, hold your breath, and press through your palms to lift your heels off the floor. Keep your legs in the same bent position as in the full squat pose, with your toes barely touching the floor (*see figure 2-5*).

Stay in this position for a few breaths, and then exhale. Hold your breath and lift your feet (*utpluti*) off the ground (*see figure 2-6*).

Then bend your knees, and bring the feet up and backward while still holding your breath out (*see figure 2-7*).

Four-Legged Staff Posture (Chaturanga-Dandasana)

Slowly lower your head, inhale, and hold your breath. Keeping your palms firmly planted, jump backward, being sure to keep your feet together and close to the floor. Land gently on your toes. Many people mistakenly jump high in this posture and land heavily on their toes, which injures the big toes. The purpose of jumping back is to move the legs backward together, so that the alignment of the legs and hips is not disturbed (as would happen if the legs were spread, crossed, or moved back one at a time). Hold this posture for three breaths (*see figure 2-8*).

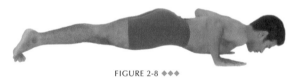

FIGURE 2-8 ◆◆◆

The Upward-Facing-Dog Pose (Urdhwa-Mukha Swanasana)

This pose strengthens the arms and shoulders and makes the spine more flexible. The pose resembles a dog stretching and is a nice anterior stretch posture that invigorates, strengthens the muscles, and makes the joints, especially the spine, supple.

As you exhale, stretch your ankles so that your toes and part of the dorsum (back of the foot) are on the floor. While inhaling slowly, stretch your body, by thrusting your chest out, arching your back, stretching your hips, and keeping your pelvis as low as possible. You may keep your chin in a chin lock (jalandhara bandha) and stay in the position for a few long, smooth inhalations and exhalations *(see figure 2-9)*.

You may also look upward upon inhalation as an additional movement in this pose *(see figure 2-10)*.

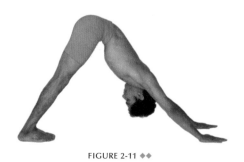

FIGURE 2-11 ♦♦

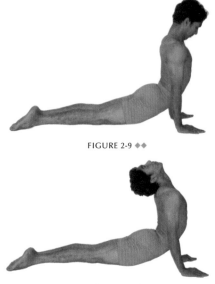

FIGURE 2-9 ♦♦

FIGURE 2-10 ♦♦

See to it that your whole body, except your toes and palms, is off the floor.

The Downward-Facing-Dog Pose (Adho-Mukha Swanasana)

Now as you slowly and deliberately exhale, raise your hips, drop your head, and press your feet into the floor. Again, you may hold this for a few breaths and concentrate on your exhalation. This is also a good position in which to do mula and uddiyana locks after a very deliberate complete exhalation *(see figure 2-11)*.

This downward-facing dog pose gives the body a full posterior stretch and is itself a useful hub pose for several poses such as the staff pose, Vasishtasana (a pose named after the Vasishta, a great Vedic sage), the plough pose, the bolt pose, and a few others.

The Jump Through (Plavana)

Inhale smoothly, hold your breath, stretch your ankles, and bend your knees slightly. Keeping your feet together (your ankles should remain nicely relaxed), bend your knees, press through your palms, and jump or hurtle your whole body through the space between your hands *(see figure 2-12)*.

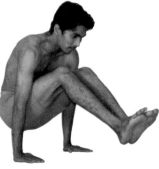

FIGURE 2-12 ♦♦♦

As you pass through your hands stretch your legs while still in motion. Hold your breath as you hold your body in the air and keep your legs stretched for five seconds *(see figure 2-13)*.

(This is the staff pose, dandasana, in lifted-up position, utpluti.) Be careful to

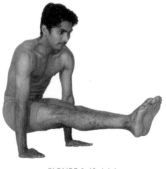

FIGURE 2-13 ◆◆◆

keep your feet together when jumping through your palms. If you do not, you will alter the alignment of the hips and become wobbly and clumsy. Your feet, especially your ankles, should be kept together right through the motion.

Staff Pose (Dandasana)

Now as you exhale slowly, lower your body onto the floor to a straight-legged seated position. This posture is the staff or stick pose (dandasana) *(see figure 2-14)*.

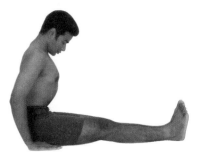

FIGURE 2-14 ◆◆

(This is an important hub posture for all seated asanas and a few others such as the *Vasishtasana*. The Vasishtasana is described in another sequence.)

Staff Pose, without Support (Niralamba Dandasana)

As you slowly inhale, raise both arms overhead; interlock your fingers while you

complete the inhalation. Lower your arms to the starting position on exhalation or stay in the posture. During every inhalation, try to stretch your back. It would be good to keep your chin locked all the while *(see figure 2-15)*.

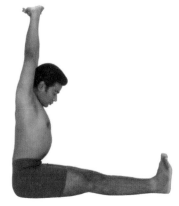

FIGURE 2-15 ◆◆

This is a nice back stretch movement. You may repeat it three times.

ASSYMMETRICAL SEQUENCE

Now you are ready to start the asymmetrical sequence. It is very versatile. The various postures and movements it consists of make the yogi fit to do the seated postures required for pranayama and meditation for long hours. Adept yogis may do all the vinyasas on one side before repeating the asana vinyasas on the other side. However, those who have limited time for practice may do each subsequence on both sides before going on to practice the next subsequence. In this way, practice on both sides at one sitting may be ensured.

In this sequence, first the movements are done for the right side, keeping the left leg straight. After completing the movements on one side the same movement will be repeated with the right leg kept straight and moving the left leg to different asana positions.

Sage Marichi Pose (Marichyasana)

The *Marichyasana* subroutine seen here involves forward bending, twisting, and also a counterpose, which stretches the front portion of the body (purva bhaga). The tibia (inner shinbone) of the right leg is kept almost vertical during a forward tilting of the pelvis. This gives the right hip joint an additional twist (especially during the forward bending) to help open the hip joint. According to my guru, this posture helps control the waistline and corrects digestive disorders such as flatulence. It is a good exercise for activating the liver and may be helpful in preventing certain ailments, such as jaundice. It is good pose for chest expansion for young adults and is said to strengthen the heart. However, it should be avoided by pregnant women. Per conventional wisdom, according to my guru, regular practice of this postural sequence will improve blood circulation (*rakta sanchara*) in the lower extremities and could prevent the onset of paralysis or nerve disorders in the lower extremities (*parsva vayu*).

To begin the Sage Marichi pose, as you exhale, slowly and smoothly bend your right knee, draw your right heel close to your right buttock (you may use your hands), and place your foot close to your right thigh. Do the chin lock (jalandhara bandha), and do three long, smooth inhalations and exhalations. This is the Marichyasana position (Marichyasana sthiti) (*see figure 2-16*).

Inhale for five seconds through a constricted throat, making a hissing sound (ujjayi). Then as you exhale smoothly, stretch your back and bend forward to hold your left foot; place your head on your left knee or shin while keeping your right leg in Marichyasana. (*see figure 2-17*).

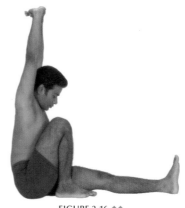

FIGURE 2-16 ◆◆

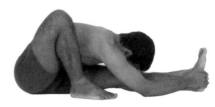

FIGURE 2-17 ◆◆

Hold this position for a number of breaths. The inhalations can be moderate, say about three to five seconds, but concentrate on extending the exhalation as much as you can. At the end of every exhalation, you may do rectal and abdominal locks for about five seconds. Release the two locks, and while inhaling, slowly return to Marichyasana sthiti.

Now from Marichyasana sthiti, while slowly exhaling, swing your right arm around your right knee; swing your left arm around your back and clasp your hands behind your back (*see figure 2-18*).

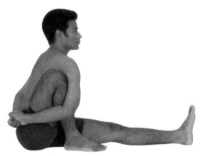

FIGURE 2-18 ◆◆

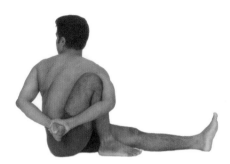

FIGURE 2-20 ◆◆

Stay in this position for three long inhalations and exhalations, tightening your grip on every exhalation. This vinyasa enhances the effect of the posture by better anchoring of the right foot, especially during forward-bending vinyasa, which follows.

In the next vinyasa inhale slowly, then as you slowly breathe out with ujjayi, stretch and bend forward, placing your face on your left knee (*see figure 2-19*).

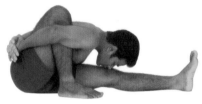

FIGURE 2-19 ◆◆

Stay in this position for a few breaths, making the exhalations especially long and smooth. During each exhalation tighten your grip so as to bend a bit more and squeeze air out of your lungs. At the end of each exhalation hold your breath out, and do rectal and abdominal locks. Return to the asana sthiti (Marichyasana sthiti) on a slow inhalation.

On the next inhalation, slowly turn your body to the left side, twisting your torso in the process (*see figure 2-20*).

Exhale slowly and stay in this position for three breaths, opening your chest on every inhalation. Also try to turn a little more on every exhalation. Thereafter as you slowly inhale, return to Marichyasana sthiti.

Proceed to the counterpose (pratikriya) in Marichyasana. Inhaling slowly, raise your arms overhead, and as you slowly exhale, lean back to place your palms on the floor about a foot behind your back. Leaning back slightly on your hands, inhale slowly and raise your trunk as high as you can for a moment. Return to the starting position on exhalation. Repeat the movement three to six times with appropriate breathing (*see figure 2-21*).

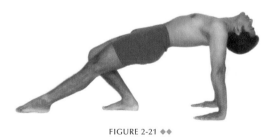

FIGURE 2-21 ◆◆

In this first subroutine in the asymmetrical seated sequence, the left leg was kept straight and the right leg was in Marichyasana sthiti. Remain in this position and proceed to the next set of vinyasas.

Half-Kingfish Pose
(Ardha Matsyendrasana)

As you exhale, place the foot of your bent right leg outside your left thigh. Now inhale smoothly and raise both arms overhead. Continue exhaling, turn to the right side, swing your right arm around your back, and hold your left thigh with your right hand. Slowly inhale as you try to turn a little more to the right side, and stretch your left hand to bring it around the outside of your bent right knee. Grasp the big toe of your right foot. Stay in this position for three to six breaths. Try to make your inhalation long and smooth (*see figure 2-22*).

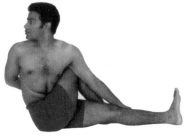

FIGURE 2-22 ◆◆◆

You may also try this pose with your hands clasped behind your back (*see figure 2-23*).

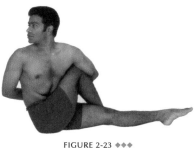

FIGURE 2-23 ◆◆◆

With your right foot well anchored, it is easier to twist your spine smoothly. Matsyendrasana and its several simpler variations—such as the *ardha Matsyendrasana*

have just seen—are excellent exercises for the spine. After holding this posture, inhale, raise both arms, and stretch your right leg to return to the staff pose (dandasana).

Half-Lotus Pose (Ardha Padmasana)

This sequence is a nice preparation for those who want to do the full lotus pose. It involves keeping the right leg in the half-lotus position, while the left leg remains stretched. According to my guru, it is very good for purifying the *apana vayu*, or neurological force operating on the lower abdomen, especially the pelvic organs. Kundalini yogis find it to be a very useful sequence in the arousal of *kundalini* (divine power). Properly done, it stimulates the pancreas, thanks to the gentle massaging of the right heel accentuated by the bandhas. This is not a sequence that should be practiced during pregnancy.

The half-lotus position involves a few more movements of the body. While you exhale in the staff pose, slowly bend your right knee, stretch your right ankle fully, and place the outer side of your right foot on your left thigh close to your groin. As you are inhaling, raise both arms overhead. This position is *ardha padmasana* (*see figure 2-24*).

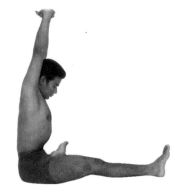

FIGURE 2-24 ◆◆

Stay in this position for three breaths. Finely adjust the posture so that you feel comfortable and well anchored. As you exhale slowly and smoothly, stretch your back and bend forward. Hold your left big toe with your right hand, and place your left hand on top of it, or hold your left heel with both hands. Place your head on your stretched-out left knee. Stay in this position for three to six breaths, making the exhalation as complete as possible. During every exhalation, try to stretch forward and bring your body down lower. You may use the bandhas, or locks, after exhalation and when holding your breath out. This is the right half-lotus posterior-stretch posture (*dakshina-ardha-padma-paschmatanasana*) (*See figure 2-25*).

This posture is the right tied-half-lotus posture (*dakshina-ardha-baddha-padmasana*).

Inhale and while exhaling smoothly and slowly, stretch your back and bend forward and place your forehead on your outstretched left knee or beyond it. You may stay in this position for a few breaths, concentrating on making the exhalations long, smooth, and as complete as possible. After some practice, you may attempt to do rectal and abdominal locks after exhalation and while holding your breath out. This vinyasa has a long name: *dakshina-ardha-baddha-padma-paschima-uttanasana*. Translated, it is the right-side-locked-half-lotus posterior-stretch posture (*see figure 2-27*).

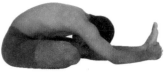

FIGURE 2-25 ◆◆

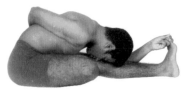

FIGURE 2-27 ◆◆◆

As you slowly inhale, stretch your arms overhead. Then during the next slow exhalation, swing your right arm behind your back and firmly grasp the big toe of your left leg. Keep your back straight, and stay in this position for three long breaths (*see figure 2-26*).

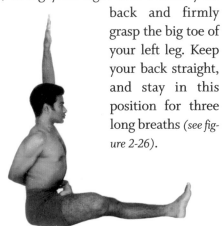

FIGURE 2-26 ◆◆

The following variation does not belong strictly in this sequence because the left leg is moved, but there is a lot to be said for keeping it in the sequence. Let us see how it works. Begin in the right tied-half-lotus pose. While exhaling, place your left palm (turned out 90 degrees) on the floor about a foot behind you. Your right hand should still be held behind the big toe of your right foot, which is placed on your left thigh. Now as you inhale, press through your left hand and the outside of your left foot, tilt to the left side, and raise your body, moving your hip. As you achieve the posture, look up (*see figure 2-28*).

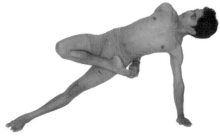

FIGURE 2-28 ◆◆◆

This posture is called the one-leg-locked half-lotus Vasishtasana (*ardha-baddha-padma Vasishtasana*), and is named after a Vedic sage called Kashyapa (*Kashyapasana*). It is considered a vinyasa of another well-known pose, the Vasishtasana. This is a very efficient posture for effecting a lateral movement of the hip and consequently stretching the hip. Stay in this position for a few breaths, lifting your body up a little bit more on every inhalation. Return to your starting position on exhalation.

Now exhaling as you lean forward, hold the inside of your left foot with your left hand. Hold your left foot firmly, and slowly inhaling, turn or twist your body to the right side, looking over your right shoulder. Stay in this position for a few breaths. This is also a variant of the half-kingfish pose (ardha matsyendrasana) (*see figure 2-29*). Return to your starting position on exhalation.

both arms overhead as in the half-lotus (ardha padmasana) position. As you keep exhaling, lean forward and hold the outside of your left foot with your right hand. Then inhale and as you exhale twist to the left side and swing your left hand from behind your back and take hold of your right thigh (*see figure 2-30*).

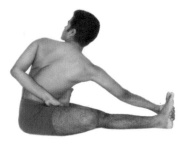

FIGURE 2-30 ◆◆

Stay in this position for a few breaths, turning even more on every exhalation. Inhale, and return to the half-lotus position.

Before you do the counterpose for the present set of half-lotus vinyasas, you can attempt another variation. Remain in the half-lotus position. Exhaling slightly, lean forward and place your palms on the floor close to your thighs. Exhale, hold your breath, and pressing down with your palms, lift your body, maintaining the half-lotus position of your right leg (*see figure 2-31*).

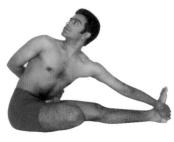

FIGURE 2-29 ◆◆

Now you can do another vinyasa of ardha matsyendrasana. Inhaling, raise

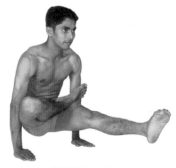

FIGURE 2-31 ◆◆◆

Once you are able to remain steady in the pose, you can attempt to stay in the position for a few breaths. Inhale, hold your breath, and slowly ease onto the floor. You may repeat the movements a few times.

Next we will consider the counterpose, or prathikriya in half-lotus. While inhaling in half-lotus, raise both arms overhead. As you breath out, place both hands behind your back about a foot away on the floor; lean back slightly. Your palms should be placed inward with the fingers pointing toward you. As you inhale, slowly press down with your palms, and lift your hip, while stretching your left ankle so that the left foot is placed on the floor. Keep your right hip relaxed, and allow your bent right leg to hang from the hip. Both the knees should be at the same level. Drop your head and look back. Exhaling, return to the starting point, and repeat the movement three times (see figure 2-32).

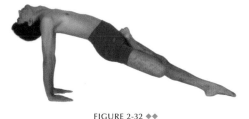

FIGURE 2-32 ◆◆

Now we will go on to the next subroutine, where the right foot is kept flush with the right thigh.

The Great Seal (Maha Mudra)

Keep your left leg stretched out and your arms raised. While exhaling, bend your right knee and place your right foot flush with your left thigh. Your right heel may touch or press against your perineum. This is maha

mudra sthiti. As the name indicates it is considered a great mudra or seal (see figure 2-33).

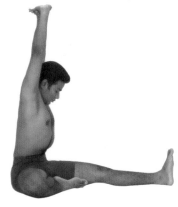

FIGURE 2-33 ◆◆

Now as you keep exhaling, stretch the back, bend forward, and grasp the big toe of your left foot with your index finger, middle finger, and thumb. This is maha mudra. Keep the chin down in jalandhara bandha. You are advised to stay in maha mudra for a long time, say about five or more minutes. At the end of every long, complete exhalation, also mula bandha and uddiyana bandha for five to ten seconds. This maha mudra, along with the bandhas, tones up the right side of the abdominal area, especially the liver (see figure 2-34).

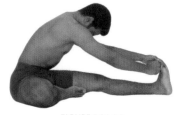

FIGURE 2-34 ◆◆

Toward the end of your stint in maha mudra, as you slowly exhale bend forward. Hold your left foot with both hands, and place your forehead on your left knee or further down on the shin. As you inhale come back to maha mudra, and repeat the movement three to six times (see figure 2-35).

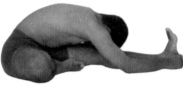

FIGURE 2-35 ♦♦

This forward bend is known as the head-on-knee pose (janusirsasana).

Now, as you exhale deeply, turn to the right. Bend forward, hold your left foot with both the hands, with your right hand on the outside of your left foot and your left hand on the inside of your left foot (see figure 2-36).

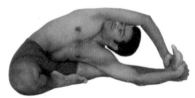

FIGURE 2-36 ♦♦♦

Stay in this position for three to six breaths, turning or twisting your body further on every exhalation. Inhale and return to the mahamudra sthiti. You now stretch your right leg and move into a staff pose.

According to my guru, many ailments of the legs respond well to this asana group. It stretches many of the joints, especially the hip and the knees and improves circulation in these joints. Runners and those who like to walk will find this asana group especially good. The lower extremities will remain in good working condition. Women who practice this sequence will find it helpful for normal delivery in childbirth. However, they should have practiced them a great

deal before pregnancy. The forward bending exercises should be avoided by pregnant women.

The Archer Pose (Akarna Danurasana)

The next few vinyasas in this group are much more difficult for ordinary practitioners but form a logical extension of the asymmetrical poses and vinyasas of the right side. The asana we take up now is called the archer pose (akarna dhanurasana).

Stretch both the legs as in staff pose (see figure 2-37).

Inhale and raise both arms overhead (see figure 2-38).

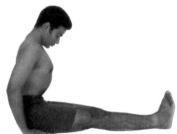

FIGURE 2-37 ♦♦

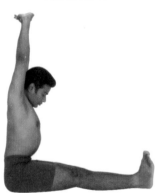

FIGURE 2-38 ♦♦

While slowly exhaling, lean forward and grasp your toes with your thumb and the next two fingers. Inhale, and on the following long, smooth exhalation, bend your right knee and slowly draw your right foot toward your right ear or beyond it (see figure 2-39).

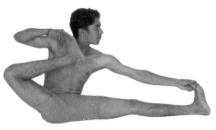

FIGURE 2-39 ◆◆◆

Stay in this position for three to six breaths, opening your hip a little more on every exhalation. This is known as akarna dhanurasana, or a posture resembling an archer with a bow drawn up to the ear, ready to shoot an arrow. As you inhale, slowly stretch your right leg into staff pose, or dandasana. This is also a good exercise for the right hip, because the femur is pushed back almost vertically, stretching the hip in an upward direction.

Heron Pose (Kraunchasana)

From dandasana, as you are exhaling slowly and smoothly, bend forward and take hold of your right foot with both hands. Inhale, and during the following exhalation, draw your right leg toward you and straight up. Try to place your forehead on your right knee while you keep exhaling (see figure 2-40).

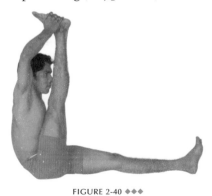

FIGURE 2-40 ◆◆◆

Stay in this position for three to six breaths. This posture is *kraunchasana*. The

tibia and femur are practically vertical. The legs are at right angles, providing a good stretch of the hamstring, thigh, and calf muscles of the upright right leg.

One-Foot-on-Head Pose (Ekapada Sirsasana)

The next vinyasas is a bit involved. Again from dandasana, as you breathe out smoothly, lean forward to grab your right foot with both hands. Inhale, and on the next exhalation, draw the leg toward the right side of your body and beyond it. Continuing the exhalation, bend your right knee and place your right foot on the back of your neck or, if possible, at about the shoulder blade. Keep your hands folded in the prayer position (anjali) (see figure 2-41).

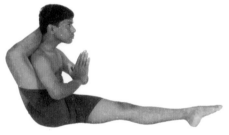

FIGURE 2-41 ◆◆◆◆

Stay in this position for three to six breaths. This posture is called the right-foot-on-head pose (dakshina-ekapada-sirsasana).

Now as you slowly exhale, bend forward and hold your left foot with both hands, keeping your head on your outstretched left knee (see figure 2-42).

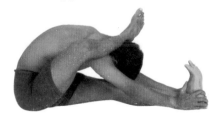

FIGURE 2-42 ◆◆◆◆

Stay in this position for three to six breaths. Try to do the abdomen and rectum locks after exhalation. This posture is known as the Skanda pose (*Skandasana*), named after Skanda, the son of Shiva. More specifically, it is called dakshina-Skandasana (*dakshina = right*), because it is done on the right side.

The next vinyasa is to lean back slowly during a long inhalation (*see figure 2-43*).

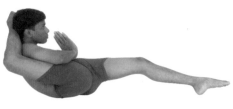

FIGURE 2-43 ◆◆◆◆

Stay in this position for three to six breaths. This pose is called *dakshina-Bhairava asana*, named after Bhairava, an aspect of Lord Shiva. Some say that Bhairava is the name of a yogi mentioned in hatha yoga texts and this pose is named after him. While exhaling, move back to ekapada sirsasana. (*See figure 2-44 for another angle.*)

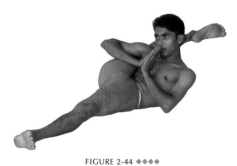

FIGURE 2-44 ◆◆◆◆

Then place your palms on the floor as you exhale, and holding your breath, lift (utpluti) your body up and balance for a few moments (*see figure 2-45*).

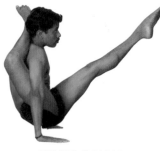

FIGURE 2-45 ◆◆◆◆◆

Stay in this position for a few breaths, breathing normally. This is the mythical moonbeam bird pose (*chakora asana*). Return to ekapada sirsasana. Finally grab your right leg with both hands, and as you inhale stretch the leg back to the staff pose (dandasana).

This group of vinyasas is very difficult to master, but with practice it becomes possible. The backward tilt of the hip joint with the tibia and thighbone almost vertical gives the maximum flexion to the right hip joint. According to conventional wisdom, this is very good for the tone of the rectal muscles and will prevent the formation of hemorrhoids. It is said to add considerable strength to the neck and shoulders, as well as create an Atlas-like capacity for carrying weight on one's shoulders.

Bent-Back-Leg Pose (Tiryang-Mukha-Ekapadasana)

The next subgroup involves keeping the right leg bent back, while the left leg remains stretched forward. From dandasana sthiti, as you exhale, bend your right leg back along your right thigh with the heel facing backward. (*see figure 2-46*).

This is tiryang-mukha-ekapadasana sthiti. Because the right leg is bent, it is also known as *tiryang-mukha-dakshina-pada-asana sthiti*,

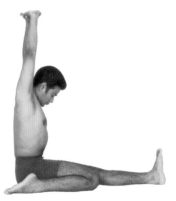

FIGURE 2-46 ◆◆

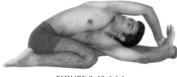

FIGURE 2-48 ◆◆◆

dakshina meaning right. Stay with your arms raised for three long smooth inhalations and exhalations.

As you slowly exhale, stretch your back thoroughly by slowly bending forward to hold your left foot. Place your forehead on your outstretched left knee (*see figure 2-47*).

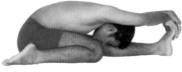

FIGURE 2-47 ◆◆

Stay in this position for about two minutes, extending your exhalation and doing the rectal and abdominal locks. This posture is known as the backward-facing one-foot posterior stretch posture (*tiryang-mukha-ekapada-paschima-uttanasana*). Because this posture pertains to the right leg it is also known as *tiryang-mukha-dakshina-pada-paschima-uttanasana*.

Inhaling, return to the starting point of the posture (asana sthiti). For the next vinyasa, as you make a long, smooth exhalation, tilt your torso to the right side, bend forward, and grasp your left foot with both the hands. The left hand should hold the

Stay in this position for three to six breaths, trying to twist a little bit more on each exhalation. Inhale, and return to asana sthiti.

Bird (Heron) Pose (Kraunchasana)

Get back to tiryang-mukha sthiti. (Another variation is to raise the right leg up on a smooth exhalation.) You may touch your right knee with your forehead. Stay in that position for three breaths, and return to the asana sthiti (*see figure 2-49*).

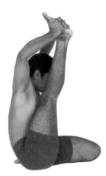

FIGURE 2-49 ◆◆◆

Now for the counterpose (pratikriya). From the asana sthiti position, exhale, lower your arms, and place your palms on the floor behind your back about a foot away from your body. Keep your chin down, and take three long ujjayi breaths. Then as you do a long inhalation, press down with your palms, stretch your left ankle outward, and lift your trunk as high as you can (*see figure 2-50*).

Exhale, come back to tiryang-mukha sthiti, and repeat the movement three to six times. This is known as the backward-facing right-foot posterior stretch posture (*tiryang-mukha-dakshinapada-purvatanasana*).

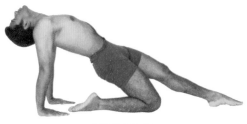

FIGURE 2-50 ◆◆

Again, this pose is very useful for preventing ailments of the leg. It improves blood circulation to the leg, facilitates the venous return of the blood, and helps prevent varicose veins. Regular practice will prevent edema of the leg.

Staying in the posture, place your palms on the floor, leaning forward slightly. Then exhale, hold your breath, and pressing down with your palms, lift your body up (utpluti) (see figure 2-51).

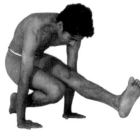

FIGURE 2-51 ◆◆◆

Stay in the raised body position for a few breaths, and as you hold your breath after inhalation, lower your body back to asana sthiti. This improves your sense of balance, strengthens your arms, and prepares you well for the next posture in the sequence.

The Monkey-God Pose (Anjaneyasana)

This posture is very involved and requires patience and repeated attempts to master. It is best to learn it under proper guidance, but I include it here as part of the entire sequence.

As you are exhaling, place your palms by your sides. Inhale, hold your breath, lift your body slighty (see the previous vinyasas), stretch your right leg all the way back. Breathe normally a few times, and then as you inhale raise both arms overhead, keeping the palms together in the gesture of prayer (anjali mudra) (see figure 2-52).

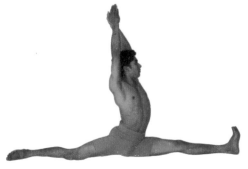

FIGURE 2-52 ◆◆◆◆◆

This posture is known as *Anjaneyasana*, named after the epic Rama devotee (in the form of a monkey) from *Ramayana*. Now as you are exhaling, lower your arms and place your palms on the floor beside your body. Inhale, and raise your arms overhead for the forward bend.

Inhale, then exhaling slowly, bend forward to place your forehead on your outstretched left knee; hold the toes of your left foot. Stay in this position for a few breaths. As you are inhaling, return to *Anjaneyasana sthiti* (see figure 2-53).

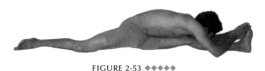

FIGURE 2-53 ◆◆◆◆◆

Then, exhaling, lift your body and bring your right leg forward to the *tiryang-mukha-asana sthiti*. Thereafter, as you inhale stretch your leg and return to the staff pose (dandasana).

ASYMMETRICAL HYBRID VINYASAS (RIGHT SIDE)

So far we have seen asanas with the left leg stretched in dandasana sthiti, while the right leg was worked in different positions. You can see that apart from dandasana sthiti, the left leg can be kept in other classical positions such as the backward-facing-foot pose (*tiryang mukha*), sage Marichi pose (Marichyasana), or half-lotus pose (*ardha padmasana*) positions, while the right leg is manipulated. All of these provide stable postures. Next, we will see some more vinyasas in which the left leg is kept in one of these positions and the right leg's position is altered.

Half-Lotus Marichi Pose (Ardha-padma Marichyasana)

Bend your right knee, as you are exhaling, and place it on your left thigh in *ardha-padmasana sthiti* (a position of half-lotus pose). Inhale, and on the next exhalation bend your left leg and draw your left foot close to your left buttock in half-lotus Sage Marichi position (*ardha-padma-Marichyasana sthiti*). Here, the right leg is in the half-lotus position and the left is in Marichi position.

Inhale and with the next exhalation, bend forward and place your forehead on the floor (*see figure 2-54*).

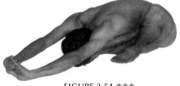

FIGURE 2-54 ◆◆◆

Stay in the position for three breaths, with very long exhalations. Inhale and return to the asana sthiti. Next, while exhaling swing your left arm around your left knee, and swing your right hand around your back to hold the left hand.

Remaining in this position, as you exhale smoothly, bend forward to place your forehead on your right knee or on the floor (*see figure 2-55*).

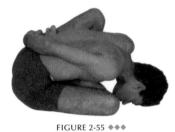

FIGURE 2-55 ◆◆◆

Stay in this position for three breaths. Return to the previous asana sthiti.

Now while exhaling, slowly twist your torso to the right and turn your head to look over your right shoulder. Stay in this position for three breaths, twisting a little more on each exhalation. After three breaths, as you inhale return to asana sthiti.

As you inhale, raise both arms overhead. While exhaling, slowly lean back and place your palms on the floor behind you, say about a foot behind your body. Press down with your hands, and while slowly inhaling, raise your trunk. Exhale and come down. Repeat these movements three times, and then return to asana sthiti on inhalation. Stretch your legs forward to dandasana sthiti.

Backward-Facing-Foot Marichi Pose (Tiryang-mukha Marichyasana)

In dandasana sthiti, exhale and place your left leg in the backward-facing-foot position (*tiryang mukha sthiti*). On the next exhalation, bend your right knee; drag your right foot close to your left thigh (*see figure 2-56*).

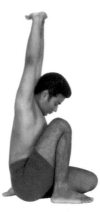

FIGURE 2-56 ♦♦

This is the asana sthiti. Stay in this position for three long inhalations and exhalations. This is another vinyasa of Marichyasana stihti.

As you exhale, slowly bend forward and place your forehead on the floor. Stay in this position for three to six breaths, concentrating on making the exhalations long and smooth. You may practice all three of the bandhas at the end of each exhalation for about five seconds.

The next vinyasa involves placing your right hand around your right knee and holding it behind your back with your left hand. This is to be done while you are exhaling smoothly (see figure 2-57).

Stay in this position for three long inhalations and exhalations.

Remaining in asana sthiti, as you breathe out slowly, turn to your left side, looking over your left shoulder (see figure 2-58).

Stay in this position for three to six smooth long breaths. On every exhalation, try to twist a little more. Then as you inhale, return to asana sthiti.

Now, let us look at the forward bend. Inhale. While exhaling, slowly bend forward and place your forehead on your left knee (see figure 2-59).

Stay in this position for three breaths, focusing on the exhalation and doing the bandhas at the end of each exhalation. Return to asana sthiti on inhalation.

Next you should do the counterpose (pratikriya). As you inhale, slowly stretch your arms overhead. While you exhale, place your palms on the floor behind your back about a foot away from your body. Press down firmly with your palms as you slowly inhale, and raise your trunk as high as you can (see figure 2-60).

Repeat the movement three times. Inhaling, raise your arms overhead. As you exhale, lower your arms.

Half-Lotus, Left-Foot-Turned-Backward Pose (Ardha-Padma-Tiryang-Mukha-Vamapadasana)

Place your right foot on top of your left thigh with your right thigh turned out to the side as you breathe out. On the next inhalation, raise your arms overhead and interlock your fingers (see figure 2-61).

This is the half-lotus, left-foot-turned-backward pose (ardha-padma-tiryang mukha vamapadasana). Stay in this position

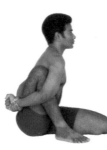

FIGURE 2-57 ♦♦

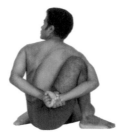

FIGURE 2-58 ♦♦

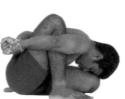

FIGURE 2-59 ♦♦♦

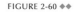
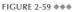

FIGURE 2-60 ♦♦

52 THE COMPLETE BOOK OF VINYASA YOGA

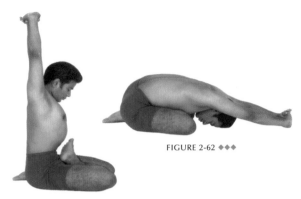

FIGURE 2-62 ◆◆◆

FIGURE 2-61 ◆◆◆

for three long inhalations and exhalations. Stretch your back on every inhalation.

Exhaling smoothly, slowly stretch your back as you place your forehead on the floor. Stay in this position for a few breaths doing the bandhas at the end of each exhalation and before starting the next inhalation. This is the half-lotus transverse left-legged posterior stretching pose (*ardha-padma-tiryang-mukha vamapada-paschima-uttanasana*). (*See figure 2-62.*)

Sage Bharadwaja Pose (Bharadwajasana)

Now we go to a well-known posture called *Bharadwajasana*, named after a Vedic sage called Bharadwaja. From the asana sthiti, exhale; swing your right arm around your back and take hold of the big toe of your right foot with your right hand. Inhale, and then on the next exhalation slowly place your left palm on the floor outside of and below your right thigh (*see figure 2-63*).

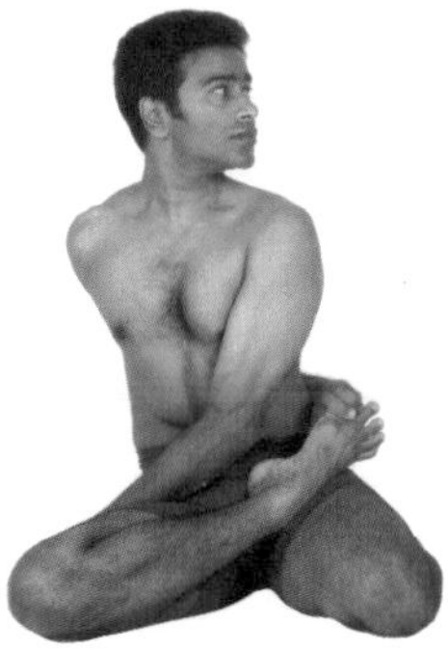

Anchor your left palm on every exhalation, as you twist more to the left side. Stay in

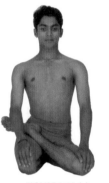

FIGURE 2-63 ◆◆◆

this position for up to five minutes. This is a very nice twisting posture.

The Great Lock (Mahabandha)

In this pose, keep your right leg bent as in the previous vinyasas, and draw your right foot inward and sit on the right heel. The heel closes the anus and presses against it. On the next exhalation bend your left knee and place it on your right thigh as in ardha padmasana (see page 42). Place your palms on your knees (*see figure 2-64*).

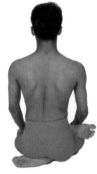

FIGURE 2-64 ◆◆   FIGURE 2-65 ◆◆

Do six long inhalations and exhalations. In this pose five bandhas, or locks, can be practiced. The rear view is shown figure 2-65.

Closing the anus with the heel is *mahabandha*. After exhalation, you can practice the rectal lock (mula bandha), followed in quick succession by the abdominal lock (uddiyana bandha) and the chin lock (jalandhara bandha). The fifth lock is the tongue lock (*jihva bandha*) in which you roll your tongue and place the tip back inside (at the end of exhalation), while closing the opening of the throat.

Half-Kingfish Pose
(Ardha Matsyendrasana)

Now you can try to do another asana, ardha Matsyendrasana. From dandasana, drag your right foot along the floor and place it by the side of your left buttock, with the entire leg remaining on the floor. This is done as you are exhaling. On the next exhalation, bend your left knee, and place your right foot on the floor beside your right knee—keeping your right leg almost vertical. Stay in this position for a few breaths. Now as you are exhaling, turn your body to the left side, and swing your left arm behind your back and take hold of your right thigh with your left hand. Stay in this position for a couple of breaths. Now as you slowly exhale, stretch your right hand and place it around the outside of your left knee to hold the big toe of the left foot (*see figure 2-66*).

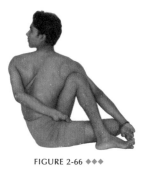

FIGURE 2-66 ◆◆◆

Stay in this position for at least three breaths, twisting your body further to the left on every exhalation. Return to asana sthiti as you breathe in.

Kingfish Pose (Purna Matsyendrasana)

The next posture in this series is the complete kingfish pose (*purna Matsyendrasana*). Just as Patanjali is considered the authoritative compiler of Raja Yoga,

Matyendra Natha is considered to be the most authoritative proponent of hatha yoga. As the legend goes, Patanjali and Matsyendranatha learned their respective yogas from Lord Shiva. This and the previous pose are named after Matsyendranatha.

This posture is similar to the previous vinyasa, ardha Matsyendrasana, except that the right foot is not free, but is kept inside the left thigh and groin (in a half-lotus position), which makes this posture many times more effective—and more difficult to practice. Stay in this position for a number of breaths, twisting a little more on every long, smooth exhalation (*see figure 2-67*). The rear view is shown in figure 2-68.

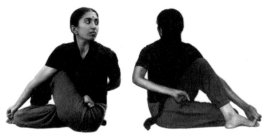

FIGURE 2-67 ◆◆◆◆◆   FIGURE 2-68 ◆◆◆◆◆

Hatha yogis credit this pose with the arousal of kundalini, whereas therapists say that regularly practiced purna Matsyendrasana can be used to temporarily prevent conception. It tones up the internal organs of the pelvic area. Next, inhale stretch both your legs in the staff pose (dandasana). You may lie down and rest for a while and get back your breath before proceeding further.

This completes the asymmetrical poses manipulating the right leg and keeping the left leg constant during different subsequences. Now you will want to repeat these movements on the left side. If you practice yogasanas for a long period, you can com-

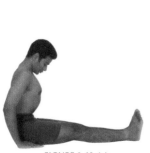

FIGURE 2-69 ◆◆

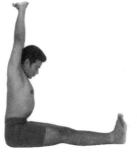

FIGURE 2-70 ◆◆

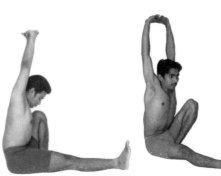

FIGURE 2-71 ◆◆   FIGURE 2-72 ◆◆

plete the whole sequence on one side and then the whole sequence on the other. Alternately, you may choose to do each subsequence on both the right and left sides before proceeding to the next subsequence.

ASYMMETRICAL VINYASAS (LEFT SIDE)

Sage Marichi Pose (Marichyasana)

Start from dandasana (*see figure 2-69*).

As you slowly inhale, raise both arms overhead; interlock your fingers while you complete the inhalation. You may repeat the movement three times (lower your arms to the starting position on exhalation) or stay in the posture, which is *niralamba dandasana* (free staff pose). During every inhalation, try to stretch your back. It is also good to perform the chin lock all the while (*see figure 2-70*).

Now, as you exhale slowly and smoothly, bend your left knee, draw your left foot close to your left buttock, and place it close to your right thigh (*see figure 2-71*).

Perform the chin lock, and do three long, smooth inhalations and exhalations. Another view is shown in figure 2-72.

This is the Marichyasa position, left side (*vama-parsva Marichyasana sthiti*).

Inhale for five seconds through a constricted throat, making a hissing sound. Then as you exhale smoothly, stretch your back and bend forward to hold your right foot with both hands. Place your head on your right knee or shin, while keeping your left leg in Marichyasana position (*see figure 2-73*).

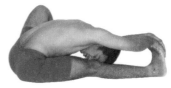

FIGURE 2-73 ◆◆◆

Stay in this position for a number of breaths. The inhalations can be moderate, about three to five seconds, but concentrate on extending the exhalations as much as you can. At the end of every exhalation, you may do rectal and abdominal locks for about five seconds. You may also hold your big toe with both hands (*see figure 2-74*).

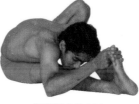

FIGURE 2-74 ◆◆◆

Release the two locks and then, while you inhale, slowly return to the starting position.

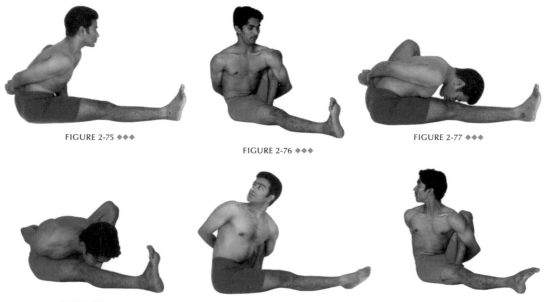

FIGURE 2-75 ♦♦♦

FIGURE 2-76 ♦♦♦

FIGURE 2-77 ♦♦♦

FIGURE 2-78 ♦♦♦

FIGURE 2-79 ♦♦♦

FIGURE 2-80 ♦♦

Now from the Marichyasana sthiti, while slowly exhaling, place your left arm around your left knee, and clasp your hands behind your back (see figure 2-75).

Stay in this position for three long inhalations and exhalations, tightening your grip on every exhalation. See figure 2-76 for another view.

In the next vinyasa, inhale slowly and then as you breathe out (ujjayi) slowly, stretch, bend forward, and place your face on your right knee (see figure 2-77).

Stay in this position, making the exhalation especially long and smooth for a few breaths. During each exhalation, tighten your grip and squeeze the air out of your lungs. At the end of each exhalation, it is good practice to hold your breath out and do rectal and abdominal locks. See figure 2-78 for another view.

Return to the asana sthiti on a slow inhalation.

On the next exhalation, slowly turn your body to the right side (see figure 2-79).

Inhale and exhale slowly and stay in this position for at least three breaths, opening your chest on every inhalation and and turning a bit more on every exhalation. Thereafter as you slowly inhale, return to the asana sthiti. See figure 2-80 for another view.

Now for the counterpose in Marichyasana. Inhaling, slowly raise your arms overhead and as you slowly exhale, lean back, and place your palms on the floor about a foot behind your back (see figure 2-81).

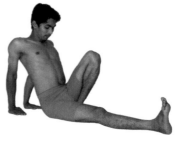

FIGURE 2-81 ♦

Leaning slightly on your hands, inhale slowly and raise your trunk as high as you can. Return to the starting position on exhalation. Repeat the movement three to six times with appropriate breathing *(see figure 2-82)*. See figure 2-83 for another view.

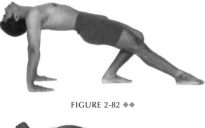

FIGURE 2-82 ◆◆

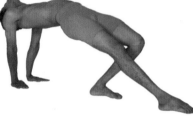

FIGURE 2-83 ◆◆

Half-Kingfish Pose (Ardha Matsyendrasana)

From Marichyasana sthiti as you are exhaling, place your left foot outside your right thigh. Now inhale smoothly and raise both arms overhead. Then as you keep exhaling, turn to the left side, bring your left arm around your back and grab your right thigh. Slowly inhale and try to turn a little more to the right side; stretch your right hand and bring it around the outside of your left knee to hold the big toe of your left foot. Stay in this position for three to six breaths *(see figure 2-84)*. See figure 2-85 for another view.

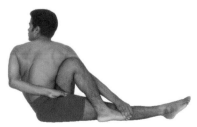

FIGURE 2-84 ◆◆◆

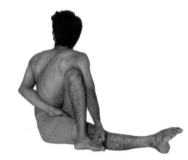

FIGURE 2-85 ◆◆◆

Try to make your inhalation long and smooth. Figure 2-86 shows the same posture twisting to the left side with the hands held behind the back.

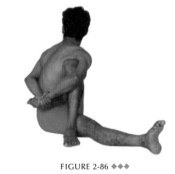

FIGURE 2-86 ◆◆◆

This is another position of ardha Matsyendrasana (half-kingfish pose). With the left foot well anchored, it helps to twist the spine smoothly. Ardha Matsyendrasana and its several simpler variations are excellent methods for twisting the spine.

Half-Lotus Pose (Ardha Padmasana)

The next subroutine in this sequence involves keeping the left leg in half-lotus position, while the right leg continues to remain outstretched and this half-lotus position affords a few more movements of the body. Now while you exhale, slowly, bend your left knee, stretch your left ankle fully, and place the outer part of your left foot on your right thigh close to your groin. Inhaling, raise both arms overhead.

This position is half-lotus position (ardha padmasana) *(see figure 2-87)*. A different angle view is given in figure 2-88.

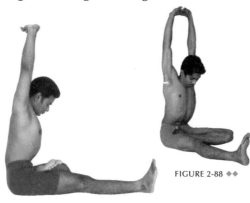

FIGURE 2-88 ◆◆

FIGURE 2-87 ◆◆

Stay in this position for a few breaths; finely adjust your posture so that you feel comfortable and well anchored. As you exhale slowly and smoothly, stretch your back and bend forward, hold your right foot with your right hand, and place your left hand on top of it. Place your head on your outstretched right knee. Stay in this position for three to six breaths, making the exhalations as complete as possible. During every exhalation try to stretch forward and bring your body down lower. You may use the bandhas, or locks, after exhalation and when holding your breath out. This is left half-lotus posterior-stretch posture (*vama-ardha-padma paschmatanasana*) *(see figure 2-89)*. Figure 2-90 is another view, in which one holds the big toe of the right leg with one's hands.

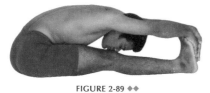

FIGURE 2-89 ◆◆

As you slowly inhale, stretch your arms overhead. Then during the next slow

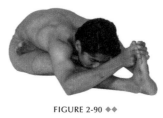

FIGURE 2-90 ◆◆

exhalation, bring your left arm behind your back and firmly hold the big toe of your left leg. Keep your back straight and stay in this position for three long breaths *(see figure 2-91)*.

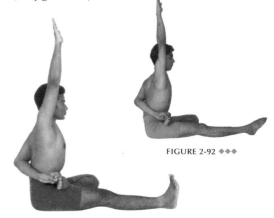

FIGURE 2-92 ◆◆◆

FIGURE 2-91 ◆◆◆

This posture is the left-tied-half-lotus posture (*vama-ardha-baddha-padmasana*). figure 2-92 is another view.

Then, inhale and while exhaling smoothly and slowly, stretch your back and bend forward. Place your forehead on your outstretched right knee or on your shin. Stay in this position for a few breaths, concentrating on making the exhalation as long, smooth, and complete as possible. After some practice, you may attempt to do rectal and abdominal locks after exhalation and while holding your breath out. This pose has a long name: *vama-ardha-baddha-padma-paschima-uttanasana*. Translated, it is left-side-tied, half-lotus posterior stretch posture *(see figure 2-93)*. Another view is shown in figure 2-94, in which you hold the big toe with your hand.

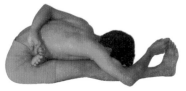

FIGURE 2-93 ♦♦♦

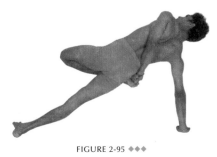

FIGURE 2-94 ♦♦♦

Although this next variation does require moving your right leg, there is a lot to be said for keeping it in the sequence. Exhaling, place your right palm, (turned out 90 degrees) on the floor about a foot behind you. Your left hand should be holding the big toe of your left foot, which is placed on your right thigh. Now as you inhale, press your right hand and the outside of the right foot, tilt your body to the right side, and raise your body, lifting your hip in particular. As you reach the posture, look up. See figure 2-95 for the rear view and figure 2-96 for the front view.

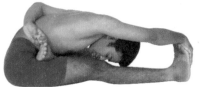

FIGURE 2-95 ♦♦♦

This posture is known as *Kashyapasana* or ardha-baddha-padma Vasishtasana. It is

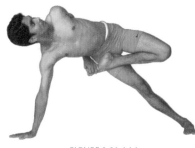

FIGURE 2-96 ♦♦♦

very useful in achieving a lateral movement and stretching the hip. Stay in this position for a few breaths, pushing your body up a little bit on every inhalation. Return to the starting position on exhalation.

Now in the ardha-baddha-padmasana position, exhale, lean forward, and grasp the inside of your right foot with your right hand. Holding your right foot firmly, slowly inhale, and turn or twist your body to the left side. Look over your left shoulder. Stay in this position for a few breaths. Return to the starting position on exhalation. This is also a variant of ardha Matsyendrasana or half-kingfish pose *(see figure 2-97)*. See figure 2-98 for another view.

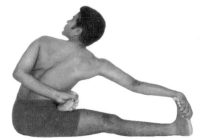

FIGURE 2-97 ♦♦

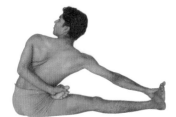

FIGURE 2-98 ♦♦

Now we go to another variant of ardha Matsyendrasana. Inhaling, raise both arms overhead as in ardha padmasana position. Now while exhaling, lean forward, and hold the outside of your right foot with your left hand. Then inhale and as you exhale, twist to the right side, reach your left hand around your back, and grab your thigh (see figure 2-99). See figure 2-100 for another view.

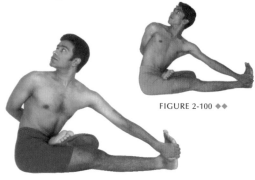

FIGURE 2-100 ◆◆

FIGURE 2-99 ◆◆

Stay in this position for a few breaths, turning more on every exhalation. Inhale, and return to the half-lotus position.

Before you do the counterpose for the present set of half-lotus vinyasas, you may attempt another variation. Remain in the half-lotus position. Exhaling slightly, lean forward, and place your palms on the floor close to your thighs. Exhale, hold your breath, pressing down with your palms, lift your body. Keep the half-lotus position of the left leg intact (see figure 2-101).

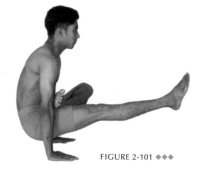

FIGURE 2-101 ◆◆◆

Stay in this position for about five seconds. Inhale, hold your breath, and slowly ease onto the floor. You may repeat the movements a few times. Once you are able to remain steady in the pose, you may attempt to stay in it for a few breaths.

Now for the counterpose, or prathikriya, in half-lotus. Inhaling, raise both arms overhead. As you keep breathing out, place both your hands behind your back about a foot away on the floor. As you inhale, slowly press down with your palms; raise your hip, while stretching your right ankle to place your right foot on the floor. Exhale, return to the starting point, and repeat the movement three times (see figure 2-102). Another view is given in figure 2-103.

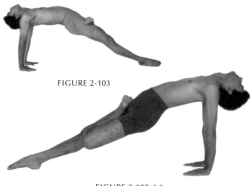

FIGURE 2-103

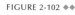

FIGURE 2-102 ◆◆

Now we go to the next subroutine, where the left foot is kept flush with the right thigh.

The Great Seal (Maha Mudra)

With your right leg outstretched, while exhaling, bend your left knee and place your left foot flush with your right thigh. The left heel may touch or press against the perineum. This is *maha mudra sthiti*, a great mudra or seal (see figure 2-104 and 2-105).

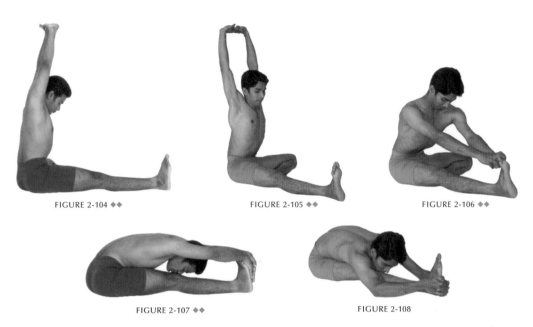

FIGURE 2-104 ♦♦   FIGURE 2-105 ♦♦   FIGURE 2-106 ♦♦

FIGURE 2-107 ♦♦   FIGURE 2-108

Now continuing to exhale, stretch your back, bend forward, and hold the big toe of your right foot with your index finger, middle finger, and thumb. This is maha mudra. Keep your chin down in jalandhara bandha. Stay in maha mudra for a long time, five minutes or more. At the end of every long, complete exhalation, also do mula bandha and uddiyana bandha for five to ten seconds. This maha mudra, along with bandhas, tones up the left side of the abdominal area, especially the pancreas (see figure 2-106).

Toward the end of your time in maha mudra, slowly exhale and bend forward. Hold your right foot with both hands, and place your forehead on your right knee, or further down on the shin. Inhaling, come back to the maha mudra position, and repeat the movement three to six times.

This position is known as janusirsasana or head-on-knee pose. See figure 2-108 for another view.

Now, deeply exhaling, turn to the left side, and bend forward. Hold your right foot with both hands; place the left hand on the outside of your foot and the right hand on the inside (see figure 2-109).

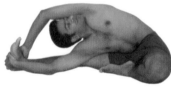

FIGURE 2-109 ♦♦♦

Stay in this position for three to six breaths, turning or twisting your body further on every exhalation. Inhale, return to the maha mudra sthiti. Now, stretch your left leg. See figure 2-110 for a rear view.

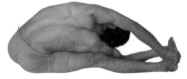

FIGURE 2-110 ♦♦♦

The Archer Pose (Akarna Dhanurasana)

Now slowly exhaling, lean forward and hold the toes of both feet with the thumbs, forefingers, and ring fingers of each hand. Inhale, and on the following smooth, long exhalation, bend your left knee and slowly pull your left foot toward your left ear (or beyond). See figure 2-111.

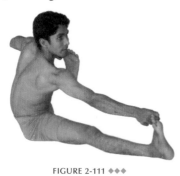

FIGURE 2-111 ◆◆◆

Stay in this position for three to six breaths, opening your hip a little more on every exhalation. This is known as akarna dhanurasana, because it resembles a bow (and arrow) drawn up to the ear. As you inhale slowly, stretch both the legs for the dandasana or staff pose.

Once again, as you are exhaling slowly and smoothly, bend forward, but hold your left foot with both hands. Inhale, and during the following exhalation, draw your left leg toward you and straight up. Try to place your forehead on your left knee (*see figure 2-112*).

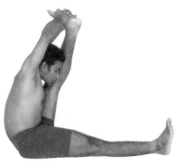

FIGURE 2-112 ◆◆◆

Stay in this position for three to six breaths, stretching and straightening your back.

One-Foot-on-Head Pose (Ekapada Sirsasana)

The next vinyasa is a bit involved. Again as you breathe out smoothly, lean forward, grab your left foot with both the hands. Inhale, and on the next exhalation, draw your leg toward the left side of your body and beyond it. Continuing the exhalation, bend your left knee and place your left leg on the back of your neck or, if possible, near your shoulder blade. Keep your hands folded in anjali (*see figure 2-113*).

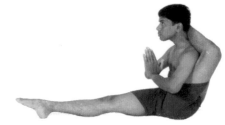

FIGURE 2-113 ◆◆◆◆

Stay in this position for three to six breaths. This posture is called *vama-ekapada-sirsasana* (left-leg-on-head pose).

Now, as you slowly exhale, bend forward and clasp your right foot with both hands, keeping your head on the stretched right knee (*see figure 2-114*).

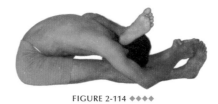

FIGURE 2-114 ◆◆◆◆

Stay in this position for three to six breaths. Try to do the abdominal and rectal locks after exhalation. This posture is known as Skandasana (*vama bhaga*, or left side), named after Skanda, the god of spiritual knowledge.

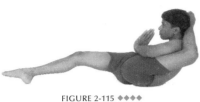

FIGURE 2-115 ◆◆◆◆

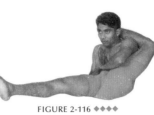

FIGURE 2-116 ◆◆◆◆

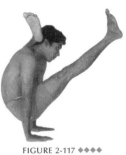

FIGURE 2-117 ◆◆◆◆

In the next vinyasa, lean back slowly during a long inhalation (see figure 2-115).

Stay in this position for three to six breaths. This pose is called the vama bhaga Bhairava asana, named after Bhairava, an aspect of Lord Shiva. See figure 2-116 for another view, with another yogi.

During the next exhalation get back to ekapada sirsasana. Now place your palms on the floor as you exhale, and holding your breath, lift (utpluti) your body up and balance for a few moments (see figure 2-117).

Stay in this position for a few breaths, breathing normally. This pose is known as chakora asana (vama bhaga). Return to ekapada sirsasana. Finally, grab your left leg with both hands and as you inhale stretch your leg back to staff pose.

Bent-Back-Leg Pose (Tiryang-Mukha-Ekapadasana)

The next subgroup involves keeping the left leg bent back, while the right leg remains stretched forward. From dandasana sthiti, exhaling, bend your left leg back and along your left thigh, with the heel facing backward (see figure 2-118).

This is known as tiryang-mukha-asana sthiti. It is a posture in which the foot is placed facing the opposite direction of the other leg. Stay in this position with your arms raised for three long, smooth inhalations and exhalations. You may practice both mula bandha and uddiyana bandhas after exhalation (see figure 2-119).

Thereafter, slowly exhale, stretch your back nicely, and slowly bend forward to hold the right foot. Place your forehead on your outstretched right knee (see figure 2-120).

Stay in this position for a long time (about five minutes), working on your exhalations and also doing the rectal and abdominal locks. This posture is known as tiryang-mukha-ekapada-paschima-uttanasana, backward-facing one-foot posterior stretch posture. Because this posture pertains to the

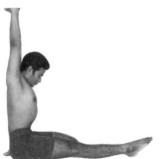

FIGURE 2-118 ◆◆

FIGURE 2-119 ◆◆

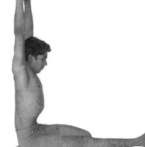

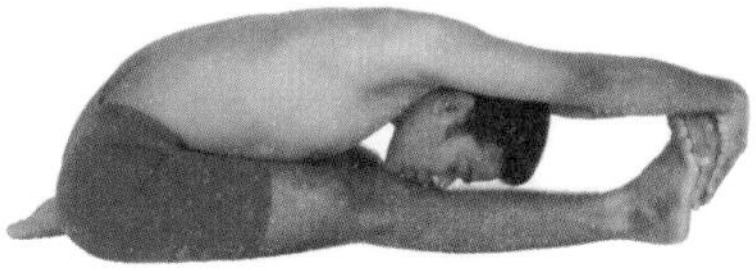

FIGURE 2-120 ◆◆

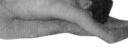

FIGURE 121 ◆◆

ASYMMETRICAL SEATED VINYASA SEQUENCE **63**

left leg, it is also known as tiryang-mukha-vama-pada-paschima-uttanasana. See figure 2-121 for another view, where one holds the heels, the body is lower, and the elbows are on the ground.

Inhaling, return to the asana sthiti.

For the next vinyasa, as you exhale long and smooth, turn to the left side, bend forward, and hold you right foot with both hands—your right hand should hold the inside of your foot and your left hand, the outside (see figure 2-122).

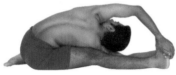

FIGURE 2-122 ◆◆◆

Stay in this position for three to six breaths, trying to twist a little bit more on each exhalation. Inhale and return to asana sthiti. See figure 2-123, which shows a fuller twist and a lower position of the body.

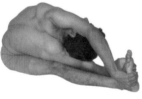

FIGURE 2-123 ◆◆◆

Now for the pratikriya, or counterpose. From the asana sthiti, while exhaling, lower your arms and place your palms on the floor behind your back about one foot away from your body. Keep your chin down, and do three long ujjayi breaths. Then as you do a long inhalation, press down with your palms, stretch your right ankle outward, and raise your trunk up as high as you can (see figure 2-124).

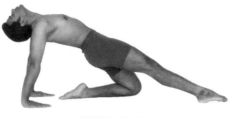

FIGURE 2-124 ◆◆

Exhale, come down, and repeat the movement three to six times. This is known as tiryang-mukha-vama-pada-purvatanasana. Also see figure 2-125.

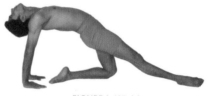

FIGURE 2-125 ◆◆

You may also do utpluti at this point: In the asana sthiti, lean forward slightly and place your palms outside your legs. Deeply exhale and hold your breath. Now pressing down with your palms, lift your body off the floor and balance on your hands, keeping the integrity of the posture intact. Stay in this position for five seconds. Inhale, hold your breath, and lower your body to the floor. This is tiryang-mukha-asana-utpluti (see figure 2-126).

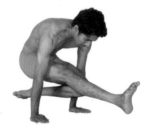

FIGURE 2-126 ◆◆◆

The Monkey-God Pose (Anjaneyasana)

While exhaling, place your palms by your side. Inhale, hold your breath, lift your body slightly, and push your left leg all the way back. This is a very complicated posture, which requires patience and slow practice. It should be practiced only with proper guidance. Breathe normally a few times, and then as you inhale raise both arms overhead (*see figure 2-127*).

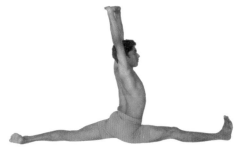

FIGURE 2-127 ◆◆◆◆◆

Stay in this position for three to six breaths. This posture is known as Anjaneyasana, the name of the epic Rama devotee (in the form of a monkey) from Ramayana. Now while exhaling, lower your arms and place your palms on the floor beside your body.

Again exhaling, slowly bend forward and place your forehead on your outstretched right knee (*see figure 2-128*).

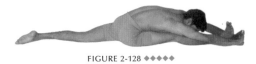

FIGURE 2-128 ◆◆◆◆◆

Stay in this position for a few breaths, and then return to Anjaneyasana sthiti. Then, exhaling, lift your body and bring your left leg forward to the tiryang-mukha-asana sthiti. Inhale and stretch your leg into dandasana again.

So far we have seen asanas with the right leg stretched in dandasana sthiti, while the left leg was worked in different positions. You can see that apart from dandasana

sthiti, the leg can be kept in other classical positions as tiryang mukha, Maricha, Matsyendra, or ardha padma, which will all provide stable postures. Here we will see some more vinyasas in which the right leg is kept in one of these positions and the left leg's position altered.

Half-Lotus Marichyasana (Ardha-padma Marichyasana)

Bend your left knee as you are exhaling, and place it on your right thigh in *ardha padmasana sthiti*. Now, inhale and on the next exhalation, bend your right knee and draw your right foot close to your right buttock for Marichyasana sthiti. Now we have *ardha-padma Marichyasana sthiti*. Inhale and while exhaling, slowly stretch your back and bend forward.

Inhale and while exhaling, bend forward and place your forehead on your left knee or the floor if possible (*see figure 2-129*).

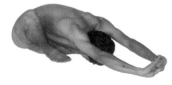

FIGURE 2-129 ◆◆◆

Stay in this position for three breaths, with very long exhalations. Inhale, and return to the asana sthiti.

Next, while exhaling place your right arm around your right knee, and hold your

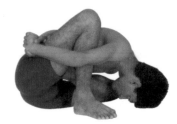

FIGURE 2-130 ◆◆◆

right hand with your left hand, placed around your back. While remaining in this position, exhale smoothly, bend forward, and place your forehead on your left knee or on the floor (see figure 2-130).

Stay in this position for three breaths. Return to previous asana sthiti. Now exhaling, slowly twist your torso to the left and turn your head to look over your left shoulder. Stay in this position for three breaths, twisting a little more on each exhalation. Return to asana sthiti after three breaths as you inhale.

Inhale, raise both arms overhead. While exhaling, slowly lean back a little and place your palms on the floor behind you, say one foot behind your body. Press down with your hands, and slowly inhaling, raise your trunk. Exhaling, come down. Repeat the movements three times, and then return to asana sthiti on inhalation. Stretch your legs forward to dandasana sthiti.

Backward-Facing-Foot Marichyasana (Tiryang-Mukha Marichyasana)

Now as you exhale place your right leg in tiryang-mukha sthiti, On the next exhalation, draw your left foot close to your right thigh, placing your right foot on the floor. This is the asana sthiti. Inhaling, stretch your arms overhead (see figure 2-131).

Stay in this position for three long inhalations and exhalations. This is another vinyasa of Marichyasana sthiti.

As you slowly and deeply exhale, gradually bend forward and place your forehead on the floor. Stay in this position for three to six breaths, concentrating on making the exhalations long and smooth. You may practice the bandhas at the end of each exhalation for about five seconds.

Returning to the asana sthiti, place your left hand around your left knee and hold it behind your back with your right hand. This is to be done while you are exhaling smoothly (see figure 2-132).

Stay in this position for three long inhalations and exhalations.

Remaining in the asana sthiti, breathe out slowly, turn to your right side, and look over your right shoulder (see figure 2-133).

Stay in this position for three to six smooth, long breaths. On every exhalation, you should try to twist a little more. Then, inhaling, return to the asana sthiti.

Now, let us look at the forward bend. Inhale and, while you breathe out, slowly

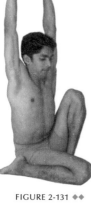

FIGURE 2-131 ♦♦

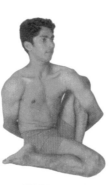

FIGURE 2-132 ♦♦

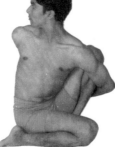

FIGURE 2-133 ♦♦

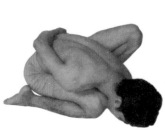

FIGURE 2-134 ♦♦♦

bend forward and place your forehead on your right knee, or, if possible, on the floor (*see figure 2-134*).

Stay in this position for at least three breaths, focusing on the exhalation and doing the bandhas at the end of each exhalation. Return to asana sthiti on inhalation.

Now do the counterpose. Inhaling, slowly stretch your arms overhead. As you exhale, place your palms on the floor behind your back, about one foot away from your body. Press firmly down on your palms, slowly inhale, and raise your trunk as high as you can (*see figure 2-135*).

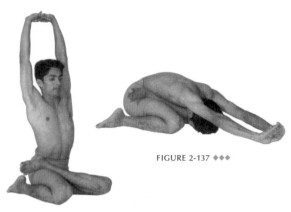

FIGURE 2-136 ◆◆

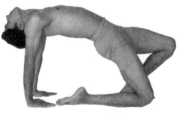

FIGURE 2-135 ◆◆

Repeat the movement three times. Inhaling, raise your arms overhead. Exhale and lower your arms.

Right Half-Lotus, Turned-Backward-Leg Pose (Dakshina-Ardha padma-Tiryang-Mukhasana)

Begin in the asana shtiti. Place your left foot on top of your right thigh as you are breathing out. On the next inhalation, raise your arms overhead and interlock your fingers (*see figure 2-136*).

This is ardha-padma-triyang-mukha vamapadasana. Stay in this position for three long inhalations and exhalations, stretching your back on every inhalation.

Exhaling smoothly, slowly stretch your back, and place your forehead on the floor. Stay in this position for a few breaths, doing

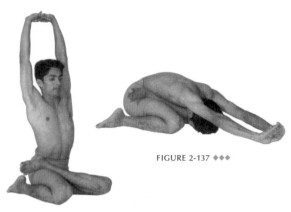

FIGURE 2-137 ◆◆◆

the bandhas at the end of each exhalation and before starting the next inhalation. This is ardha-padma-tiryang-mukha vamapada-paschima-uttanasana. Translated this would be half-lotus transverse left-legged posterior stretching pose (*see figure 2-137*).

Sage Bharadwaja Pose (Bharadwajasana)

Now we go to a classic posture called Bharadwajasana, named after an epic sage called Bharadwaja. It is a very nice twisting posture. From asana sthiti, exhaling, extend your left arm around your back and grab the big toe of your left foot with your left hand. Inhale and then on the next exhalation, slowly place your right palm on the floor outside of and below your left thigh (*see figure 2-138*).

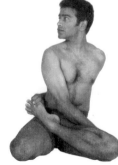

FIGURE 2-138 ◆◆◆

Anchoring your right palm, on every exhalation, twist more to the right side. Stay in this position for a long period, about five minutes. See figure 2-139 for another view.

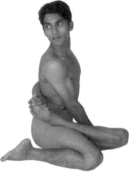

FIGURE 2-139

The Great Lock (Mahabandha)

Next will be mahabandha, or the great lock. Keep your left leg bent, draw your left foot inside of your left leg, and sit on the left heel, thereby closing the anus. On the next exhalation, bend your right knee and place it on your left thigh as in ardha padmasana. Place your palms on the knees (see figure 2-140).

Do six long inhalations and exhalations. In this position five bandhas, or locks, can be practiced. The rear view is shown in figure 2-141.

Closing the anus with the heel is the mahabandha. After exhalation you can practice the mula bandha, or rectal lock, followed in quick succession by uddiyana bandha, or abdominal lock, and the chin-down position, jalandhara bandha, or the chin lock. The fifth lock is tongue lock (jihva bandha), in which you roll your tongue and place the tip back, closing the opening of the throat.

Another variation is to raise your left leg up and pull it toward you on smooth exhalation. You may touch your left knee with your forehead. Stay in this position for three breaths, and return to asana sthiti (see figure 2-142).

This is another variation of kraunchasana.

Half-Kingfish Pose (Ardha Matsyendrasana)

Now we will go to another asana, ardha Matsyendrasana. While exhaling, drag your left foot along the floor and place it by the side of your right buttock, with the entire leg remaining on the floor. On the next exhalation, bend your right knee and place your right foot on the floor by the side of your left knee. Stay in this position for a few breaths. Now as you are exhaling, turn your body to the right side, stretch your right arm around your back and hold your left thigh with your right hand. Stay in this position for a couple of breaths. Now as you slowly exhale, stretch your left hand and place it around the outside of your right

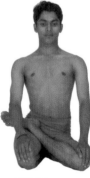

FIGURE 2-140 ♦♦

FIGURE 2-141 ♦♦

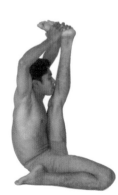

FIGURE 2-142 ♦♦♦

knee to hold the big toe of your right foot (*see figure 2-143*).

Stay in this position for at least three breaths, twisting your body further right on every exhalation. Return to asana sthiti as you breathe in. The front view is shown in figure 2-144.

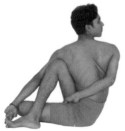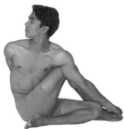

FIGURE 2-143 ◆◆◆   FIGURE 2-144 ◆◆◆

Complete Kingfish Pose (Purna Matsyendrasana)

This posture is similar to the previous vinyasa, ardha Matsyendrasana, except that the right foot is not free, but is kept inside the left thigh and groin, making this position much more effective and difficult to practice (*see figures 2-145 and 2-146*).

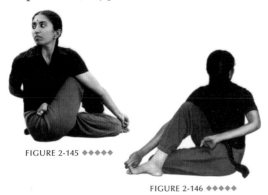

FIGURE 2-145 ◆◆◆◆◆

FIGURE 2-146 ◆◆◆◆◆

After completing the series, fully or in an adapted version, you may return to samasthiti before lying down in savasana for samasthiti. The rest pauses are dictated by the condition of your breathing. If your breathing cannot be done long and smoothly, it may be time to take rest for a short period, just two to three minutes, before proceeding to the return series.

RETURN SERIES

From dandasana (*see figure 2-147*), exhale, hold your breath, and lift your body to dandasana-utpluthi (*see figure 2-148*).

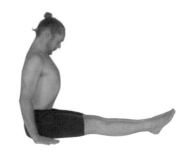

FIGURE 2-147 ◆◆

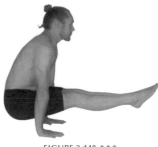

FIGURE 2-148 ◆◆◆

Bend your knees, keeping your feet together. Do not cross your legs (*see figure 2-149*).

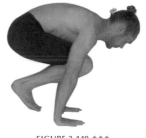

FIGURE 2-149 ◆◆◆

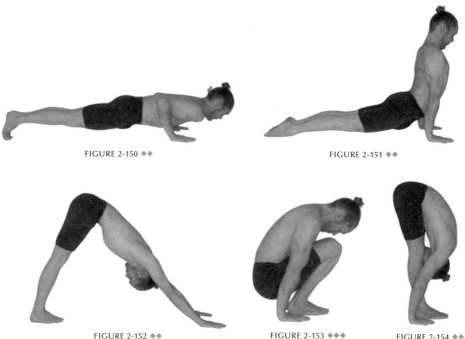

FIGURE 2-150 ◆◆

FIGURE 2-151 ◆◆

FIGURE 2-152 ◆◆

FIGURE 2-153 ◆◆◆

FIGURE 2-154 ◆◆

Take a short inhalation, balance yourself nicely by leaning forward a little and keeping your head down, and hurtle backward smoothly, close to the ground. Land on your big toes. Keep your upper body horizontal. This is chaturanga dandasana, or the four-legged staff pose *(see figure 2-150).*

From dandasana, while inhaling, press down with your palms to arch your back and push the chest forward. Stay in this position for a breath in this upward-facing-dog pose *(see figure 2-151).*

As you exhale, raise your hip and drop your head to the downward-facing-dog position *(see figure 2-152).*

Stay in this position for a breath.

Now inhale and after the next exhalation, hold your breath and gently jump forward, keeping your body close to your thighs and your head down. Land gently between your hands in utkatasana (the hip stretch pose). *(See figure 2-153).*

Keeping your forehead on your knees, as you slowly inhale, press your palms and feet and straighten your knees to come to forward stretch pose. You may try to keep your forehead on your knees as you straighten them *(see figure 2-154).*

On the next inhalation, return to tadasana-samasthiti. This completes the return routine from dandasana.

3

SEATED
POSTERIOR STRETCH
SEQUENCE

IN THE PREVIOUS chapter, we discussed the sequence of several seated-posture vinyasas in which the seated position was asymmetric. In the asymmetric sequence, one leg is kept straight, for the most part, and the other is manipulated in a logical progression of vinyasas. It is time to go into a popular sequence, where the postures are basically symmetrical, and in which both the legs are kept straight while the upper body is worked. The posterior portions of the lower extremities are difficult to exercise. They contain considerable muscle tissue that requires special efforts to work on. Stretching the legs and trying to touch the toes while sitting could be awkward for many people. This seated posterior stretch sequence will help to uniformly stretch the heels, ankles, calves, hamstrings, thighs, and gluteal muscles, and then go on to stretch the back, spine, shoulders, and neck. It improves blood circulation (rakta sanchara) to the posterior portion of the body and helps to maintain good health and vigor. One feels a certain lightness of the lower limbs, which itself is a good feeling. Those who are interested in the esoteric aspects of yoga will find that this sequence is an invariable aid in the arousal of the mystic energy (kundalini). Regular practice makes the body light and the mind calm. According to my guru, the main pose in this sequence, which is the posterior stretching pose (*paschimatanasana*, or *adho-mukha-paschimatanasana*) will not provide the intended benefits if it is attempted merely from a seated position without the movements facilitated by vinyasa krama.

THE LEAD SEQUENCE OF VINYASAS

The posture from which the actual sequence starts is the hub pose—the staff pose (dandasana). However, according to the classical vinyasa method, all poses are led from the standing samsthiti; therefore, the first pose in this sequence will be tadasana, or the hill pose. This is the first vinyasa. Keep your feet together, back straight, and shoulders slightly thrown back (see figure 3-1). A side view of the same pose is shown in figure 3-2.

Now close your eyes and watch how you balance for a minute. Then watch—just watch—for a minute the movement of your breath inside your chest.

The next vinyasa involves keeping the head down in jalandhara bandha (the chin lock). Do smooth, long throat breathing (ujjayi) three times with your mind closely following your breath. Then, as you slowly inhale, raise your arms overhead and inter-lock your fingers (see figure 3-3). The side view is shown in figure 3-4.

Inhalation should last for at least five seconds, but you can go as long as ten seconds if your breathing is smooth and slow. The movement of your arms and your breathing should be synchronized, that is, you should complete your inhalation at the same moment that you complete your arm movement. Your mind should closely follow your breath, resulting in your body, mind, and breath functioning in unison.

After completing the movement, stay in position with your body fully stretched for a second, holding your breath in. Then keeping your hands free and slowly exhaling (five to ten seconds), bend forward and place your palms by the sides of your feet and place your face on your knees (or on your shins if possible), again synchronizing your exhalation with the movement of your upper body (see figure 3-5).

As mentioned, this back-stretching vinyasa goes by the name uttanasana. You

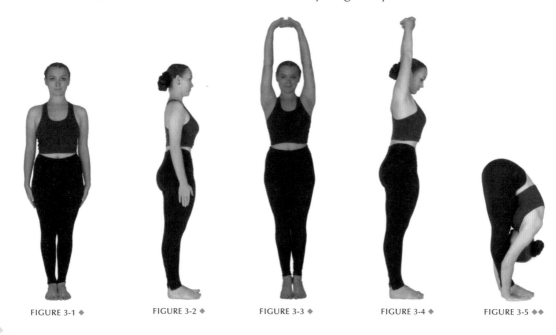

FIGURE 3-1 ◆   FIGURE 3-2 ◆   FIGURE 3-3 ◆   FIGURE 3-4 ◆   FIGURE 3-5 ◆◆

may want to stay in this posture for a few breaths, say three to six. In this position, the inhalations will be short, say about three to five seconds, but the exhalations can be quite long, up to ten seconds or more. This pose provides a good stretch of the posterior portions of the body, the thigh and calf muscles along with the hamstrings, the entire back, neck, shoulders, and arms. Let us look at the next vinyasa in the sequence.

Take a short inhalation, and as you are breathing out for five to ten seconds, bend your knees smoothly and squat on your haunches (*see figure 3-6*).

This position is known as utkatasana. As you lower your trunk, bending your knees and also breathing out slowly, you can draw in your lower abdomen and then your stomach to facilitate the downward movement of your body, without the tummy obstructing movement. You can also do all the three bandhas (chin, rectal, and abdominal locks) while in this posture. Again, this posture helps arouse kundalini. It is a very good toning exercise for the pelvic muscles and organs.

Now let us consider the movement to the next vinyasa. Take a short breath, about three to five seconds, and hold the breath in. Then as you hold the breath, raise your heels, lean forward a bit, and gently jump back, stretching your legs and landing on your toes. This posture is known as the four-legged staff pose (*chaturanga-dandasana*). See figure 3-7.

Be careful: many people jump high and land heavily and painfully on their toes. The reason one jumps back is to facilitate bringing back both legs at the same time symmetrically, rather than using the other, asymmetrical, option of placing one leg after

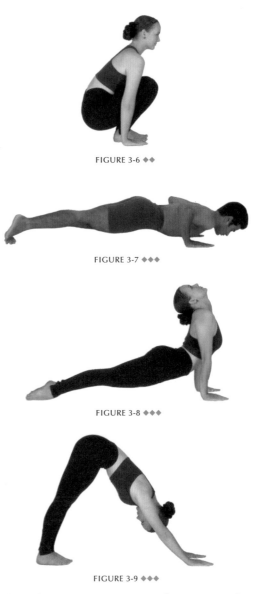

FIGURE 3-6 ♦♦

FIGURE 3-7 ♦♦♦

FIGURE 3-8 ♦♦♦

FIGURE 3-9 ♦♦♦

the other. You can stay in this posture for long time, breathing in and out with a chin lock (jalandhara bandha), taking equal time for inhalation and exhalation. Or else you can proceed to the next vinyasa. This pose strengthens the wrists and arms and also is said to remove impurities from several joints.

The next movement in this sequence is the famous upward-facing-dog pose (urdhwa-mukha swanasana). Exhale smoothly and slowly in chaturanga-dandasana, and as you inhale (five to ten seconds), raise your trunk and arch your spine. You may keep your chin in jalandhara bandha if you wish to stay in this posture. Or you can arch your back while moving up. See figure 3-8 for the position of the feet and the toes.

This is an excellent movement for the spine. Regular practice will prevent kyphosis (hunchback). Digestion will improve. This gives overall strength to the whole body and tones up all the muscles and joints in the anterior portion of the body.

Now while exhaling (five to ten seconds) and pressing down with your palms, push your feet back to the floor, simultaneously raising your hips to resemble a dog stretching and looking downward (see figure 3-9).

Here too you can stay in this position for a long time, doing long, smooth ujjayi inhalations and exhalations. At the end of each exhalation, you can hold your breath out for three to five seconds and draw in your rectum and abdomen, thus practicing all the three locks (bandhas). This is known as the downward-facing-dog pose (adhomukha swanasana). It is a very important hub posture.

Now the next movement. Exhale slowly, hold your breath, and raise your head. Slightly bend your knees, and jump through your hands and balance on your hands (see figure 3-10).

Then exhaling lower your trunk to dandasana, or the staff posture (see figure 3-11).

Dandasana is the starting posture for all sitting yoga asanas. Stay in this position for a few breaths, stretching your back during every inhalation and also pulling up your waist.

Now, as you inhale slowly (five to ten seconds), raise your arms overhead and interlock your fingers (see figure 3-12).

This position is known as the staff without support pose (niralamba dandasana).

On the next inhalation lie on your back. You may stay in this position for three breaths. Stretch your body, from the toes to the fingers, thoroughly on every inhalation (see figure 3-13).

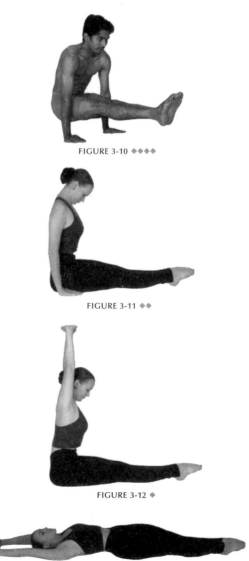

FIGURE 3-10 ◆◆◆◆

FIGURE 3-11 ◆◆

FIGURE 3-12 ◆

FIGURE 3-13 ◆◆

THE POSTERIOR STRETCH
(Paschimatanasana)

Release the lock to keep your hands free and, exhaling deeply, sit up and in one movement stretch forward and hold your toes. Your head or forehead will be on your knees, with your back somewhat rounded like the back of a turtle *(see figure 3-14)*.

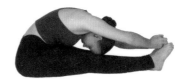

FIGURE 3-14 ◆◆◆

This posture is the posterior stretching posture *(paschimatanasana)*. This curving of the back stretches the spine out.

Now inhaling smoothly, return to the niralamba dandasana position (as shown in figure 3-12). Again exhaling slowly (five to ten seconds), bend forward, clasp your toes or your feet with your hands from above, but stretch your neck a little more and place your face on your knees *(see figure 3-15)*.

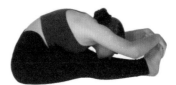

FIGURE 3-15 ◆◆◆

In this vinyasa, the neck starts stretching.

Again inhaling, return to niralamba dandasana very slowly. Once again exhaling slowly and smoothly, bend forward, clasp your toes or feet, and stretching your neck place your chin on your knees *(see figure 3-16)*.

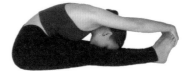

FIGURE 3-16 ◆◆◆

Now the neck is stretched completely.

Return to niralamba dandasana on a slow inhalation. Now exhaling slowly and very deeply, stretch fully forward and place your face between your shins, and hold your feet as shown in figure 3-17.

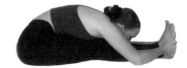

FIGURE 3-17 ◆◆◆

You may stay in this vinyasa of paschimatanasana for a long time with short inhalations (three to five seconds), but very long exhalations (five to ten, or even fifteen, seconds). After you complete every exhalation you may do both the abdominal and rectal locks. During every inhalation, relax your grip, but on every exhalation stretch forward and lower your trunk

down slightly. Yoga texts recommend *vaseth*, which means one should stay in this posture for a long time. Even a stay of five minutes has a tonic effect on the posterior muscles, the abdominal muscles, and the pelvic organs, because of the rectal and abdominal locks.

Exhaling this time hold your hands out and turn the palms outward. Then on the next exhalation, bend forward and clasp your feet, but keep your hands extended beyond your feet *(see figure 3-18)*. Another view is shown in figure 3-19.

On the following exhalation, bend forward to paschimatanasana. Stay in this

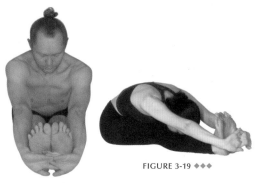

FIGURE 3-18 ◆◆◆

FIGURE 3-19 ◆◆◆

position for three breaths, and return to niralamba dandasana sthiti.

To work more on your shoulders, from niralamba dandasana, as you smoothly exhale, cross your hands and hold the outsides of your feet with the opposite hands (see figure 3-20).

You may stay in this vinyasa for a few breaths. You can feel a good stretch of your shoulders and neck in this vinyasa.

The next vinyasas will involve twists of the torso. From niralamba dandasana, as you exhale turn to the right side. Inhale

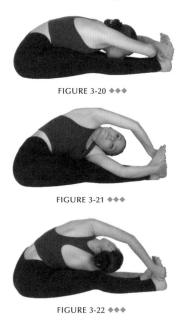

FIGURE 3-20 ◆◆◆

FIGURE 3-21 ◆◆◆

FIGURE 3-22 ◆◆◆

briefly in the same position, and exhaling slowly, smoothly, and completely, bend forward and down, and clasp your right foot with your left hand and your left foot with your right hand. Stay in this position for three to six breaths, twisting your body during every exhalation (see figure 3-21).

Now return to niralamba dandasana on a slow inhalation, and repeat the previous movement on the left side with the appropriate breathing as mentioned (see figure 3-22).

Seated Forward Stretch, without Support (Niralamba Paschimatanasana)

Other hand variations can also be practiced. Here, too, return to dandasana every time, and bend forward and hold your feet with your hands in different ways. This helps to stretch different parts of the arms and shoulders. You may also attempt to bend forward without holding your feet. In one such variation, you start from niralamba dandasana and, after inhaling, exhale long and smoothly, while bending forward. You do not hold any part of your legs, but stretch your hands along the floor, beyond your feet (see figure 3-23). This is one vinyasa of niralamba paschimatanasana.

The next variation is to keep your hands interlocked and behind your back, while in niralamba dandasana. You will move down your hands to interlace your fingers while you exhale. Now, after a smooth long inhalation when you freely expand your chest, breathe out slowly, stretch your back, and swing your arms over your back as you place your face on your knees or shins (see figure 3-24).

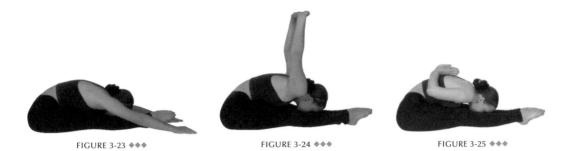

FIGURE 3-23 ◆◆◆   FIGURE 3-24 ◆◆◆   FIGURE 3-25 ◆◆◆

Stay in this positon for at least three breaths.

Another example is to keep your hands in a salute behind your back and bend forward without the help of your hands. From niralamba dandasana, while slowly exhaling, bring your arms down and place them behind your back. Join your palms and slowly turn the joined palms in anjali, but behind your back. Now, inhale, expand your chest, and during the next long, smooth exhalation slowly bend forward (*see figure 3-25*). This is yet another variation of niralamba paschimatanasana.

THE TURTLE POSE (KURMASANA)

The next vinyasa in the series is a difficult one called kurmasana, or the turtle posture. While exhaling, keep your legs slightly ajar, and on the next deep exhalation bend forward and push your hands through and under your thighs (*see figure 3-26*).

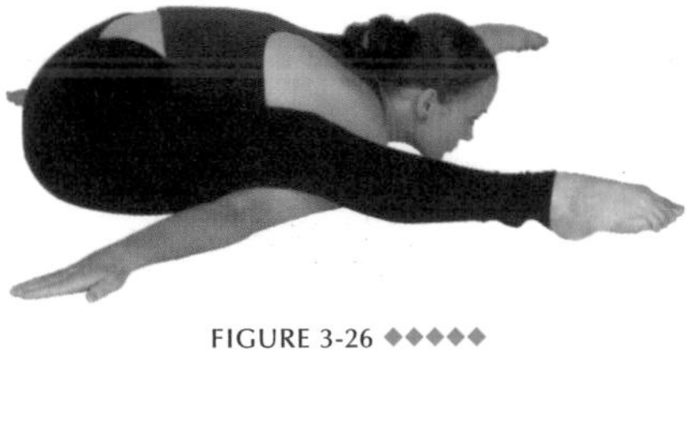

This posture looks like a turtle waddling along the beach. You can stay in this position for a few breaths, doing short inhalations and very long, smooth exhalations.

Turtle-in-its-shell Pose (Akunchita Kurmasana)

In the next variation of kurmasana, you breathe out and bring your legs closer to your body and also move your arms around your back and hold them together (*see figure 3-27*).

This is the kurmasana, which has withdrawn into its shell. Stay in this position for a number of breaths, concentrating on the exhalations.

Now in the same turtle pose, as you are exhaling lift your legs a little off the floor and place your feet over your head. Stay in this position for three to six breaths (*see figure 3-28*)

This is *akunchita kurmasana*, or a turtle in its shell.

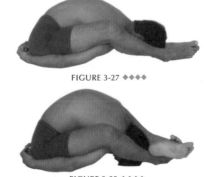

FIGURE 3-27 ◆◆◆◆

FIGURE 3-26 ◆◆◆◆◆

FIGURE 3-28 ◆◆◆◆

THE ANTERIOR STRETCH POSE
(PURVA TANASANA)

Now let us move to the next posture, which is the counterpose to paschimatanasana. It is called *purva tanasana*, or anterior stretching posture. We have done a number of forward-stretching movements, and this counterpose provides some relief to the posterior part of the body and also helps balance the stretching of the front of the body. Remain in niralamba dandasana, and while exhaling place your palms behind your back on the floor. Now as you slowly inhale, raise (pump) your body up, stretch the anterior portion of your body, and drop your head back, placing your feet firmly on the floor (*see figure 3-29*).

Repeat the movement three to six times.

The previous pose is the classical counterpose (pratikriya) for the posterior stretch (paschimatanasana vinyasa). The next asana that follows is named after a great sage, Vasishta. Remain in the staff pose (dandasana), and while exhaling, slowly turn to the right side, taking your left hand off the floor and placing it on your left side. During the next inhalation, press down with your right hand and anchor the outside of the right foot and

slowly lift your body laterally, moving the pelvis up and toward the left side of your body. As you complete the movement, stretch your left arm up as well, turning your head up. As you complete the movement, place your left foot on the floor beside your right foot (*see figure 3-30*).

Stay in this position for three breaths, gently nudging your pelvis laterally and up with every inhalation. Then return to the staff pose (dandasana) as you slowly exhale.

The same movement can be done on the left side. As you exhale, slowly turn to the left, raising your right arm and placing it on the right side of your body. Now as you are exhaling, press down with your right palm and lift your body laterally. You can raise your right arm as high as possible, and turn your head. As you lift your pelvis up, stretch your right leg and place your right foot on the floor beside your left foot (*see figure 3-31*).

Stay in this position for six slow, smooth breaths. As you exhale, give a gentle nudge to your pelvis, giving it an extra lateral stretch. Exhaling slowly, return to your starting position, the staff pose (dandasana).

You could see that the three poses, paschimatanasana, purvatanasana, and Vasishtasana, work on the pelvic joint

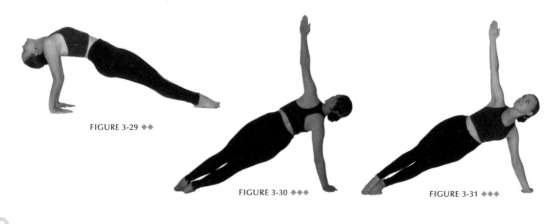

FIGURE 3-29 ◆◆

FIGURE 3-30 ◆◆◆

FIGURE 3-31 ◆◆◆

effectively. The paschimatanasana tilts the pelvis forward, virtually folding it over the thighs. Purvatanasana helps to open up the pelvis with the forward thrust of the pelvis, and performing Vasishtasana on either side gives the pelvis a lateral stretch. Both the pratikriyas, the anterior stretch and Vasishtasana, are also very effective because the movements are virtually "in the air," making it much easier to manipulate the joint. Further, in these two poses, the body is very well anchored with the palms and feet firmly planted on the floor.

Vasishta, whose name the asana bears, was one of the seven great spiritual seers of the Vedas. References to him abound in epics such as the Ramayana. It is customary to invoke his blessings during the Sun Worship performed by millions of Indians every day at dawn, midday, and dusk. One of his well-known works is the *Yoga Vaasishta* (meaning the *Yoga of Vasishta*). It is a voluminous work, and through fables and debates it explains great spiritual truths and yogic accomplishments. According to Indian mythology, the seven great seers, of whom Vasishta is one, are given an exalted place in the seven constellations.

Table Pose (Catushpada-Peetam)

Now keeping the palms in the same position as purvatanasana, while slowly exhaling, bend your knees and draw your feet close to your buttocks. While slowly inhaling, press down with your palms and feet to lift and stretch your body until it is horizontal. This is called the table pose (*catushpada-peetam*) (*see figure 3-32*).

This is an easy pose, but is a very effective stretch. It also gives some relief to the knees, which have been stretched all along.

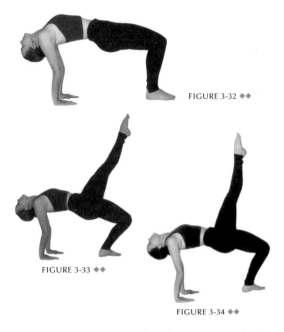

FIGURE 3-32 ◆◆

FIGURE 3-33 ◆◆

FIGURE 3-34 ◆◆

Remaining in catushpada-peetam, inhale slowly and raise your right leg as you raise your trunk (*see figure 3-33*).

Toward the end of the movement, give a gentle nudge to your lower back, thereby stretching the small of your back and also lifting your leg a little further (*see figure 3-34*).

Exhale, come down, and repeat the movement three to six times.

Repeat the movement raising your left leg (*see figure 3-35*).

Repeat the movement several times, lifting your pelvis a little more at the end of each inhalation (*see figure 3-36*).

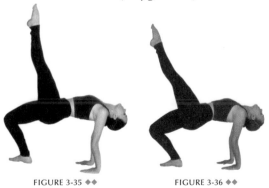

FIGURE 3-35 ◆◆   FIGURE 3-36 ◆◆

Boat Pose (Navasana)

Exhaling, return to the starting position, the table pose. Now lean back on your hands, and stretch your legs up in front of your face (*see figure 3-37*).

This is called *navasana vinyasa*, or the boat posture vinyasa. This is also known as *salamba navasana*, or the boat pose with support.

The next movement will be navasana. From the previous position, as you inhale, stretch your arms forward and stay in this position for in this pose for a few breaths, balancing on your buttocks (*see figure 3-38*).

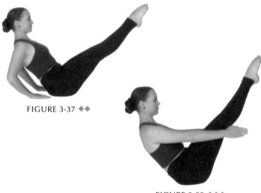

FIGURE 3-37 ◆◆

FIGURE 3-38 ◆◆◆

Some call this *purna navasana*, or the complete boat pose.

Upward-Looking, Posterior Stretch Pose (Urdhwa Paschimatanasana)

Now from this position, you may attempt to hold your legs and, smoothly exhaling, draw your legs toward you, at the same time stretching your upper body so that you can place your face on your knees or shins (*see figure 3-39*).

This posture is named *urdhwa paschimatanasana*, or upward-looking posterior stretch pose. Stay in this position for a short while with smooth inhalations and exhala-

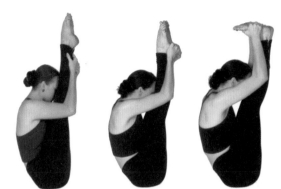

FIGURE 3-39 ◆◆◆   FIGURE 3-40 ◆◆◆   FIGURE 3-41 ◆◆◆

tions. After a few breaths, slowly bend your knees slightly on exhalation, stretch your arms a little more, and grab your heels and stretch your knees (*see figure 3-40*).

Place your forehead on or beyond your knees. Stay in this position for a few breaths. Then, again bend your knee slightly, hold the soles of your feet, and again stretch your knees (*see figure 3-41*).

Stay in position for a few breaths, stretching your back and gently balancing on your buttocks. Then return to niralamba dandasana as you inhale slowly. Exhaling, lower your arms to dandasana.

Inhale, lie down, and rest, breathing normally and following your breath, rather than allowing your mind to wander or falling asleep (*see figure 3-42*).

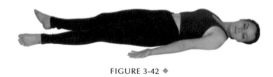

FIGURE 3-42 ◆

Keep all your joints loose—toes, ankles, knees, hips, spine, neck, shoulders, elbows, wrists, knuckles, and fingers. You may slowly direct your attention to all the joints in the order mentioned and make sure that

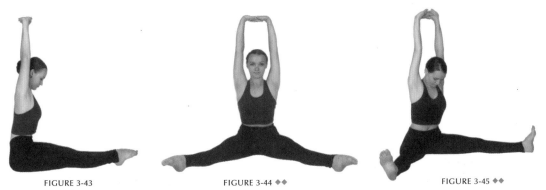

FIGURE 3-43 | FIGURE 3-44 ◆◆ | FIGURE 3-45 ◆◆

all these joints are relaxed, along with the connecting muscles. Then turn your attention to the breath inside your chest, and keep watching it during the rest period, which may be two to three minutes. Take care to see that your mind is coaxed back to your breath every time you become aware that your mind is wandering.

This completes the sequence of vinyasas of the seated posterior stretch. The next group of vinyasas will require you to open your hip joints in seated obtuse angle and straight angle sequences, which commence from the staff pose. This group has the *upavishta konasana* (seated-angle posture) as the main posture. You may take a rest in savasana, as mentioned earlier, or proceed without the break. It depends upon how your breath is—whether it is smooth or hurried.

Seated-Angle Pose (Upavishta Konasana)

From the staff pose, while slowly inhaling, raise both arms overhead for niralamba dandasana (*see figure 3-43*).

Exhale slowly and then as you are inhaling spread your legs. Depending upon how supple your hip joints are, find a convenient angle between 90 and 120 degrees at which you can sit (*see figure 3-44*). figure 3-45 shows another angle of the same asana sthiti.

Stay in the preceding position for three long inhalations and exhalations. Then while on the next smooth long exhalation, slowly bend forward (*see figure 3-46*).

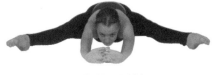

FIGURE 3-46 ◆◆◆

Stay in this position for three breaths, or if you wish, inhale raise your trunk back to the asana sthiti, and then as you exhale bend forward.

The next vinyasa will require you to spread your arms as you bend forward on a smooth long exhalation and hold the big toes of the both feet (*see figure 3-47*).

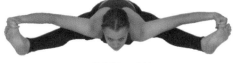

FIGURE 3-47 ◆◆◆

You may keep the feet straight without flexing the dorsa of your feet (*see figure 3-48*).

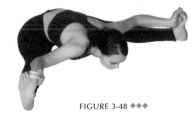

FIGURE 3-48 ◆◆◆

SEATED POSTERIOR STRETCH SEQUENCE 81

Again stay in this position for three to six breaths; pull your wrists forward, stretch, lower, and flatten your trunk in the process. Stretching well, you may able to place your chin on the floor (*see figure 3-49*).

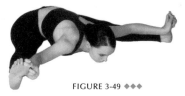

FIGURE 3-49 ◆◆◆

You may keep your feet straight without flexing the dorsa of your feet.

The next vinyasa will involve bending forward without support from your hands. Exhaling, move your hands back to the back salute (prishtanjali). Again as you slowly and smoothly breathe out with a hissing sound, stretch, and bend forward and place your face on the floor (*see figure 3-50*).

Again stay in this position for at least three breaths, stretching your torso on every exhalation and pulling your body up from the waist. You will feel a strong pull in your hips.

The next move also is a forward bend, but to the right side (*see figure 3-51*), which is done on again a very smooth long exhalation.

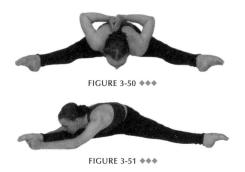

FIGURE 3-50 ◆◆◆

FIGURE 3-51 ◆◆◆

As you turn and lower your trunk, you will experience a healthy stretch of your left

hip and also a good turn in your right hip. Raise your trunk on inhalation, and bend forward on exhalation. Do this three to six times. Inhale and return to asana sthiti.

Now you can do the same movement on the left side, while exhaling (*see figure 3-52*).

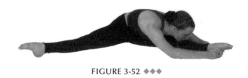

FIGURE 3-52 ◆◆◆

Stay in this position for three to six breaths, or move up and down with appropriate breathing

Inhale and while exhaling, slowly look over your left shoulder and lower your trunk to the right side. Clasp your right foot with both the hands, with your right hand on the sole and your left hand on the dorsum of your foot (*see figure 3-53*).

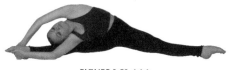

FIGURE 3-53 ◆◆◆

Stay in this position for three to six breaths, and on the next inhalation slowly come back to asana sthiti.

Now you may repeat the movement on the left side with the appropriate breathing (*see figure 3-54*).

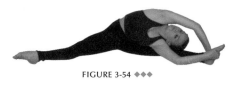

FIGURE 3-54 ◆◆◆

And then return to asana sthiti, while slowly inhaling.

The next two vinyasas are quite involved, requiring a very high degree of twisting of the spine and also the hip joint. It is better to be very cautious while trying these vinyasas. As you are exhaling, from the asana sthiti, turn on your right side and slowly ease your trunk down, and clasp your right foot with both hands (*see figure 3-55*).

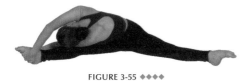

FIGURE 3-55 ◆◆◆◆

Stay in this position for three to six breaths, twisting a little more on each exhalation. Return to asana sthiti while you are inhaling.

Now you may repeat this upavishta konasana vinyasa on the left side, and then return to asana sthiti (*see figure 3-56*).

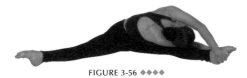

FIGURE 3-56 ◆◆◆◆

Now for the counterpose for upavishta konasana. As you are breathing out, place your hands on the floor about a foot behind your back. Then as you slowly inhale, press down with your palms,

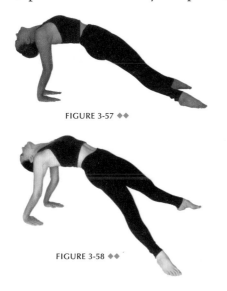

FIGURE 3-57 ◆◆

FIGURE 3-58 ◆◆

stretch your ankles, and raise your trunk, especially your hip until you are able to place your feet on the floor (*see figure 3-57*).

You may repeat the movement three to six times, very slowly lowering your trunk on slow, smooth exhalations. For clarity another view is shown in figure 3-58.

Straight-Angle Pose (Samakonasana)

Now we can look at another complicated asana in which the hip joint opens up considerably. From upavishta konasana, while you are exhaling, place your palms on the floor a little way behind your back. Keeping your chin down and slowly inhaling, spread your legs a little more, in stages, until your legs are 180 degrees apart. This is called *samakonasana* (salamba), or straight-angle posture with support (*see figure 3-59*).

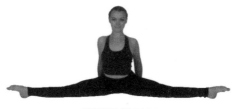

FIGURE 3-59 ◆◆◆◆

Stay in this position for three to six breaths, trying to keep your back erect on every exhalation.

Figure 3-60 shows the same asana from the back view with the palms placed in front for support.

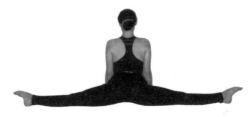

FIGURE 3-60 ◆◆◆◆

SEATED POSTERIOR STRETCH SEQUENCE **83**

In the next vinyasa, as you slowly exhale, stretch your back and bend forward, placing your entire torso on the floor, still keeping your legs spread out at 180 degrees (see figure 3-61).

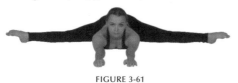

FIGURE 3-61

Stay in this position for three to six breaths. While inhaling, return to asana sthiti.

You may try another variation. Place your hands in front of you on the floor while you are exhaling. Then, as you hold your breath, press down with your palms and lift up your body, trying to keep your legs spread out as before (see figure 3-62).

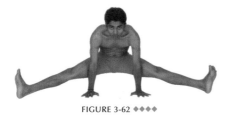

FIGURE 3-62 ◆◆◆◆

Return to the asana sthiti on inhalation. Repeat the movements three to six times.

In samakonasana, keeping your legs anchored, as you inhale, raise both arms overhead. Now as you slowly exhale, move your hands behind your back and hold the palms in back salutation (prishtanjali). (See figure 3-63).

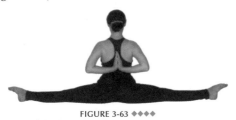

FIGURE 3-63 ◆◆◆◆

Stay in position for three to six breaths.

Baddha Konasana

From samakonasana, slowly exhale, bend both your knees and keep the sides of your feet abutting each other close to the perineum (see figure 3-64).

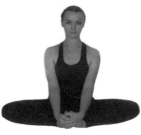

FIGURE 3-64 ◆◆◆

This posture is called *baddha konasana*. It gives good relief to the knees, which have been kept stretched throughout this sequence, but still maintains the hip extension. Stay in this position for several minutes, concentrating on long, slow breathing (ujjayi). Baddha konasana with chin lock is shown in figure 3-65.

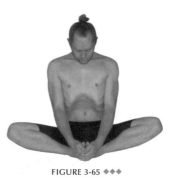

FIGURE 3-65 ◆◆◆

Another vinyasa is to support yourself with your hands, and as you are exhaling open your feet further by lowering your thighs further down (see figure 3-66).

Now, you may stay with your feet spread, but remove the support by placing your palms on your knees. In all these positions, the chin lock is maintained (see figure 3-67).

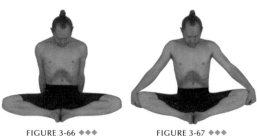

FIGURE 3-66 ◆◆◆   FIGURE 3-67 ◆◆◆

While in baddha konasana, exhale, place your palms on the floor just behind you. Inhale, and as you slowly exhale, press down with your palms, lift your body up, and sit on your heels. Now hold your feet and stay in that position for a long time, doing long smooth inhalations and exhalations (see figure 3-68).

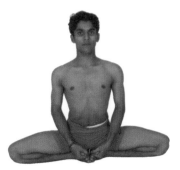

FIGURE 3-68 ◆◆◆◆

You may attempt to do all the three bandhas in the posture, which is called mula bandhasana. As you raise your body, the pelvis is stretched and the hip joint is pulled up.

With this the seated hip opener sequence is completed.

OTHER SEATED POSTURES

Lotus Position (Padmasana)

This is perhaps the best occasion to consider other seated postures arising out of dandasana. From the staff pose, exhale, bend your right knee and place your right leg on your left thigh close to the left side of your groin. Inhale, and during the following exhalation, bend your left knee and place your left foot on your right thigh close to your groin (see figure 3-69). This position is the lotus pose. The side view is shown in figure 3-70.

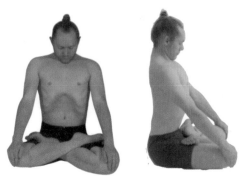

FIGURE 3-69 ◆◆◆   FIGURE 3-70 ◆◆◆

Stay in this position for twelve breaths. This is one of the most important seated poses.

The Accomplished Pose (Siddhasana)

From dandasana while exhaling, bend your right knee, stretch your ankle, and place your heel below your genitals, pressing the perineum. During the next exhalation, similarly bend your left knee and place your heel on the hollow of your right ankle (see figure 3-71).

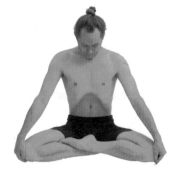

FIGURE 3-71 ◆◆

Keep your back straight and stay in this position for twelve long inhalations and exhalations. This is *siddhasana*.

You may repeat the same posture with the left foot on the floor *(see figure 3-72)*.

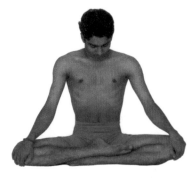

FIGURE 3-72 ♦♦

Cow-Head Pose (Gomukhasana)

Now bend your right knee and place your right foot beside your left buttock on the floor. During the following exhalation, bend your left knee and place it beside your right buttock. Keep your palms on your feet, and keep your back erect *(see figure 3-73)*.

Stay in this position for six long inhalations and exhalations. This is *gomukhasana*, or cow-head pose. Inhaling, you may stretch your legs to dandasana.

You may repeat the pose with the left leg bent first *(see figure 3-74)*.

Yoganarasimhasana Pose

The posture attributed to Lord Narasimha, or the man-lion incarnation of the Lord, is the next one. From dandasana, as you are exhaling, bend your knees and draw your feet close to your buttocks, with the right foot placed in front of the left buttock and the left foot in front of the right buttock. Inhaling, place your arms on your knees and stretch your arms in front of you. Inhale, and then exhale through your throat with a hoarse sound, like a lion roaring. As you roar, stick your tongue out, squint your eyes, and look at the middle of your eyebrows; spread your fingers as well *(see figure 3-75)*.

As you exhale, you may start drawing in your tummy and rectum, ending the exhalation with the abdominal and rectal locks in place. Hold on to the locks for about five seconds as you also hold your breath out. After you complete the "roar," roll your tongue back, and close your mouth and your eyes as well; keep your fingers together. Then inhale slowly through your throat, this time making the typical ujjayi sound. Breathe out as before. Repeat this several times. You may repeat the same procedure, changing the position of your legs *(see figure 3-76)*.

Then return to samasthiti.

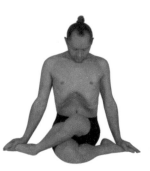

FIGURE 3-73 ♦♦

FIGURE 3-74 ♦♦

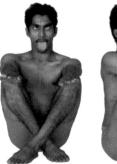

FIGURE 3-75 ♦♦

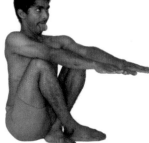

FIGURE 3-76 ♦♦

4

ON
ONE LEG
YOGASANAS

THIS SEQUENCE WILL involve standing on one leg and doing a number of vinyasas. These are generally known as austerity postures (tapas asanas). Dedicated sages doing penance (*tapasvins*) resorted to these endurance postures during the ancient Puranic (epic) age. Several sages and devotees used to stand on one leg and meditate on their chosen Lord, to have His vision, to listen to their master's voice, or to get the boon they desired from him.

Start the sequence from samasthiti *(see figure 4-1)*.

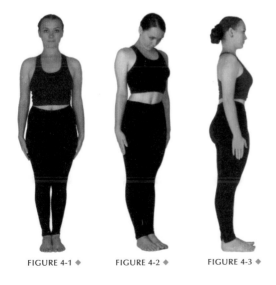

FIGURE 4-1 ◆   FIGURE 4-2 ◆   FIGURE 4-3 ◆

Keep your feet and ankles together and your shoulders thrown slightly back. Watch your balance closely and continually *(see figures 4-2 and 4-3)*.

Take a few long ujjayi breathes. Now you may start doing the sequence, one vinyasa after another.

POSTURE OF BHAGIRATA
(BHAGIRATASANA)

Exhaling slowly, bend your right knee and place your right foot so that it abuts your thigh and the heel is against the left side of your groin. Inhaling, raise both arms laterally overhead, and keep your palms together in anjali *(see figure 4-4)*; stay in this position for three to six breaths, balancing on your left leg.

This is known as *Bhagirathasana*, named after a royal sage, Bhagiratha. The great river Ganges bears his name as Bhagirati (one brought by Bhagiratha) because, according to legend, he was instrumental in bringing the great river from the heights of the Himalayas to the Gangetic plains.

Exhale and lower your right leg—returning to samasthiti.

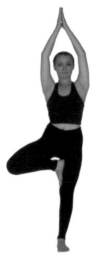

FIGURE 4-4 ◆◆

Now exhaling, bend your left knee and place your left foot against the inside of your right thigh, with the heel abutting your groin. Inhale, raise your arms overhead, and keep your palms together in the anjali gesture *(see figure 4-5)*.

Stay in this position for three to six long inhalations and exhalations, maintaining your balance effortlessly. Again, this is Bhagiratasana, balancing on the right leg.

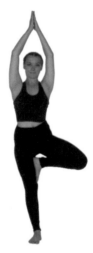

FIGURE 4-5 ◆◆

THE TREE POSE (VRIKMASANA) AND ITS VINYASAS

The next vinyasa is also known as vrikshasana, or the tree pose. Once again from samasthiti, as you breathe out, bend your right knee and place your foot on your left thigh very close to your groin in the half-lotus position. Inhale slowly as you raise both arms overhead, and balance in the posture *(see figure 4-6)*.

Stay in this position for three long inhalations and exhalations.

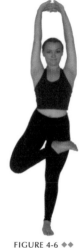

FIGURE 4-6 ◆◆

The next vinyasa will involve bending forward and placing your palms by the side of your left foot and your forehead on your right knee. Stay in this position for a few breaths, and then while slowly inhaling, return to the tree pose.

Now as you exhale, bend your right knee and lower your body until your bent right knee touches the floor. Keep your arms overhead in anjali *(see figure 4-7)*.

Stay in this position for a few breaths. Another variation of the hand position is shown in figure 4-8.

This is called the horse pose *(vatayasana)*. Stay in this position for three long breaths. Then as you inhale, return to the starting position.

Again remaining in vrikshasana, exhale, lower your arms to shoulder level. Inhale, and then start exhaling slowly. While you exhale, slowly draw in your stomach and also your rectum, and start to squat, bending your right knee. The left leg remains in half-lotus position. Take care not to raise

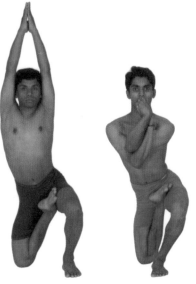

FIGURE 4-7 ◆◆◆   FIGURE 4-8 ◆◆◆

your arms overhead, keep them laterally at shoulder level, or use one of the other hand variations mentioned.

Now as you are exhaling, lower both arms but bring the right arm around from behind to hold your right big toe. You may use the left hand to affect a good grip. Stay in this position for three long inhalations and exhalations (*see figure 4-10*).

Now slowly raise your left arm, while you concentrate on a very slow smooth ujjayi inhalation (*see figure 4-11*).

your left heel off the floor and also to maintain your balance. Exhaling slowly and paying attention will help you to relax and do the posture (*see figure 4-9*).

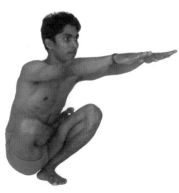

FIGURE 4-9 ◆◆◆◆

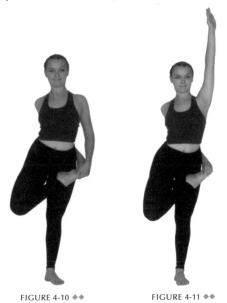

FIGURE 4-10 ◆◆   FIGURE 4-11 ◆◆

Stay in this position for three long breaths.

Stay in this position for a few breaths, drawing in both your rectum and your abdomen during every exhalation. Inhaling slowly, raise your body to return to the tree pose.

This vinyasa can be done with different positions of the arms as we have seen with respect to utkatasana, or the full squat pose in the first chapter. You may keep

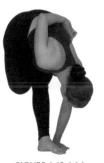

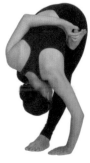

FIGURE 4-12 ◆◆◆   FIGURE 4-13 ◆◆◆

Exhaling smoothly, stretch your back and bend forward, maintaining good balance. Place your outstretched left hand on the floor *(see figure 4-12)*, beside your left foot. Stay in this position for three breaths.

While in the forward bend position, exhale still more deeply, bend forward further, and place your forehead on your stretched left knee *(see figure 4-13)*.

Stay in this position for three breaths. Return to the starting position, the tree pose (vrikshasana).

While in vrikshasana, as you are inhaling, stretch your left arm in front of you at shoulder level. Stay in this position for a breath. Now exhaling slowly and deeply (with your right leg still in half-lotus position), slowly squat on your haunches *(see figure 4-14)*.

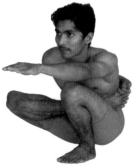

FIGURE 4-14 ◆◆◆

Stay in this position for three breaths, concentrating on your exhalation. Inhaling, raise your trunk. While you are exhaling, lower your arms and your right leg back to samasthiti.

TREE POSE AND VINYASAS
(LEFT KNEE BENT)

Now this minisequence may be repeated with the left leg in the half-lotus position. From samasthiti, while you are exhaling, bend your left knee and place your left foot on your right thigh, very close to your groin. Inhaling, raise both arms overhead and interlock your fingers. Stay in this position for three long inhalations and exhalations. This is vrikshasana (vama bhaga), or the tree pose, left side *(see figure 4-15)*.

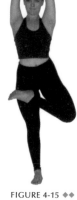

FIGURE 4-15 ◆◆

The next vinyasas will involve bending forward and placing your palms by the side of your right foot and your forehead on your left knee. Stay in this position for a few breaths, and then while slowly inhaling, return to the tree pose.

Now as you exhale, bend your left knee and lower your body until your bent left knee touches the floor. Keep your hands in the position shown in figure 4-16, the horse pose (vatayasana).

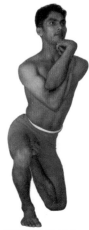

FIGURE 4-16 ◆◆◆

Stay in this position for three long breaths. Then as you inhale, return to the starting position.

Again remaining in vrikshasana, exhale, lower your arms to shoulder level. Inhale, and then start exhaling slowly. While you exhale, slowly draw in your stomach and rectum, and start to squat, bending your left knee. The right leg remains in the half-lotus position. Take care not to raise your right heel off the floor and to maintain your balance. Exhalating and paying attention will help you to relax and do the posture (*see figure 4-17*).

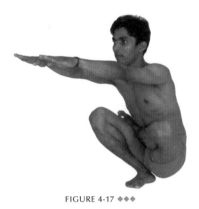

FIGURE 4-17 ◆◆◆

Stay in this position for a few breaths, drawing in both your rectum and your abdomen during every exhalation. Inhaling slowly, raise your body to return to the tree pose.

Locked Half-Lotus in Tree Pose (Ardha-Baddha-Padmasana in Vrikshasana)

Now let us consider the locked half-lotus vinyasa in tree pose (*ardha-baddha-padmasana in vrikshasana*). This is a left locked half-lotus in tree pose. Exhaling slowly, lower your arms, but bring the left arm behind your back to hold the big toe of your left foot. You may use your right hand to facilitate a good enough grip (*see figure 4-18*).

Stay in this position for three long inhalations and exhalations.

Now while inhaling, raise your right arm overhead with the left hand still holding your left foot (*see figure 4-19*).

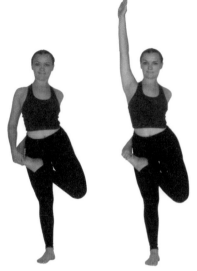

FIGURE 4-18 ◆◆   FIGURE 4-19 ◆◆

Again stay in this position for three long inhalations and exhalations.

As you exhale completely but slowly, stretch your back and place your right hand beside your right foot (*see figure 4-20*).

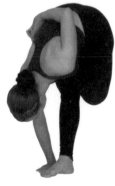

FIGURE 4-20 ◆◆◆

Try to relax and maintain your balance. Stay in this position for three long inhalations and exhalations.

Continuing to stay in the same position, exhale more deeply and bend forward further to place your forehead on your stretched right knee (*see figure 4-21*).

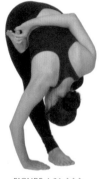

FIGURE 4-21 ◆◆◆

Stay in this position for three long breaths. As you inhale, slowly return to vrikshasana sthiti. On the next exhalation, lower your raised right arm and release the lock on your left foot.

While in vrikshasana, as you are inhaling, stretch your right arm in front of you at shoulder level. Stay in this position for a breath. Then exhaling slowly and deeply (with the left leg still in half-lotus position,) slowly squat on your haunches (*see figure 4-22*).

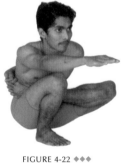

FIGURE 4-22 ◆◆◆

Stay in this position for three breaths, concentrating on your exhalation. Inhaling, raise your trunk. While you are exhaling, lower your arms and the left leg to return to samasthiti.

STANDING MARICHI

In the next vinyasa group, the leg position is changed. Remaining in samasthiti, as you exhale, slowly bend your right knee and raise your leg up and bring it up against your chest. The right thigh will be close to your chest (*see figure 4-23*).

Inhale, and on the following exhalation, embrace your right leg around the knee and stay in this position for three breaths. The leg position resembles Marichyasana sthiti.

Inhaling, release your grip, but on the following exhalation slightly bend forward, place your right arm around your bent right leg and bring your left arm around your back to take hold of your right hand with your left hand (*see figure 4-24*).

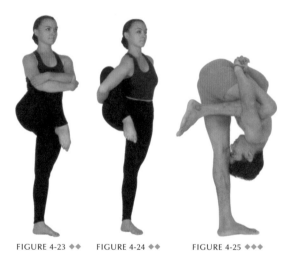

FIGURE 4-23 ◆◆   FIGURE 4-24 ◆◆   FIGURE 4-25 ◆◆◆

Stay in this position for three breaths. On every exhalation, tighten your grip, squeezing as much air out of your lungs as possible.

This time, as you exhale slowly and maintain balance, bend forward gradually until you touch your stretched left knee with your forehead. Stay in this position for three long inhalations and exhalations (*see figure 4-25*).

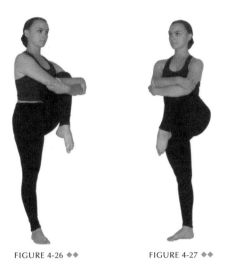

FIGURE 4-26 ◆◆   FIGURE 4-27 ◆◆

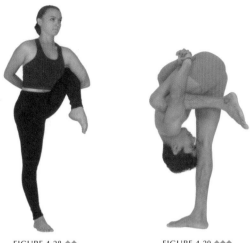

FIGURE 4-28 ◆◆   FIGURE 4-29 ◆◆◆

Then while inhaling, return to the starting sthiti. During the following exhalation, lower your right leg and your arms.

Now, for the left side. Remaining in samasthiti, as you exhale, slowly bend your left knee, raise your leg up and bring it against your chest, holding the leg with your hands. The left thigh will be close to your chest. Now inhale, and on the following exhalation, embrace the left leg around the knee and stay in this position for three breaths (see figure 4-26).

The leg position resembles that of Marichyasana sthiti. Another view is shown in figure 4-27.

Inhaling, release your grip, but on the following exhalation bend slightly forward, place your left arm around your bent left leg, and bring your right arm around your back to take hold your left hand with your right hand (see figure 4-28).

Stay in this position for three breaths. On every exhalation, tighten your grip, squeezing as much air out of your lungs as possible.

Now as you exhale slowly and balance carefully, bend forward gradually until you touch your outstretched right knee with your forehead. Stay in this position for three long inhalations and exhalations (see figure 4-29).

Then while inhaling, return to the starting sthiti. During the next exhalation, lower your left leg and your arms.

STRETCHED LEG-ARM SEQUENCE (UTTITA PADANGUSHTASANA)

From samasthiti while exhaling, slowly stretch your right leg in front of you up to the hip level and grasp your big toe with your right hand. Keep your left hand on your waist to help you balance (see figure 4-30).

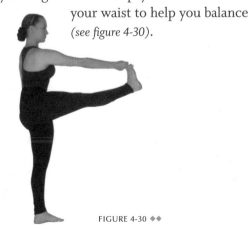

FIGURE 4-30 ◆◆

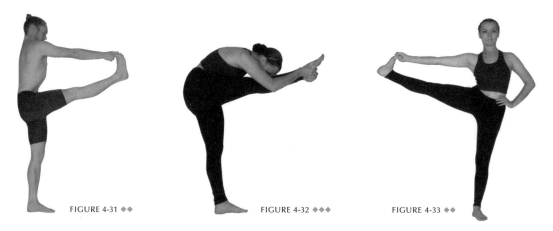

FIGURE 4-31 ◆◆   FIGURE 4-32 ◆◆◆   FIGURE 4-33 ◆◆

Stay in this position for three long inhalations and exhalations. This position has a pretty long name: *dakshina uttita hasta padangushtasana* (right-stretched hand and toe pose).

You could also practice the uddiyana bandha or abdomen lock after exhalation (*see figure 4-31*).

Now as you are exhaling, stretch forward and hold your right foot with both hands. Inhale and on the next exhalation, bend forward and place your forehead on your outstretched right knee (*see figure 4-32*).

Stay in this position for three long inhalations and exhalations. Then return to your starting position on inhalation. This vinyasa is known as the raised-right-leg, forward stretch pose (*dakshina uttita-pada paschimatanasana*).

On the next exhalation, while holding the big toe of your right leg with your right hand, slowly swing your leg to the right side up to waist level (*see figure 4-33*).

Stay in this position for three long inhalations and exhalations. Inhaling, swing your leg in front of you.

Standing in uttita padangushtasana; slowly exhale and squat on your haunches. Keep your left hand on your waist to maintain some balance (*see figure 4-34*).

Remember not to raise your heel. Stay in this position for three long inhalations and exhalations. Remaining in this utkatasana variation, with your right leg outstretched, slowly exhale; while exhaling, swing your right leg to the right side as you continue to hold the right big toe with your right hand (*see figure 4-35*).

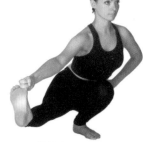

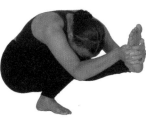

FIGURE 4-34 ◆◆◆   FIGURE 4-35 ◆◆◆   FIGURE 4-36 ◆◆◆

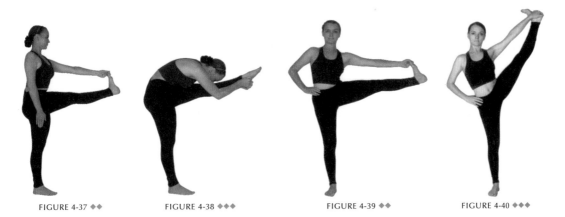

FIGURE 4-37 ♦♦   FIGURE 4-38 ♦♦♦   FIGURE 4-39 ♦♦   FIGURE 4-40 ♦♦♦

Maintain your balance, and do not raise your left heel off the floor. Stay in this position for three breaths.

Now as you slowly exhale, bend forward and hold your right foot with both hands and place your forehead on your outstretched right knee *(see figure 4-36)*.

Stay in this position, balancing with awareness for three long, smooth breaths. Return to the utkatasana variation, and then during the next inhalation stand up to uttita padangushtasana sthiti. On the next exhalation, lower your leg and arms.

From samasthiti, while exhaling slowly, stretch your left leg in front of you up to hip level. Keep your right hand on your waist to help you balance *(see figure 4-37)*.

Stay in this position for three long inhalations and exhalations. *Vama uttita hasta padangushtasana* (left-stretched hand and toe pose) is the name of the pose.

Now as you are exhaling, stretch forward and take hold of your left foot with both hands. Inhale and on the next exhalation, bend forward and place your forehead on your outstretched left knee *(see figure 4-38)*.

Stay in this position for three long inhalations and exhalations. Then return to your starting position on inhalation.

In the next exhalation, while holding the big toe of your left foot with your left hand, slowly swing your leg to the left side up to waist level *(see figure 4-39)*.

Stay in this position for three long inhalations and exhalations. Then as you are exhaling, raise your left leg further up, to about 135 degrees *(see figure 4-40)*.

Stay in this position for three breaths. Inhaling, lower your leg to hip level, and then swing the leg back in front of you.

Now as you stand in uttita padangushtasana, slowly exhale and squat on your haunches *(see figure 4-41)*.

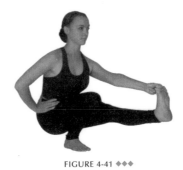

FIGURE 4-41 ♦♦♦

Do not raise your heel. Stay in this position for three long inhalations and exhalations. Remaining in this utkatasana variation, with your left leg outstretched, slowly exhale; while exhaling, swing your left leg to the left side as you continue to hold the left big toe with your left hand *(see figure 4-42)*.

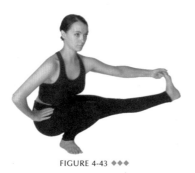

FIGURE 4-43 ◆◆◆

stretch your right leg backward and bend forward with your arms stretched overhead (*see figure 4-44*).

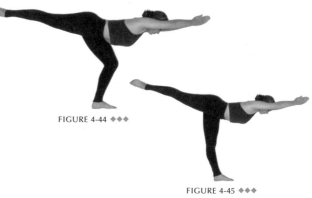

FIGURE 4-44 ◆◆◆

FIGURE 4-45 ◆◆◆

Maintain your balance, and do not raise your left heel off the floor. Stay in this position for three breaths.

Now as you slowly exhale, bend forward and take hold of your left foot with both hands and place your forehead on your outstretched left knee (*see figure 4-43*).

Stay balanced for three long inhalations and exhalations.

Now from this virabhadra position, inhale slowly, straighten your left knee, and balance with the left leg straight (*see figure 4-45*).

The upper body is kept horizontal. Stay in this position for three long inhalations and exhalations.

From this virabhadra variation, while you are exhaling, slowly raise your right leg as high as you can while lowering your upper body to place your palms on the floor beside your left foot (*see figure 4-46*).

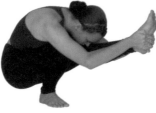

FIGURE 4-42 ◆◆◆

Stay in this position, balancing with awareness, for three long and, smooth breaths. Inhale and return to the standing position. On the next exhalation, lower the your leg and also the arms.

WARRIOR POSE SEQUENCE (VIRABHADRASANA)

Following are a series of variations on the *virabhadrasana*, or warrior pose.

From samasthiti, while inhaling, raise your arms overhead. Then as you are exhaling, bend your knees slightly and lower your trunk. Now on the next inhalation, keeping your left knee bent, raise and

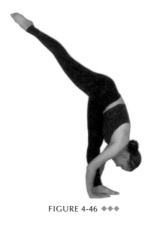

FIGURE 4-46 ◆◆◆

Stay in this position for three to six breaths. Inhaling, return to samasthiti.

Now, from samasthiti, inhale and raise your arms overhead. Then as you are exhaling, bend your knees slightly and lower your trunk. On the next inhalation, keeping your right knee bent, raise and stretch your left leg backward and bend forward with your arms stretched overhead (*see figure 4-47*).

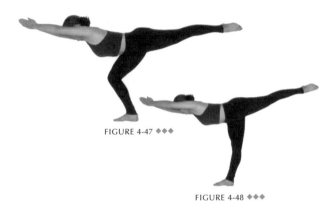

FIGURE 4-47 ◆◆◆

FIGURE 4-48 ◆◆◆

Stay balanced for three long inhalations and exhalations.

Now from this virabhadra position, while inhaling, slowly straighten your right knee and balance with your right leg straight (*see figure 4-48*).

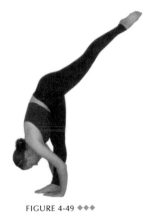

FIGURE 4-49 ◆◆◆

Your upper body should be horizontal. Stay in this position for three long inhalations and exhalations.

From this virabhadra variation, while you are exhaling, slowly raise your left leg as high as you can, lowering your upper body to place your palms on the floor beside your right foot (*see figure 4-49*).

Stay in this position for three to six breaths. Inhaling, return to samasthiti.

THE CONQUEROR OF THE THREE WORLDS SEQUENCE (Trivikramasana)

In samasthiti, while exhaling bend your right leg and take hold of the big toe with your right hand. As you are inhaling, stretch your right leg as high and as close to your body as possible. Keep your left arm along your left side (*see figure 4-50*).

Stay in this position for three long inhalations and exhalations. Then lower your right leg as you are exhaling. This pose is well known as *Trivikramasana* and is named after one of the ten incarnations of Lord Vishnu.

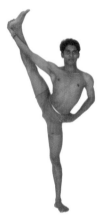

FIGURE 4-50 ◆◆◆◆

The Sage Durvasa Pose and Variations

While remaining in samasthiti, exhale slowly, slightly bend your left knee, and rounding your back, pull the right leg up and place it behind your neck or shoulder blade. You will be crouching a bit in this pose (*see figures 4-51 and 4-52*).

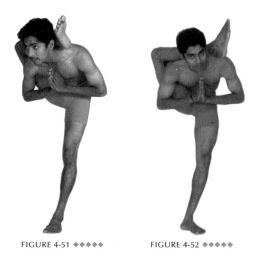

FIGURE 4-51 ◆◆◆◆◆   FIGURE 4-52 ◆◆◆◆◆

Stay in this position for three long inhalations and exhalations. Lower your leg as you slowly exhale. This posture is known as *Durvasasana*, named after a rishi, or sage, found in epics, such as the *Mahabharata*.

Remaining in the Durvasa pose, exhale, stretch your arms, and slowly bend forward without raising your left heel or bending your left knee. Place your palms beside your left foot. Stay in this position for a few breaths (*see figure 4-53*).

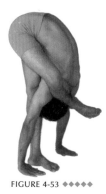

FIGURE 4-53 ◆◆◆◆◆

This pose is known as the *Richikasana*, named after a sage.

From this position, as you are exhaling, slowly bend your knee, and gingerly squat without raising your left heel (*see figure 4-54*).

Now place your palms on the floor while you exhale. Stay in this position for a few breaths. Then exhale completely, hold your breath, and pressing down with your hands, lift your body up and stay balanced on you hands (*see figure 4-55*).

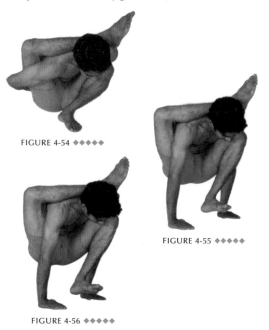

FIGURE 4-54 ◆◆◆◆◆

FIGURE 4-55 ◆◆◆◆◆

FIGURE 4-56 ◆◆◆◆◆

You may use a mat for a proper grip on the floor (*see figure 4-56*).

You may stay in this position for a few moments or even a few breaths and then lower your trunk and place your left foot on the floor.

Dancing Shiva Pose (Natarjasana)

From samasthiti, while exhaling, take hold of your right foot with your right hand and pull it behind your back. Stretch your left hand in front of you (*see figure 4-57*).

Stay in this position for six long inhalations and exhalations, balancing on your left foot. Inhale, lower your right leg and left arm to return to samasthiti. This is called *Natarajasana*, named after the dancing Shiva.

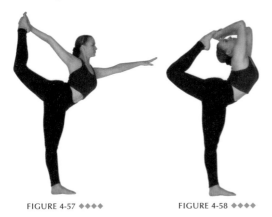

FIGURE 4-57 ◆◆◆◆   FIGURE 4-58 ◆◆◆◆

Now hold your right foot behind your back with both hands, arching your spine in the process *(see figure 4-58)*.

Stay in this position for three long inhalations and exhalations, pulling your right leg up, arching your back, and lifting your chest on every inhalation. Exhaling, return to samathiti, by lowering your arms and right leg. This is also considered a vinyasa of Natarajasana.

Conqueror of the Three Worlds (*Trivikramasana*)

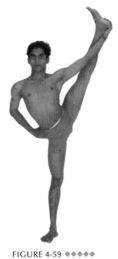

In samasthiti, while exhaling bend your right leg and hold the left big toe with your left hand. As you are inhaling, stretch your left leg as high and as close to your body as possible. Keep your right arm along your right side or on your waist *(see figure 4-59)*. Stay in this position for three long inhalations and exhalations. Then lower

FIGURE 4-59 ◆◆◆◆◆

your left leg as you exhale. As mentioned, this pose is well known as Trivikramasana and is named after one of the ten incarnation of Lord Vishnu.

Remaining in samasthiti, exhale slowly, bend your right knee, and rounding your back, pull your left leg up, and place it behind your neck or shoulder blade. You will be crouching a bit in this pose *(see figures 4-60 and 4-61)*.

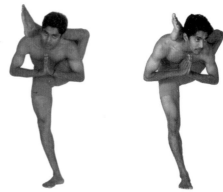

FIGURE 4-60 ◆◆◆◆◆   FIGURE 4-61 ◆◆◆◆◆

Stay in this position for three long inhalations and exhalations. Lower your leg as you slowly exhale. As mentioned previously, this is posture is known as Durvasasana

Remaining in the Durvasasana pose, as you exhale, stretch your arms and slowly bend forward without raising your right heel or bending your right knee. Place your palms beside your right foot. Stay in this position for a few breaths *(see figure 4-62)*.

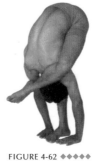

FIGURE 4-62 ◆◆◆◆◆

This pose is known Richikasana (asana named after sage Richika).

Starting from this position, as you exhale, slowly bend your right knee, and squat carefully without raising your right heel (see figure 4-63).

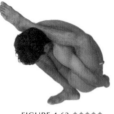

FIGURE 4-63 ◆◆◆◆◆

Place your palms on the floor while you exhale. Stay in this position for a few breaths. Then exhale completely, hold your breath, and pressing down with your hands, lift your body up and stay balanced on you hands (see figure 4-64).

You may use a mat to maintain a proper grip on the floor (see figure 4-65).

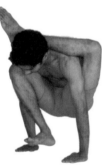 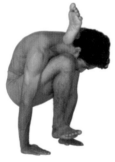

FIGURE 4-64 ◆◆◆◆◆   FIGURE 4-65 ◆◆◆◆◆

You may stay in this position for a few moments or even a few breaths and then lower your trunk and place your left foot on the floor.

Dancing Shiva Pose (Natarajasana)

From samasthiti, while exhaling, hold your left foot with your left hand and pull it behind your back. Stretch your right hand out in front of you (see figure 4-66).

Stay in this position for six long inhalations and exhalations, balancing on your right foot. Inhale, and lower your left leg and right arm to return to samasthiti. As mentioned earlier, this is called Natarajasana, after the dancing Shiva.

Now take hold of your left foot behind your back with both hands, arching your spine in the process (see figure 4-67).

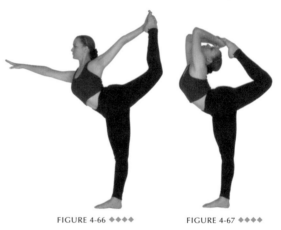

FIGURE 4-66 ◆◆◆◆   FIGURE 4-67 ◆◆◆◆

Stay in this position for three long inhalations and exhalations, pulling your left leg up, arching your back, and lifting your chest on every inhalation. Exhale, and return to samathiti by lowering your arms and left leg. This is also considered a vinyasa of Natarajasana.

This completes the sequence of asana vinyasas requiring balancing on one leg. This sequence produces a tremendous sense of balance. It requires very close attention and in the process helps the practitioner to attain a high degree of concentration, which is required for meditation and other yogic accomplishments.

5

THE
SUPINE
SEQUENCE

LYING-DOWN POSES, or supta asanas, enable many people who otherwise could not practice yoga to do many useful yogic exercises. The sequence starts from the lying-down position. One can achieve this position in three ways. One could sit down first, then lie down on one's back and start from there. But in vinyasa krama, one must start from samasthiti and go through a certain series of vinyasas (which we have already seen), come to the staff pose (dandasana), and then lie down. There is also an involved procedure by which one goes through the plough posture (*halasana*) and rolls down to the lying-down position. We will record all the vinyasas leading up to dandasana and proceed from there.

The simplest procedure is to start straight from the staff pose (*see figure 5-1*).

Then inhaling, raise and stretch your arms overhead (*see figure 5-2*).

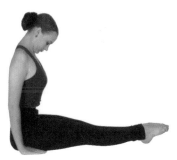

FIGURE 5-1 ◆◆

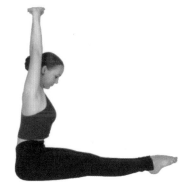

FIGURE 5-2 ◆◆

Exhale and then as you are inhaling, round your back and lie down on it, without raising your feet off the floor (*see figure 5-3*)

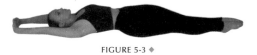

FIGURE 5-3 ◆

Then you may lower your arms on exhalation (*see figure 5-4*).

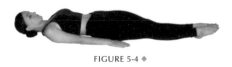

FIGURE 5-4 ◆

You are now in the lying-on-back pose (*supta asana*). This and its variations (*vinyasas*) are the starting pose for all lying-down poses.

LEAD SEQUENCE

The more classical progression to supta asana is to get to the staff pose through the sequence of vinyasas that were discussed earlier. For the sake of completeness, the names of the postures/vinyasas are given here:

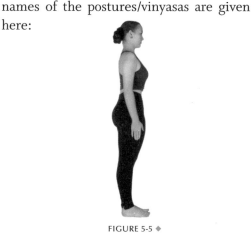

FIGURE 5-5 ◆

1. **SAMASTHITI** (*see figure 5-5*)

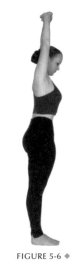

FIGURE 5-6 ◆

2. **TADASANA-SAMASTHITI**, arms raised (movement while inhaling) (*see figure 5-6*)

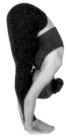

FIGURE 5-7

3. **UTTANASANA**, forward bend (movement while exhaling) (*see figure 5-7*)

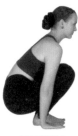

FIGURE 5-8

4. **UTKATASANA**, hip stretch (movement while exhaling) (*see figure 5-8*)

Here, press your palms down while inhaling, and pressing with your big toes, raise your heels (*see figure 5-9*).

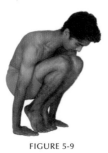

FIGURE 5-9

Then exhale completely, hold your breath, press down with your palms, and lift your body up, bending your knees and balancing on your hands *(see figure 5-10)*.

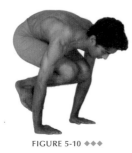

FIGURE 5-10 ◆◆◆

Take a short breath, and while holding your breath, jump backward to achieve the next vinyasa.

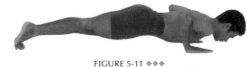

FIGURE 5-11 ◆◆◆

5. **CHATURANGA DANDASANA**, four-legged staff pose (while holding your breath after inhalation) *(see figure 5-11)*

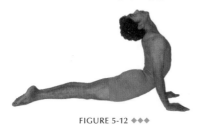

FIGURE 5-12 ◆◆◆

6. **URDHWA-MUKHA SWANASANA**, upward-facing-dog pose (movement while inhaling) *(see figure 5-12)*

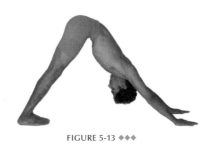

FIGURE 5-13 ◆◆◆

7. **ADHO-MUKHA SWANASANA**, downward-facing-dog pose (movement while exhaling) *(see figure 5-13)*

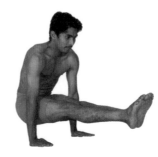

FIGURE 5-14 ◆◆◆

8. **DANDASANA UTPLUTHI**, jumping and balancing in staff pose (while holding your breath after exhalation) *(see figure 5-14)*

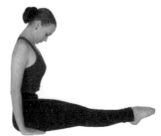

FIGURE 5-15 ◆◆

9. **DANDASANA**, the staff pose (movement while exhaling) *(see figure 5-15)*

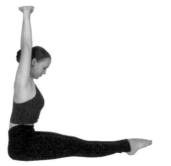

FIGURE 5-16 ◆◆

10. **NIRALAMBA DANDASANA**, unsupported staff pose (movement while inhaling) (*see figure 5-16*)

FIGURE 5-17 ◆

11. **SUPTA ASANA**, lying supine (movement while inhaling) (*see figure 5-17*)

FIGURE 5-18 ◆

12. **SUPTA ASANA**, lying supine and lowering the arms (movement while exhaling) (*see figure 5-18*)

LEAD SEQUENCE (ADVANCED)

The third approach is a little bit more involved. Up to the downward-facing-dog pose (*see figure 5-19*), the procedure is the same.

Then while exhaling, lower your head to touch the floor, even as you stretch your ankles, raise your heels and remain on your toes (*see figure 5-20*).

Thereafter, inhale and exhale completely, and raise your head slightly, keeping

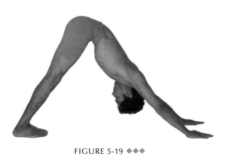

FIGURE 5-19 ◆◆◆

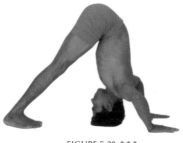

FIGURE 5-20 ◆◆◆

your chin locked. Flexing and rolling your neck, gently place the back of your neck and head on the floor, and you will be in halasana, or the plough pose (*see figure 5-21*).

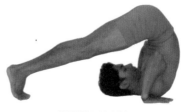

FIGURE 5-21 ◆◆◆

Caution: This involves a very high degree of flexion of the neck. You should have practiced the shoulder stand (pages 123–125) and plough posture (pages 123–124) and be very comfortable in those poses before attempting this vinyasa sequence.

Now stretch your arms overhead as you inhale and hold your toes (*see figure 5-22*). Then exhale, and on the next inhalation slowly roll your body down to the lying-down position (*see figure 5-23*)

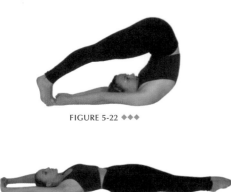

FIGURE 5-22 ◆◆◆

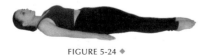

FIGURE 5-23 ◆

Lower your arms on exhalation (*see figure 5-24*).

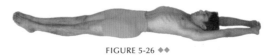

FIGURE 5-24 ◆

POND GESTURE (TATAKAMUDRA)

Stay in the lying-down position for one or two breaths. Exhale completely. Anchor your heels, tailbone, arms, and back; press down through your palms and draw in the rectum; pull the lower abdomen in and toward your back. Hold the locks for five to ten seconds. Your chin should be kept locked as well. When you draw the rectal and abdominal muscles inward and backward, the marks of the ribs and the pelvis bordering the abdominal cavity will be apparent. Because this resembles a pond, it is called pond gesture, or *tatakamudra* (*see figure 5-25*).

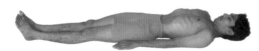

FIGURE 5-25 ◆◆

These are actually the three locks in the lying-down position. They are a very good way to start the practice of the bandhas. Inhale, and relax the locks. Repeat this exercise three to six times.

Inhaling, lift your arms overhead and keep your fingers interlocked and your palms turned outward. Stay in this position for a breath. As you start exhaling, draw in your rectum and your abdomen as in the previous vinyasas. Maintain the locks for five to ten seconds and then release them. This is a variation of tatakamudra (*see figure 5-26*).

FIGURE 5-26 ◆◆

Because your rib cage is pulled up in the arms raised position, the abdominal lock could be more effective. As you are inhaling, release the locks. You may repeat the procedure three to six times. Then as you exhale, lower your arms to supta asana sthiti

BELLY TWIST (JATARAPARIVRITTI)

As you inhale, spread your arms laterally along the floor up to shoulder level. Anchoring your pelvis, especially your tailbone, move your legs to the right side one at time until they are at an angle of 45 to 60 degrees. On the next exhalation, raise your head slightly off the floor, turn your head to the left side, and place your left cheek on the floor (*see figure 5-27*).

Stay in the pose for three to six breaths. At the end of each exhalation, you may do rectal and abdominal locks as in tatakamudra.

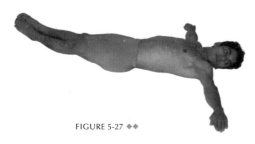

FIGURE 5-27 ◆◆

Inhaling, bring your legs back to the lying-down position even as you straighten your head.

During the next exhalation, you may do the same procedure on the other side *(see figure 5-28)*.

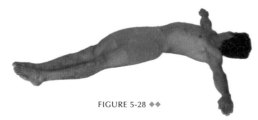

FIGURE 5-28 ◆◆

Stay in this position for three to six breaths and then return to asana sthiti, as you did on the other side.

PELVIC FLOOR POSES
(APANASANA)

Slowly exhaling, bend your right knee and bring your right thigh up against your ribs. Inhale and again while exhaling, gently raise your head, embrace your bent right leg with both hands, and lower your head *(see figure 5-29)*.

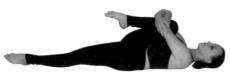

FIGURE 5-29 ◆◆

Stay in this position for three long inhalations and exhalations. On every exhalation, tighten your grip around your right leg and gently press your right thigh against your lower abdomen. This is *dakshina pada apanasana* (right side pelvic pose) Return to supta asana sthiti as you are inhaling.

The next step will involve raising your head and placing your forehead on your right knee as you exhale, even as you press your thigh against your lower abdomen *(see figure 5-30)*.

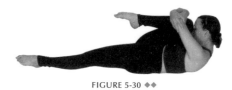

FIGURE 5-30 ◆◆

During the inhalation, relax your grip a little bit, dropping your head back to the floor. Repeat the movement three to six times. Then inhaling, stretch your right leg all the way down. This is *dakshina pada pavanamuktasana* (right-side wind-relieving pose) *(see figure 5-31)*.

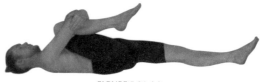

FIGURE 5-31 ◆◆

In this sequence, you may raise your head and position your head, forehead, face, or chin in various ways, each requiring a greater movement and rounding of your spine.

Figures 5-32 through 5-34 show different head positions.

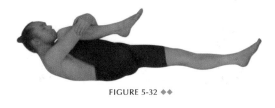

FIGURE 5-32 ◆◆

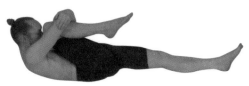

FIGURE 5-33 ◆◆

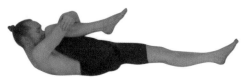

FIGURE 5-34 ◆◆

Slowly exhaling, bend your left knee and bring your left thigh up against your chest. Inhale and again while you are exhaling, gently raise your head, embrace your bent left leg with both hands, and lower your head (see figure 5-35).

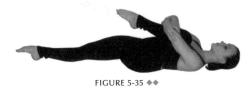

FIGURE 5-35 ◆◆

Stay in this position for three long inhalations and exhalations. On every exhalation, tighten your grip around your left leg and gently press your left thigh against your lower abdomen. This is *vama pada apanasana* (left side pelvic pose). Return to supta asana sthiti as you are inhaling.

The next step involves raising your head and placing your forehead on your left knee as you exhale, even as you press your

thigh against your lower abdomen (see figure 5-36).

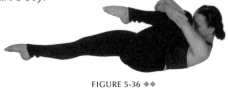

FIGURE 5-36 ◆◆

During the inhalation, relax your grip a little bit, lowering your head back to the floor. Repeat the movement three to six times. Then inhaling, stretch your left leg all the way down. This is *vama pada pavanamuktasana* (left side wind-relieving pose)

Now while exhaling, bend your right knee and place your right foot on your left thigh close to your groin in the half-lotus position. Inhale and on the next exhalation, slowly bend your left leg, slightly raise your head, and embrace your bent left leg with both hands. Inhaling, slowly lower your head back to the floor (see figure 5-37).

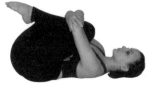

FIGURE 5-37 ◆◆◆

Stay in this position for three to six breaths. On each long, deep exhalation, press your bent left leg against your right foot, which will press against the left side of your lower abdomen.

Now as you exhale, while you press your left leg, raise your head and place it on your left knee (see figure 5-38).

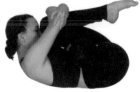

FIGURE 5-38 ◆◆◆

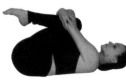

FIGURE 5-39 ◆◆◆

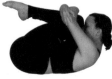

FIGURE 5-40 ◆◆◆

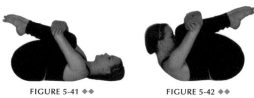

FIGURE 5-41 ◆◆

FIGURE 5-42 ◆◆

Return to asana sthiti while inhaling. Repeat the movement three to six times. Then stretch both your legs all the way out on the floor as you smoothly inhale.

Now exhaling, bend your left knee and place your left foot on your right thigh close to your groin in the half-lotus position. Inhale and on the next exhalation, slowly bend your right leg, slightly raise your head, and embrace your bent right leg with both hands. Inhaling, slowly drop your head back to the floor (see figure 5-39).

Stay in this position for three to six breaths. On each long, deep exhalation, press your bent right leg against your left foot, which will press against the right side of your lower abdomen.

Now as you exhale and press down with your right leg, raise your head and place it on your right knee (see figure 5-40).

Return to asana sthiti while inhaling. Repeat the movement three to six times. Thereafter, stretch your legs all the way out on the floor as you smoothly inhale.

Deeply exhaling, bend both your knees this time. Raise your head slightly, and smugly embrace both your legs with both hands. Inhaling, drop your head back to the floor (see figure 5-41).

Stay in this position for three to six breaths. Keep every exhalation very long, smooth, and complete, and press your thighs against your lower abdomen during every exhalation. This is called *apanasana*, or the pelvic region pose.

Staying in apanasana, as you are exhaling, press your thighs against your lower abdomen; also raise your head and place your forehead on your knees (see figure 5-42).

Inhaling, return to the asana sthiti. Repeat this three to six times. Concentrate on your exhalations. Make them as complete as possible so that your thighs could press against your pelvic area. This is called *pavanamuktasana,* or wind releaser.

Once again, round your back, raise your head in pavanamuktasana and place your head on your knees. Stay in this position for three breaths (see figure 5-43).

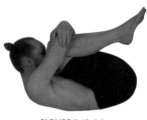

FIGURE 5-43 ◆◆

Return to the apanasana position. This time when you raise your head on exhalation, place your face on your knees and stay in this position for three long inhalations and exhalations (see figure 5-44).

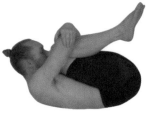

FIGURE 5-44 ◆◆

The next vinyasa requires that you place your chin on your knees at the completion of the movement (*see figure 5-45*).

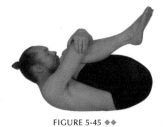

FIGURE 5-45 ◆◆

Stay in this position for another three breaths before returning to the apanasana position. Then, inhaling, stretch your legs in the lying-down position, or supta asana.

DESK POSE (Dwipadapitam)

From the supta asana sthiti, while exhaling, bend both your knees and draw your legs close to your body. Keep your feet together and place them close to your buttocks. As you are slowly inhaling, press down through your palms, your feet, and the back of your head and neck, slowly lifting your hips as high as you can. You should keep your feet together (*see figure 5-46*).

Exhaling, lower your trunk. Repeat the movement slowly so that you can feel the stretch in every vertebra. This posture is called *dwipadapitam*, meaning a two-legged seat or a desk.

Please note: Moving into this pose and other variations of the desk pose should be done on inhalation. However, there are some exceptions. In the introductory chapter I explained that in langhana kriya some expansive movements are done during exhalation, rather than on inhalation. Persons who are obese, older, or stiff may use langhana kriya because the exhalation will relax their muscles and create less pressure in their abdomen. It is a trade-off between expanding your chest and working on your internal thoracic muscles and doing the exercises without much pressure.

In this vinyasa, try to hold your ankles with your hands. Then as you are inhaling, slowly lift your chest and raise your waist as high as you can (*see figure 5-47*).

Exhaling, lower your trunk. You may repeat the movement three to six times, stretching your spine, hips, and shoulders.

The next position will be another hasta, or hand vinyasa. As you exhale, raise your body slightly, stretch your hands under your body, and clasp your left ankle with your right hand and your right ankle with your left hand. Then as you slowly inhale, arch your spine, raising your hips (*see figure 5-48*).

While you are exhaling come down. Repeat the movement three to six times.

This time when you are inhaling, raise your hips and arch your spine in dwipadapitam; also raise your arms, interlock your fingers, and keep your hands in front of your face. Exhaling, lower your trunk and

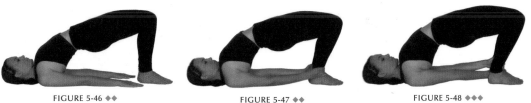

FIGURE 5-46 ◆◆   FIGURE 5-47 ◆◆   FIGURE 5-48 ◆◆◆

arms. Repeat the movement three times (*see figure 5-49*).

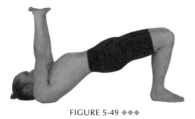

FIGURE 5-49 ◆◆◆

This vinyasa will involve raising your arms overhead while you are inhaling. Exhale and during the following inhalation, raise your waist as high as you can. While you are exhaling, return to the starting position. Repeat the movement three times (*see figure 5-50*).

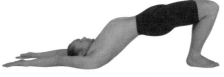

FIGURE 5-50 ◆◆◆

Now let us look at some leg movements that stretch your hip a little more. Keep your feet in the initial dwipadapitam position. As you inhale, stretch your right leg all the way down, while keeping your left leg bent. Now press down with your arms, the back of your head and neck, and your left

foot; slowly raise your trunk and your right leg as high as you can. As you reach the end of the movement, give a very gentle nudge to your right hip and the tailbone (*see figure 5-51*).

Exhaling slowly, return your right leg to an outstretched position on the floor. You may repeat the movement three to six times.

As you are lowering your trunk for the last time in the previous vinyasa (which you do as you are exhaling), bend your right knee and place your right foot on your left thigh close to the left side of your groin in the half-lotus position. Then as you breathe out, raise your body slightly and slip your right arm under your back and clasp the big toe of your right foot with your right hand. Hold your left ankle with your left hand (*see figure 5-52*).

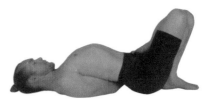

FIGURE 5-52 ◆◆

Wait for one or two breaths. While you are inhaling, press down with your left foot, the back of your head, and your neck. Lift your trunk as high as you can. Try to keep both your knees at the same level, by relaxing and keeping your right hip loose (*see figure 5-53*).

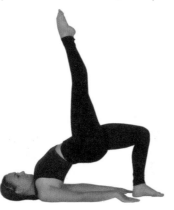

FIGURE 5-51 ◆◆◆

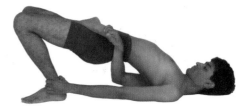

FIGURE 5-53 ◆◆◆

As you exhale, lower your trunk. Repeat the movement three to six times.

After completing the previous vinyasas, while inhaling stretch your right leg, keeping your left leg bent. As you are slowly inhaling, press down with your left foot, the back of your head and neck, and your right foot (your right ankle is stretched so that your right foot is on the floor at the end of the movement), and lift your hips as high as you can, arching your spine nicely in the process (*see figure 5-54*).

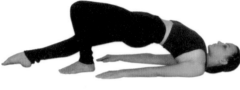

FIGURE 5-54 ◆◆

While you are exhaling, lower your trunk and return to the starting position. Repeat the movement three to six times.

Now let us look at some movements of the left leg. As you inhale, stretch your left leg, which was kept bent; on the following exhalation, bend your right leg and place your right foot just behind your right buttock. Now press down with your arms, the

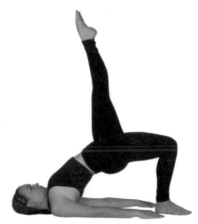

FIGURE 5-55 ◆◆◆

back of your head, and your neck, slowly raising your trunk and left leg as high as you can. As you reach the end of the movement, give a very gently nudge to your left hip (*see figure 5-55*).

Exhaling slowly, lower your trunk while keeping your left leg stretched out on the floor. You may repeat the movement three to six times.

As you are lowering your trunk for the last time (while exhaling), bend your left knee and place your left foot on your right thigh close to the right side of your groin in the half-lotus position (*see figure 5-56*).

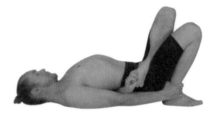

FIGURE 5-56 ◆◆

Then as you breathe out, raise your body slightly and slip your left arm underneath your body and clasp the big toe of your left foot with your left hand. Hold your right ankle with your right hand. Wait for one or two breaths. While you are inhaling, press down with your right foot, the back of your head, and your neck, and raise your trunk as high as you can. Keep both your knees at the same level, by relaxing and keeping your left hip loose (*see figure 5-57*).

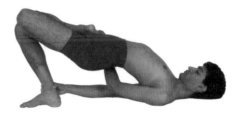

FIGURE 5-57 ◆◆◆

As you exhale, lower your trunk. Repeat the movement three to six times.

After completing the previous vinyasa, while inhaling stretch your left leg, keeping your right leg bent. Now, as you are slowly inhaling, press down with your right foot, the back of your head and neck, and your left foot (your left ankle should be stretched so that your left foot is on the floor), raise your hips as high as you can, arching your spine thoroughly in the process (see figure 5-58).

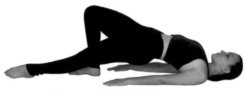

FIGURE 5-58 ◆◆

While you are exhaling, lower your trunk and return to the starting position. Repeat the movement three to six times.

From the previous position, as you inhale stretch your right leg so that you are back to supta asana. Now pressing down with your arms, the back of your head, and your neck, slowly arch your entire trunk (from your neck to your feet). (See figure 5-59.)

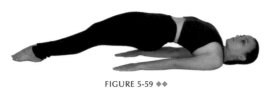

FIGURE 5-59 ◆◆

As you exhale, slowly lower your trunk. Repeat the movement three to six times. This is called *madhya sethu*, or the mid-region-bridge pose.

Remaining in supta asana, as you are inhaling, slowly stretch your arms and swing them overhead all the way to the floor. Interlock your fingers, and turn your palms outward. Exhale. As you are inhaling, pressing down through your heels, and anchoring your back of your head and neck, arch your body from your neck to your heels. This is a vinyasa of the center bridge, or madhya sethu (see figure 5-60).

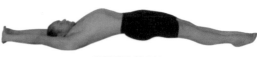

FIGURE 5-60 ◆◆◆

This time, anchoring your buttocks, arch your torso and place the crown of your head on the floor (see figure 5-61).

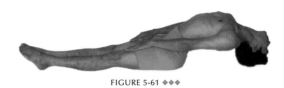

FIGURE 5-61 ◆◆◆

You may use your palms to press down, and lift and arch your torso. Now press down through your forearms, and lift your legs up as much as possible, pivoting your buttocks (see figure 5-62).

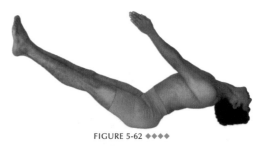

FIGURE 5-62 ◆◆◆◆

This is raised-leg pose (*uttana-padasana*). Stay in this position for three breaths, and then lower your torso and your legs to assume supta asana.

Now bend your knees slightly and draw your feet inward a bit. Place your palms near your shoulders. Inhale and hold your breath; press down through your palms and feet, and lift your waist and buttocks as high as possible, arching your whole body, from your crown to your feet, which should be well anchored in the process. Stretch your arms, and place your hands on the sides of your thighs. This is the bridge pose (*sethubandasana*). *(See figure 5-63.)*

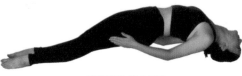

FIGURE 5-63 ◆◆◆◆

People with stiff necks should do this posture only after preparing their neck with many of the arm and neck exercises mentioned in the "Hasta Vinyasas" section of the first chapter. Stay in this position for three breaths. Then place your palms by the sides of your shoulders, and exhaling slightly, lift your head and lower your body to the floor to supta asana.

You have been keeping your head and neck on the floor for several vinyasas. Now exhaling, bend your knees as in the desk pose. On the next exhalation, place your palms by the sides of your neck and below your shoulders, with your palms turned inward toward your feet. Inhale slowly, hold your breath, and pressing down through your palms and your feet, raise your trunk and arch your body as much as you can *(see figure 5-64)*.

As you are exhaling return to the starting desk pose sthiti. Repeat the movement three to six times. Then as you are exhaling,

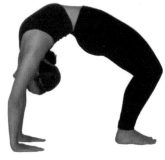

FIGURE 5-64 ◆◆◆

stretch your legs and arms beside your body, back in supta asana sthiti. This posture is called the upward-looking bow posture (*urdhwa dhanurasana*). Some experts call it the half-wheel pose (*ardha chakrasana*).

As a variation, you can bring your palms closer to your feet during exhalation and keep your back arched. Stay in this position for three breaths, stretching and lifting your tailbone at the end of the inhalation *(see figure 5-65)*.

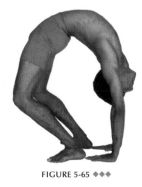

FIGURE 5-65 ◆◆◆

This is known as the wheel pose (*chakrasana*), because your body makes a circle—almost, that is. Return to the desk pose on exhalation and then return to supta asana sthiti.

DESK POSE—
ADVANCED VARIATIONS
(Dwipadapitam Vinyasas)

Remain in the lying-down position (supta asana). Exhaling, slowly draw up your feet and place them close to your buttocks. Keep your forearms on the floor close to your body. We have already seen some simpler variations of the desk pose. Here you can work to stretch your spine a bit more by proper anchoring, especially by holding your ankles.

Hold your ankles with your hands. Inhaling, lift your body up, and arch your spine as much as possible. Your thighs should be horizontal (see figure 5-66).

Stay in this position for three breaths, and while exhaling slowly lower your torso.

The next vinyasa will involve your holding your right ankle with your left hand and your right ankle with your right hand. Your fingers and palms should grip your ankles. Stay in this position for a breath, and then as you inhale, slowly raise your trunk, arching your spine, opening your chest and your shoulders in the process. Stay in this position for three breaths, and gently nudge your tailbone up at the end of each exhalation. Then as you are exhaling, return to the starting position (see figure 5-67).

This time, hold your left ankle with both hands. Stay in this position for a breath. Then while you are inhaling, press down through your left foot, the back of your head, and your neck, and lift your body as high as you can, arching your spine thoroughly in the process (see figure 5-68).

You will be pulling your right hip with the straight leg lifted up. Stay in this position for three breaths, gently lifting your

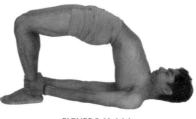

FIGURE 5-66 ◆◆◆

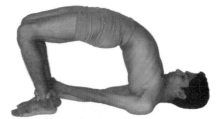

FIGURE 5-67 ◆◆◆

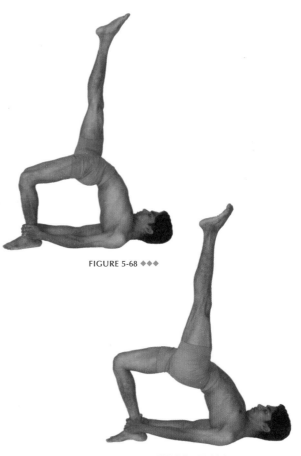

FIGURE 5-68 ◆◆◆

FIGURE 5-69 ◆◆◆

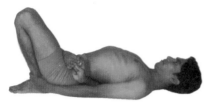

FIGURE 5-70 ◆◆◆

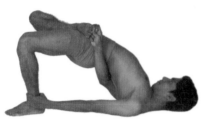

FIGURE 5-71 ◆◆◆

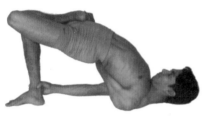

FIGURE 5-72 ◆◆◆

your back and clasp your right big toe (see figure 5-70).

Also hold your left ankle with your left hand. Inhaling, lift your trunk as high as you can (see figure 5-71).

Stay in this position for three breaths, and then while exhaling lower your trunk to the starting position.

You may repeat the same movement on the other side (see figure 5-72).

LEG AND ARM LIFTS

We have seen a number of vinyasas involving arching of your spine in the lying-down position. Normally back-bending exercises are associated with such positions as bow pose or cobra pose. But here you can see that because your body is well anchored with your neck and your feet on the floor, it is much easier to control the extent of the arching of your spine, whereas in the face-down poses it is more difficult to control the back arch. So for therapy or teaching older people, some of the vinyasas in this group could prove to be very useful and highly beneficial.

We can now see some more vinyasas in the lying-down position, in which your trunk is mostly on the ground, but your arms and legs are manipulated to achieve different postures and benefits. From supta asana sthiti, as you are inhaling raise your right arm overhead all the way to the floor (see figure 5-73).

tailbone a bit at the end of every exhalation. Stay in this position for three breaths, and while exhaling lower your trunk; bend your right knee to return to the starting position.

Hold your left ankle with both hands. As you inhale, press down through the back of your head, neck, and right foot, and lift your body as high as you can, experiencing a nice stretch up to your tailbone (see figure 5-69).

Stay in this position for three breaths. On the next exhalation, return to the asana sthiti.

As you are exhaling, bend your right knee and place your right foot on your left thigh, close your groin. Exhaling, lift your body slightly, swing your right arm behind

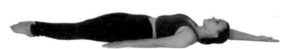

FIGURE 5-73 ◆

Stay in this position for three long inhalations and exhalations.

Then as you are breathing out, raise your right arm and your right leg—your arm to the level of your shoulder and the leg to the level of your right hip (see figure 5-74).

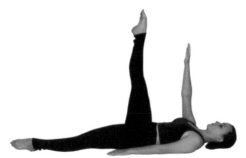

FIGURE 5-74 ◆◆

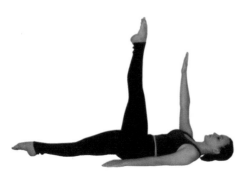

FIGURE 5-75 ◆◆

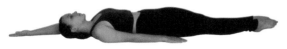

FIGURE 5-76 ◆

Inhaling, return to the stating position. You may repeat the movement three to six times.

The next vinyasa will involve again movement of an arm and a leg. Exhaling, raise your right arm and your left leg to 90 degrees (see figure 5-75).

While you are inhaling, lower your right arm overhead and bring your leg all the way down, stretching it right across your body. Return to the starting position. Now as you are exhaling, lower your right hand to be back to supta asana.

As you breathe in, stretch your left arm overhead all the way down to the floor (see figure 5-76).

Stay in this position for three long inhalations and exhalations stretching the left side of your body.

After stretching your left side, as you breathe out, raise your left arm and your left leg vertically (see figure 5-77).

Stay in this position for three long inhalations and exhalations. Repeat the movement three times. Then lower your left arm overhead and your left leg all the way down, in the process slowly and deliberately stretching the entire left side of your body.

Now for parivritti, or across-the-body movement. As you are exhaling, raise your left arm and your right leg to a vertical position (see figure 5-78).

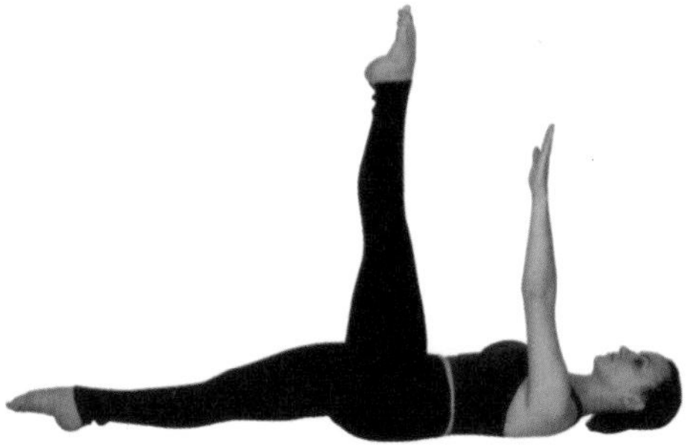

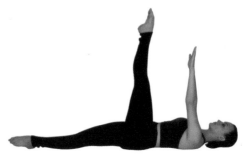

FIGURE 5-77 ◆◆

FIGURE 5-78 ◆◆

Return to the starting position on inhalation. Repeat the movement three times, every time as you come down stretch right across your body. Lower your left arm on exhalation.

This time, inhaling raise both arms overhead, stretching your body as you move your arms up (see figure 5-79).

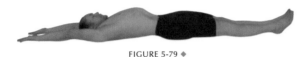

FIGURE 5-79 ◆

As you exhale the next time, raise both arms and legs vertically (see figure 5-80).

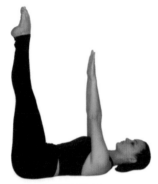

FIGURE 5-80 ◆◆◆

As you inhale, lower your arms overhead and bring your legs all the way down, stretching your body all the way. Repeat the movement three to six times. This pose is known as *urdhwa-prasarita-pada-hastasana* (stretched-up legs and arms pose). My guru used to jocularly call it the "U" pose.

Another vinyasa requires that you stop at midpoint as you come down. This will require you to keep your arms and legs at about 45 degrees (see figure 5-81).

Stay in that position for one breath and continue to move down while you are inhaling, until you are in supta asana sthiti. Exhaling, lower your arms.

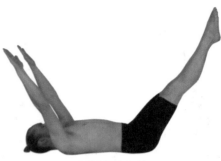

FIGURE 5-81 ◆◆◆

Now, pressing down with your arms, raise your legs to 90 degrees. Stay in this position for three long inhalations and exhalations (see figure 5-82).

My teacher used to call this the "L" form. Inhaling, you lower your legs back so that you are in supta asana sthiti.

In this vinyasa, from the previous position, while exhaling bring your legs further up and hold your feet with both your hands (see figure 5-83).

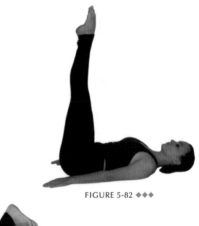

FIGURE 5-82 ◆◆◆

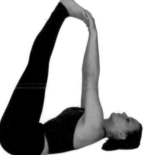

FIGURE 5-83 ◆◆◆

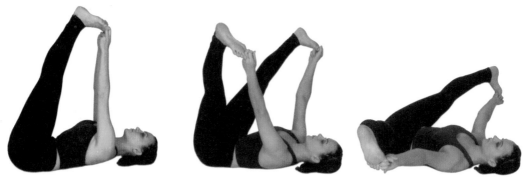

FIGURE 5-84 ◆◆◆   FIGURE 5-85 ◆◆◆   FIGURE 5-86 ◆◆◆

Stay in this position for six long inhalations and exhalations.

Remaining in the same position, clasp your big toes with your hands (*see figure 5-84*) and stay in this position for six long inhalations and exhalations.

Now holding your big toes as in the previous vinyasa, while slowly inhaling, spread your legs to about 90 degrees (*see figure 5-85*).

Stay in this position for three long inhalations and exhalations. Alternately, exhale, close your legs, and inhaling spread your legs, and repeat the movement three times. My guru used to call this the "V" formation.

In this vinyasa, while holding your toes, spread your legs as much as possible and lower your legs as far down as possible (*see figure 5-86*).

Stay in this position for six long breaths. Return to the starting position.

In the next vinyasa, you will hold your right big toe with your right hand, but while you are inhaling, lower your right leg all the way down to the floor and keep your left hand close to your left leg on the floor (*see figure 5-87*).

Exhaling, bring your leg up and inhaling slowly, lower your leg. Repeat the movement three to six times. The name of this pose is *supta dakshina-parsva-padangushtasanam*, supine right-foot-to-fingers pose.

Return to the position wherein you are holding your right big toe with your right hand, with your right leg vertical. Your left leg is on the floor. Now as you are exhaling, pull your right leg down and bend your knee, still holding your toe. Raise your head slightly and as you exhale further, bring your right leg down close to your body while placing your right hand behind your head (*see figure 5-88*).

Stay in this position for three long inhalations and exhalations. This pose is called *supta ardha-parivarta-dakshina-padasanam*, supine half-crossed-right-leg pose.

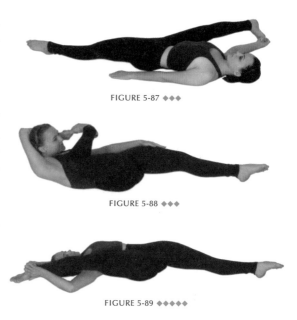

FIGURE 5-87 ◆◆◆

FIGURE 5-88 ◆◆◆

FIGURE 5-89 ◆◆◆◆◆

The next vinyasa is quite involved and is known as *supta Trivikramasana*. From the asana sthiti, using your right hand lower your right leg all the way down as you slowly exhale. You will do well to hold your right foot with both hands after reaching the pose (*see figure 5-89*).

Stay in this position for six to twelve breaths. Inhaling, you may return to asana sthiti. On the next inhalation, lower your leg all the way down to supta asana, or the supine position.

This time, raise your head slightly and place your right leg behind your right shoulder (*see figure 5-90*).

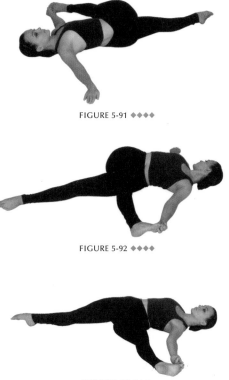

FIGURE 5-91 ◆◆◆◆

FIGURE 5-92 ◆◆◆◆

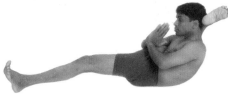

FIGURE 5-90 ◆◆◆◆◆

FIGURE 5-93 ◆◆◆

Stay in this position for three breaths and then return to the supta asana sthiti, while you are inhaling. This is dakshina Bhairava asana.

Now, as you are exhaling once again raise your right leg, but hold your right big toe with your left hand. On the next inhalation sweep the right leg laterally to the level of your right shoulder. Again inhale, and as you are breathing out, lower your right leg to your left side all the way to the floor (*see figure 5-91*)

Stay in this position for a breath, and during the next exhalation, raise your head slightly, turn to right, and place the right side of your face on the floor (*see figure 5-92*).

Stay in this position for six long breaths, maintaining a good twist to your right hip. Thereafter, inhaling raise your leg back to

asana sthiti. This is another complicated variation of the stomach twist (jatara-parivritti).

As we saw earlier, in this vinyasa, you will hold your left big toe with your left hand, but while you are inhaling, lower your right leg all the way down to the floor and keep your right hand close to your right leg on the floor. Inhale and then during the next smooth inhalation slowly lower your left leg to the left side all the way to the floor (*see figure 5-93*).

Exhaling, bring your leg up and inhaling slowly, lower your leg. Repeat the movement three to six times. The name of the pose is *supta vama-parsve-padangushtasanam*, supine left-foot-to-fingers pose.

Return to the position in which you are holding your left big toe with your left hand, with your left leg vertical. Your right leg should be on the floor. Now as you are exhaling, pull your left leg down and bend your knee, still holding your toe. Raise your head slightly, and as you are exhaling further, bring your leg down close to your body while placing your left hand behind your head (see figure 5-94).

Stay in this position for three long inhalations and exhalations. This is called *supta ardha-parivarta-vama-padasanam*, supine half-crossed-left-leg pose.

The next vinyasa is supta Trivikramasana. From asana sthiti, pull up your left leg and lower it over your head all the way down to the floor as you exhale slowly. You should hold your left foot with both hands (see figure 5-95).

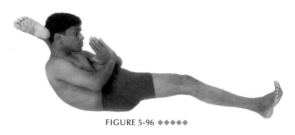

FIGURE 5-96 ◆◆◆◆◆

Since you have done Bhairava asana on each side, you can try to keep both your feet behind your shoulders. Remaining in Bhairava asana, place your left leg behind your shoulder. This is the yoga reclining pose (*yoganidrasana*). See figure 5-97.

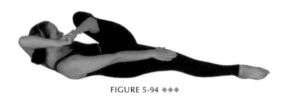

FIGURE 5-94 ◆◆◆

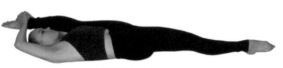

FIGURE 5-95 ◆◆◆◆◆

Stay in this position for six to twelve breaths. Inhaling, return to asana sthiti. On the next inhalation, lower your leg all the way down to supta asana, or the supine position.

This time, raise your head, slightly, place your left leg behind your left shoulder (see figure 5-96).

Stay in this position for three breaths and then return to the supta asana sthiti while you are inhaling. This is vama Bhairava asana.

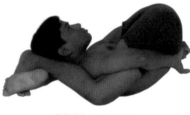

FIGURE 5-97 ◆◆◆◆◆

Stay in this position for three breaths and then return to supta asana sthiti. The next figure shows the same pose with the left leg first and then the right leg (see figure 5-98).

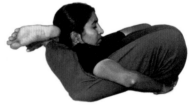

FIGURE 5-98 ◆◆◆◆◆

Return to supta asana sthiti on inhalation.

Now, as you are exhaling, once again raise your left leg, but hold your left big toe with your right hand. On the next inhalation, sweep your left arm laterally to the level of your left shoulder. Again inhale and as you are breathing out, use your right hand to lower your left leg to your right side all the way to the floor (*see figure 5-99*).

Stay in this position for a breath, and during the following exhalation, raise your head slightly, turn it to the left, and place the left side of your face on the floor (*see figure 5-100*).

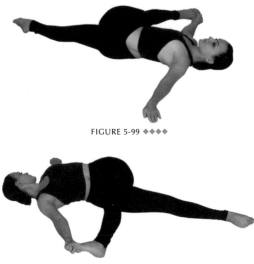

FIGURE 5-99 ◆◆◆◆

FIGURE 5-100 ◆◆◆◆

Stay in this position for six long breaths, maintaining a good twist to your left hip. These two vinyasas are variations of the stomach twist (jataraparivritti). Then, inhaling raise your leg back to asana sthiti. Now exhaling, you may lower your arm and leg to supta asana sthiti.

As you are exhaling, raise both legs to hip level. This is urdhwa-prasarita-pada asana, which we saw earlier (*see figure 5-101*).

During the next inhalation, spread your arms laterally along the floor to the level of your shoulders (*see figure 5-102*).

Now turn your right hand up. Inhale and while you exhale, slowly lower both your legs and land your feet on your open right palm, twisting your hips significantly

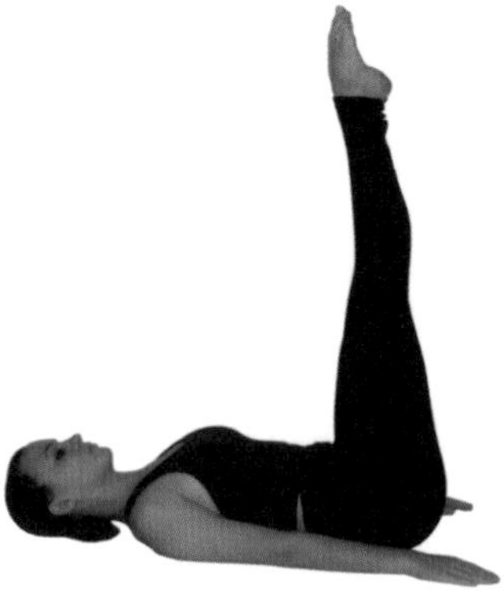

FIGURE 5-101 ◆◆◆

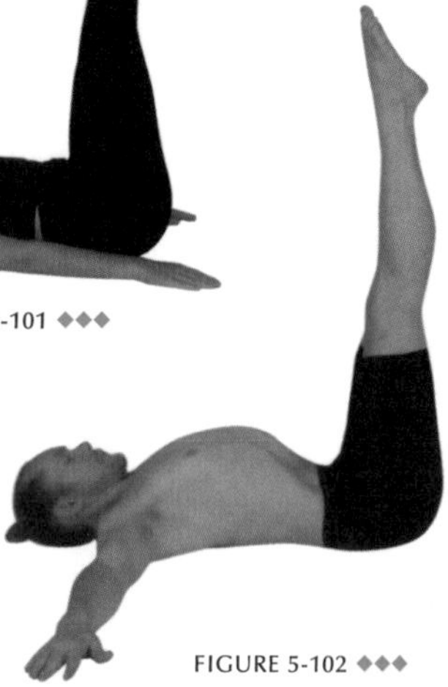

FIGURE 5-102 ◆◆◆

in the process. On the next exhalation, slightly lift your head, turn to your left side, and place the left side of your face on the floor (*see figure 5-103*).

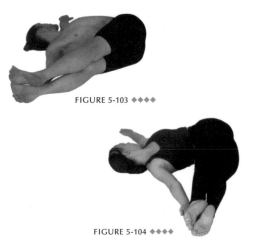

FIGURE 5-103 ◆◆◆◆

FIGURE 5-104 ◆◆◆◆

Stay in this position for three to six breaths. Inhaling, you may turn your right palm down, and pressing both your hands, lift both your legs back to the starting position. You may place your toes or the dorsa of your feet on your palm as another vinyasa (see figure 5-104).

This is another variation of stomach twist (jataraparivritti).

From asana sthiti, now turn your left palm up, and during the next exhalation, pressing down with your arms, slowly raise your legs to the "L" form, and in one motion, twist your hips and lower your legs onto your open left palm (see figure 5-105).

Alternately, you may place your toes or the dorsa of your feet on your palm (see figure 5-106).

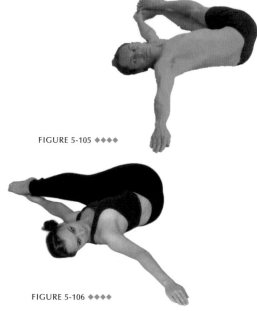

FIGURE 5-105 ◆◆◆◆

FIGURE 5-106 ◆◆◆◆

This is another difficult vinyasa of the stomach twist (jataraparivritti). Stay in this position for three to six breaths. Inhaling, lift your legs up to asana sthiti. On the next inhalation, stretch your legs down and also lower both your arms while you are exhaling. In another version, the twisting to the side just described is done alternately. You lower your legs to the right side on the first exhalation, return to the asana sthiti on the next inhalation, and

then do the same movements on the left side. You can do the vinyasas alternately three to six times. However, if you become short of breath, you may rest between each set of movements.

We have so far seen vinyasas while lying down. In these the first set involved bending your knees while your whole back was on the floor. The second set involved basically arching your spine and lifting your chest up. The third set involved keeping your back on the ground, but moving your leg/legs, especially working on your hip joint. This set is the hip opener for you, while lying down.

The next set of vinyasas will involve lifting not only your legs but also your back. This requires the ability not only to raise your legs but also to raise your waist to reach the famous pose, the shoulder stand, or *sarvangasana* (all-body-parts pose). It is considered one of the important innovations of yoga, and is given the pride of place among the greatest of asanas. Therapeutically, it is one of the most important yoga poses. However, regrettably, it is one of the least popular asanas in the West. Sarvangasana, or the shoulder stand, has a variety of variations and movements.

SHOULDER STAND/ALL–BODY-PARTS POSE (SARVANGASANA)

Even though all the vinyasas we have considered so far under the category of supine poses can be reckoned to be preparatory for the shoulder stand, three of them are considered essential before going in for the shoulder stand pose in the vinyasa method of yoga practice. They are:

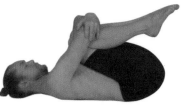

FIGURE 5-107 ◆◆

1. Apanasana, or the pelvic pose *(see figure 5-107)*

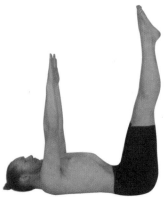

FIGURE 5-108 ◆◆

2. Urdwa-prasarita-pada-hastasana ("U" formation) *(See figure 5-108)*

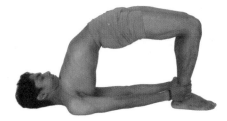

FIGURE 5-109 ◆◆

3. Dwipadapitam, the desk pose *(see figure 5-109)*

How does one get to the shoulder stand pose? You can reach supta asana or supine pose *(see figure 5-110)* by going through the vinyasas explained at the beginning of the chapter.

Then as you are exhaling, pressing down with your arms, the back of your head, and your neck, lift your trunk up and support your back with your hands *(see figure 5-111)*.

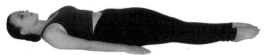

FIGURE 5-110 ◆

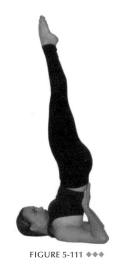

FIGURE 5-111 ◆◆◆

Your palms should be kept together with your fingers pointing up.

Another more involved approach is to proceed from the hub pose, the downward-facing-dog (DFD) pose *(see figure 5-112)*.

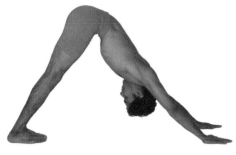

FIGURE 5-112 ◆◆

You may have proceeded to the DFD pose by following the vinyasa krama. Then from the DFD posture, while exhaling,

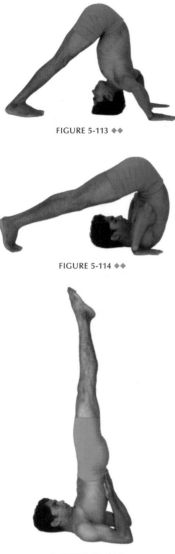

FIGURE 5-113 ◆◆

FIGURE 5-114 ◆◆

FIGURE 5-115 ◆◆◆

Then while you are inhaling, supporting your back with both your hands, raise your trunk up to the shoulder stand (*see figure 5-115*).

There is another variation in the sequence just described. Again start from the downward-facing-dog position with your chin locked (jalandhara bandha). See figure 5-116.

Exhaling, stretch your ankles, thigh muscles, calf muscles, waist, and back. Maintain the chin lock, and tuck your chin against your sternum. Lower your body,

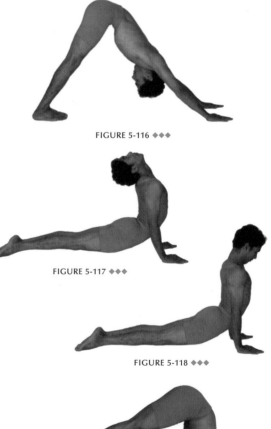

FIGURE 5-116 ◆◆◆

FIGURE 5-117 ◆◆◆

FIGURE 5-118 ◆◆◆

stretch your ankles, and standing on your toes, slowly lower your head and place your crown on the floor (*see figure 5-113*).

Now keep your chin nicely tucked in (locked) and continuing the exhalation, place the back of your head and neck on the floor, as you stretch your ankles, while pressing with your big toes. You are now in plough pose (*see figure 5-114*).

Stay in this position for a few breaths.

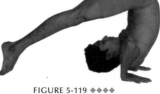

FIGURE 5-119 ◆◆◆◆

arch your spine, and bend back to the upward-facing-dog pose (urdhwa-mukha swanasana). *(See figure 5-117.)*

Stay in this position for a breath, and on the next exhalation do a chin lock (jalandhara bandha). *(See figure 5-118.)*

Stay in this position for a breath. Now exhaling, and maintaining the chin lock, raise your buttocks, lower your upper body, and round your back nicely until the back of your head and the back of your neck are just above the floor *(see figure 5-119)*.

Ease gently into the plough pose. Stay in this position for a few breaths. Stretch your arms, and exhaling, raise your legs and your torso to assume the shoulder stand position *(see figure 5-120)*.

Being an antigravity posture, sarvangasana is a great innovation of the yogis. It affords one the opportunity to do many vinyasas. There are many therapeutic benefits of sarvangasana when done with several vinyasas. *Sarvanga* means "all parts of the body." Traditional yogis believe that it is a staple asana in everyday practice. The first vinyasa you can do is to bend your right knee to touch the right side of your forehead, rounding your back in the process *(see figure 5-121)*.

Keep your left leg straight. It is best to have both your ankles thoroughly stretched. This movement is done as you are exhaling. Inhaling, straighten your right leg. You may repeat the movement three to six times, unhurriedly. If your balance is not good, you should adjust the position of your hands supporting your back at the completion of each movement. If you become short of breath, stay in the shoulder stand for a few breaths and then resume the movements. The name of this vinyasa is *dakshina pada akunchanasana*, or the right-leg contraction pose.

The left-side contraction, vana pada akunchasana, is done similarly, by bending your left leg and rounding your back while you are exhaling. You may repeat the movement three to six times *(see figure 5-122)*.

Now remaining steady in the shoulder stand, you should support your back well. Slowly exhaling, round your back, and bend both your knees and place them on your forehead *(see figure 5-123)*.

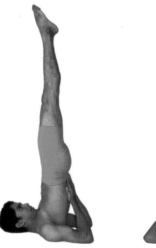

FIGURE 5-120 ◆◆◆

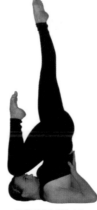

FIGURE 5-121 ◆◆

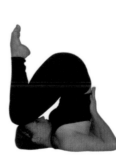

FIGURE 5-122 ◆◆

FIGURE 5-123 ◆◆◆

Here you may stay in this position for three to six breaths. You may also stretch your legs back to a shoulder stand while inhaling, and repeat the movement three to six times. Because the pose is inverted, when you stretch your leg up, you get a very good traction for your spine; the upward movement pulls your spine up, while gravity pulls your spine down. This pose is called *akunchanasana*, or the contraction pose.

This time around, as you exhale, bend your knees, but as you lower your legs, gently twist your torso to the right, so that your knees are on the right side of your head on the floor. Stay in this position for three to six breaths, making the exhalations as complete as possible. This is right-side contraction pose (*dakshina parsva akunchanasana*). (*See figure 5-124.*)

You may also practice the rectal and abdominal locks at the end of each exhalation. Inhaling, return to the shoulder stand position. From the shoulder stand position, do the same vinyasa on the left side (*see figure 5-125*).

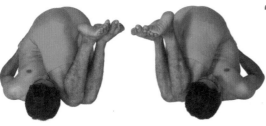

FIGURE 5-124 ◆◆◆   FIGURE 5-125 ◆◆◆

Instead of bending your knees and lowering them, you may lower your right leg all the way down, keeping your knee straight. Your left leg should be straight and up. Exhaling while in the shoulder stand, slowly lower your right leg to the floor (*see figure 5-126*).

While you inhale slowly, raise your leg all the way up. You may repeat this three to six times, but each time before you start the movement, see that your torso is well supported, your legs are straight, and your breathing is not hurried. This pose is called *ekapada sarvangasana*. Some call it *ekapada halasana*. Either way, you may call it the one-legged shoulder stand or one-legged plough pose.

Once again see that your shoulder stand is straight, and your back well supported. Then while you are slowly exhaling with the hissing sound in your throat, indicating that you are doing ujjayi, lower your left leg all the down, over your head (*see figure 5-127*).

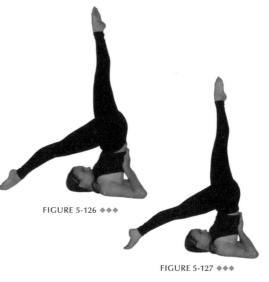

FIGURE 5-126 ◆◆◆

FIGURE 5-127 ◆◆◆

Inhale, and return to the shoulder stand. Repeat the movement three to six times.

The next vinyasa is a little more involved. While in the shoulder stand, as you are exhaling slowly, bend your right knee and place your right foot on your left thigh close to your groin in the half-lotus position. You may use your left hand to position your right foot on your left thigh. Inhale, and on the next exhalation, swing your right hand around your back and clasp the big toe of your right foot with your right hand. Now you have your right leg in the locked half-lotus (ardha baddha padma) position. Inhale, and while very slowly exhaling, lower your stretched left leg to the plough position. During the next inhalation, stretch your left arm and clasp your left big toe (see figure 5-128).

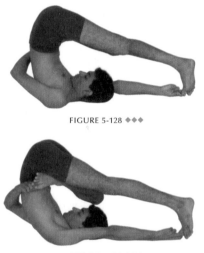

FIGURE 5-128 ♦♦♦

FIGURE 5-129 ♦♦♦

Stay in this position for six long inhalations and exhalations. Inhaling, raise your left leg and trunk, and stretch your right leg to return to the shoulder stand.

Now you may repeat the same pose on the left side (see figure 5-129).

This time, from the shoulder stand position, as you slowly breathe out, lower your legs over your head, all the way to the floor. You may now stretch your arms on the floor. This is halasana, or the plough pose (see figure 5-130).

Stay in this position for six to twelve breaths. The inhalations will be short, but you may concentrate on your exhalation, making it long and smooth.

In the next move, staying in the plough pose, as you slowly inhale, sweep your arms all along the floor, and clasp your big toes. Stay in this position for three breaths. Alternately, you can sweep your arms down on exhalation and bring them up on inhalation; repeat this pair of movements three to six times with the appropriate breathing, as already explained (see figure 5-131).

In this vinyasa, as you keep holding your toes and inhaling, rock back a little. Now as you slowly exhale, raise your head so that you are able to touch your knees with your forehead (see figure 5-132).

Inhaling, lower your head and as you exhale, raise your head to touch your knees. Here the weight, which was in the region of your neck, is shifted to your back so that you are able to raise your head.

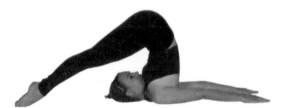

FIGURE 5-130 ♦♦♦

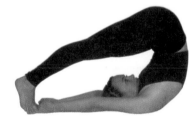

FIGURE 5-131 ♦♦♦

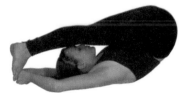

FIGURE 5-132 ♦♦♦

Repeat the movement three to six times. This pose is *urdhwa-mukha paschimatanasana*, or the upward-facing posterior stretch pose. It is a mirror image of the classical paschimatanasana, the seated forward stretch pose, but so much more difficult and different from paschimatanasana.

A more involved variation of this upward facing paschimatanasana requires holding the sides of your feet. In this case, your back is stretched more. Exhaling, raise your head to touch your knees (*see figure 5-133*) and inhaling lower your head.

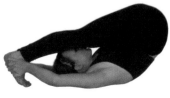

FIGURE 5-133 ◆◆◆

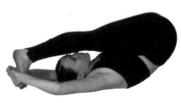

FIGURE 5-134 ◆◆◆

Repeat the movement three to six times. This time, bend your knees slightly while you are exhaling. Then, interlock your fingers and turn your palms outward. As you inhale, stretch your hands beyond your feet. During the next inhalation, straighten your knees, pushing with your hands in the process. Stay in this position for three breaths. During every exhalation try to raise your head and place your forehead on your knees. This is another variation of urdhwa-mukha paschimatanasana (*see figure 5-134*).

Return to the shoulder stand as you slowly inhale. Firmly supporting your back, spread your legs (*see figure 5-135*).

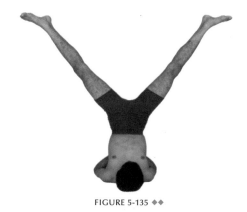

FIGURE 5-135 ◆◆

Without allowing your legs to lean forward, stay in this position for three long inhalations and exhalations. Alternately, you may close your legs on exhalation and spread your legs on inhalation. This pose is the upward triangle pose (*urdhwa konasana*).

Remaining in the previous urdhwa konasana vinyasa, as you slowly exhale bend both your knees, and keep your feet joined (*see figure 5-136*).

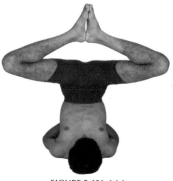

FIGURE 5-136 ◆◆◆

Again, you may stay in this position for three to six breaths. This is *urdhwa baddha konasana*, upward locked-angle pose.

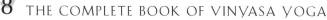

Inhaling, you may return to urdhwa konasana.

From the urdhwa konasana position, while exhaling slowly, lower your legs over your head, all the way down to the floor. Stay in this position for three breaths. During the next inhalation, sweep your arms in a circular motion along the floor, and clasp the big toes of both your feet with both your hands (*see figure 5-137*).

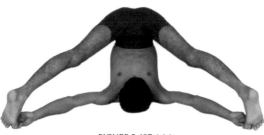

FIGURE 5-137 ◆◆◆

Stay in this position for six long inhalations and exhalations. These three vinyasas help to open your hips nicely. Because of the antigravity effect and because the movements are done without constraint, these vinyasas are very good for relaxing and stretching your hip joints. Inhaling, return to urdhwa konasana position.

From the shoulder stand position with your legs spread, bend your right knee and place your right foot on your left thigh close to your groin. You may use your left hand to pull your foot into position, supporting it with your right hand. Then inhale, and while you are exhaling again, bend your left leg and place your left foot on your right thigh close to your groin. Now you have your legs locked in the lotus pose position (*see figure 5-138*).

Stay in this position for six to twelve long inhalations and exhalations. This pose is

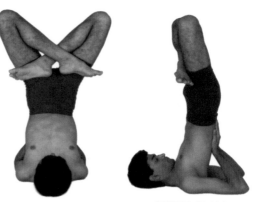

FIGURE 5-138 ◆◆◆   FIGURE 5-139 ◆◆◆

urdhwa padmasana, or the upward lotus pose. The side view is shown in figure 5-139.

From the upright lotus pose, while you are exhaling, slowly bend your waist and lower your legs locked in the lotus position. Try to keep your legs as close to your chest as possible. Stay in this position for six breaths, concentrating on very smooth, long exhalations (*see figure 5-140*).

This is called *akunchita urdhwa padmasana* (drooping lotus pose).

Remaining in this pose, balance on the back of your neck and head. Exhaling fully, swing your arms around your legs, embrace your lower extremities with your hands, and clasp your hands (*see figure 5-141*).

Stay in this position for six to twelve breaths, again concentrating on your exhalation. After every exhalation, you can do all the

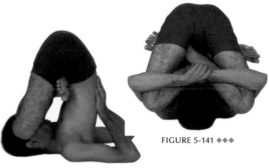

FIGURE 5-141 ◆◆◆

FIGURE 5-140 ◆◆◆

three bandhas for which this pose is ideally suited. Your heels press against your pelvic region and invigorate your pelvic organs. All the elements necessary to work on the pelvic region is available in this pose: gravity to move the organs up within the body, full exhalation to facilitate the movement of the pelvic organs, the position of the feet to apply positive gentle pressure on these organs, and the ability to use the very effective mula and uddiyana bandhas. This pose is called *pindasana*, or the fetus pose. Many people who practice this, when they are able to do it correctly mention that they feel a certain secure feeling while in this posture breathing very smoothly. The side view is shown in figure 5-142.

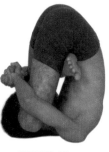

FIGURE 5-142 ◆◆◆

Inhaling move your hands back and support your back. During the next inhalation, bring your legs up to urdhwa padmasana, keeping your legs still in the lotus position. During the following exhalation, twist your torso to the right and stay in this position for three breaths (*see figure 5-143*).

The next move will involve your twisting further to the right, but lowering your right knee so that it is close to your right ear (*see figure 5-144*).

Stay in this position for three breaths. As you are inhaling, return to urdhwa padmasana.

This process is then repeated on the left side. Exhaling, slowly twist your waist to the left (*see figure 5-145*).

Stay in this position for three breaths.

From the same position, while exhaling twist further left as you lower your left leg so that your left knee touches your left ear (*see figure 5-146*).

Stay in this position for three breaths, and then while inhaling return to upright lotus position.

As a counterpose for the forward bend you have done in the lotus position, you can bend your waist back in the sarvangasana-padmasana position. This movement should be done while you are inhaling. Stay in this position for three breaths, and return to the starting position (*see figure 5-147*).

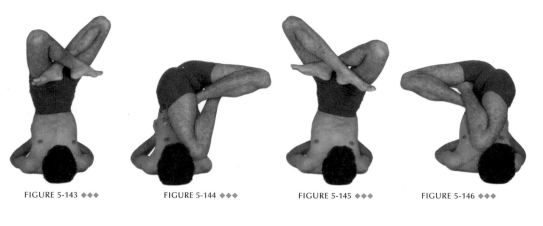

FIGURE 5-143 ◆◆◆   FIGURE 5-144 ◆◆◆   FIGURE 5-145 ◆◆◆   FIGURE 5-146 ◆◆◆

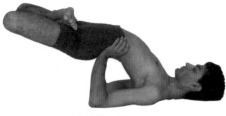

FIGURE 5-147 ◆◆◆

Inhaling, stretch your legs to return to the shoulder stand. You may now attempt another variation of shoulder stand. In this one the hand support is dispensed with. As you are inhaling, stretch your trunk further up, and lean over a little, almost to the point of overbalancing. Balancing well on the following inhalation, stretch your arms up and place them along your thighs (see figure 5-148).

Stay in this position for six to twelve breaths, trying to stretch your back a little more and straighten it. By carefully maintaining your balance and stretching your spine, you will be able to close the gap between your body and your upstretched arms (see figure 5-149).

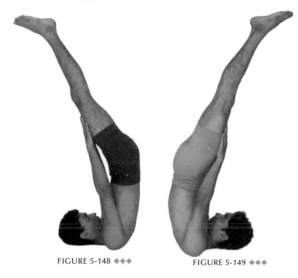

FIGURE 5-148 ◆◆◆   FIGURE 5-149 ◆◆◆

This is a vinyasa of the unsupported shoulder stand (niralamba sarvangasana).

Remaining in this position, slowly inhale and lower your upstretched right arm to the floor. Stay in this position for a breath and during the following exhalation, slowly lower you right leg to land your right big toe on your right palm. Hold your right big toe with your fingers; stay in this position for three breaths, concentrating on your exhalation and also stretching your back (see figure 5-150).

During the next inhalation, raise your right leg back to sarvangasana. Exhaling, raise your right arm to return to the starting position. In a similar way, you can do the movements on the left side (see figure 5-151).

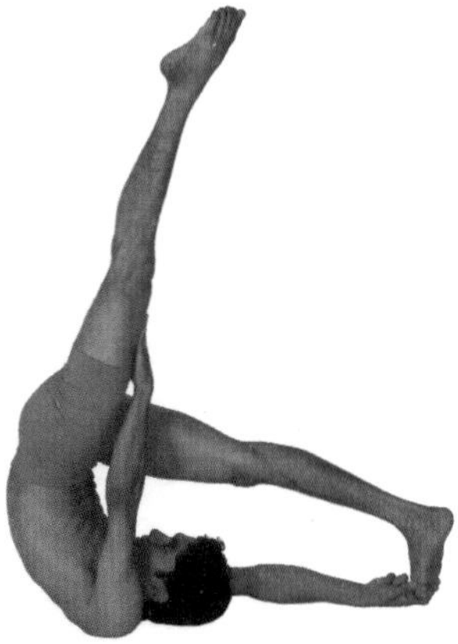

FIGURE 5-150 ◆◆◆

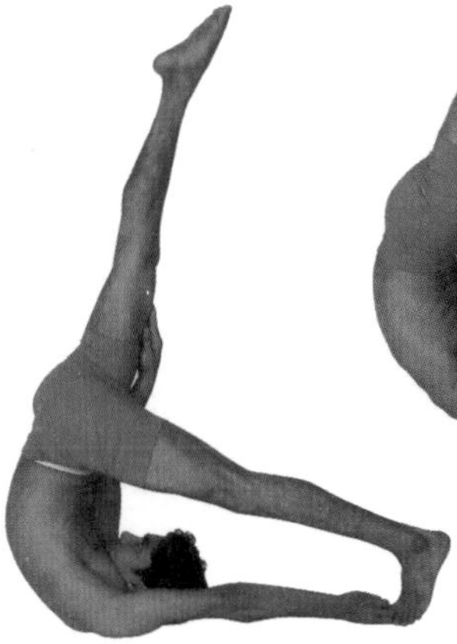

FIGURE 5-151 ◆◆◆

From the previous position, while inhaling, lower your arms over your head. Stay balanced for three long inhalations and exhalations (see figure 5-152).

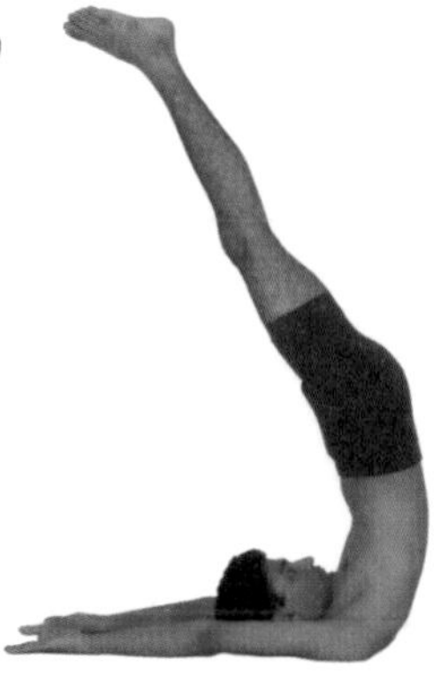

FIGURE 5-152 ◆◆◆

This is another variation of the shoulder stand without support.

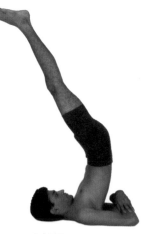

FIGURE 5-153 ◆◆◆

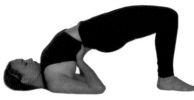

FIGURE 5-155 ◆◆◆

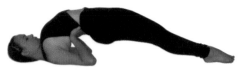

FIGURE 5-156 ◆◆◆

From this position, while balancing on the back of your neck, inhale and bring your arms behind your neck and clasp your elbows (see figure 5-153).

Again, stay in this position for three long inhalations and exhalations. Then exhaling, support your back with your hands and straighten your legs, returning to the shoulder stand.

So far we have seen a number of vinyasas in the shoulder stand position and the plough pose. In all these, your back is either straight or rounded. The following vinyasas help to arch your back and open up or lift your chest. First, we start from plough pose, which is done by lowering your legs from shoulder stand (see figure 5-154).

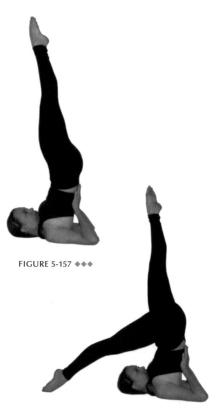

FIGURE 5-157 ◆◆◆

FIGURE 5-158 ◆◆◆

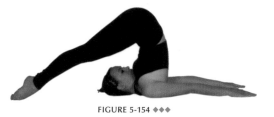

FIGURE 5-154 ◆◆◆

From the plough, supporting your back with both your hands, bend your knees

and lift your legs to akunanasana. Stay in this position for a breath, and during the next inhalation, supporting your back with your hands arch your spine and gently land your feet behind your elbows, with your knees still bent *(see figure 5-155)*.

Wait for a breath and during the next inhalation, stretch your legs, straightening your knees and keeping your feet firmly planted on the floor *(see figure 5-156)*.

This pose is called *uttana-mayurasana*, or the stretched peacock pose. Stay in this position for six breaths, then return to the shoulder stand, first going through the intermediate stage *(see figure 5-157)*.

Again while in the shoulder stand, exhaling slowly, lower your right leg all the way to the floor for a one-legged plough pose *(see figure 5-158)*.

Then inhale and hold your breath. Next, bend your left knee, and arching your spine lower your left leg, landing softly on your left foot. Your right leg should follow the movement and become vertical. Stay in this position for three breaths *(see figure 5-159)*.

Then as you are inhaling, stretch your left leg, straightening your left knee. Stay in this position for three breaths. This is *dakshina-pada uttanamayurasana* (right-side peacock stretch pose). *(See figure 5-160.)*

Exhaling, bend your left knee and pull your left leg toward you until it is in position *(see figure 5-161)*.

Exhaling, hold your breath, and pressing down through your elbows, round your back, lift your left leg, and return to ekapada halasana. While you inhale again, lift your right leg up to return to the shoulder stand.

The same procedure can be followed using your left leg. Figure 5-162 shows the one-legged plough pose, which is done while exhaling.

Figure 5-163 shows the intermediate stage, and figure 5-164 shows the final position of the vinyasa.

Then return to shoulder stand position.

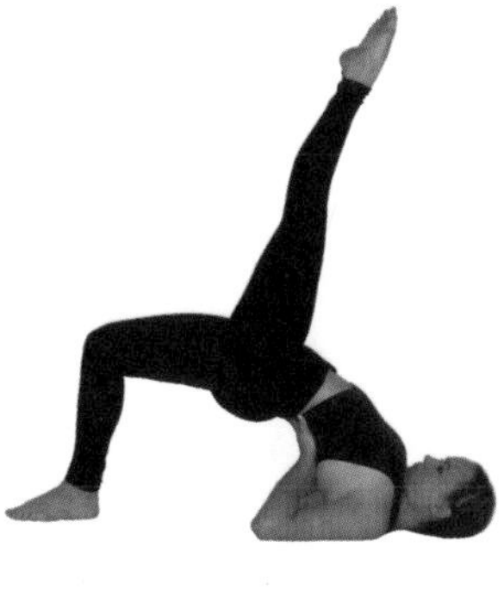

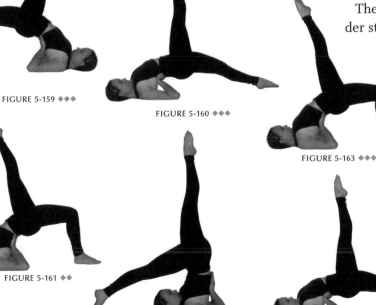

FIGURE 5-159 ◆◆◆

FIGURE 5-160 ◆◆◆

FIGURE 5-161 ◆◆

FIGURE 5-162 ◆◆◆

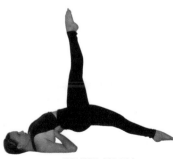

FIGURE 5-163 ◆◆◆

FIGURE 5-164 ◆◆◆

CIRCULAR AMBULATION IN THE PLOUGH POSE (SARVANGASANA-MANDALA)

The next sequence is known as *mandala*, or circular ambulation. From the plough pose *(see figure 5-165)*, while supporting your back, slowly move your legs to your right to about 45 degrees, while you are exhaling *(see figure 5-166)*.

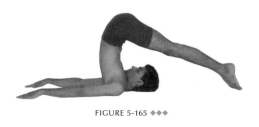

FIGURE 5-165 ◆◆◆

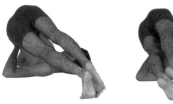

FIGURE 5-166 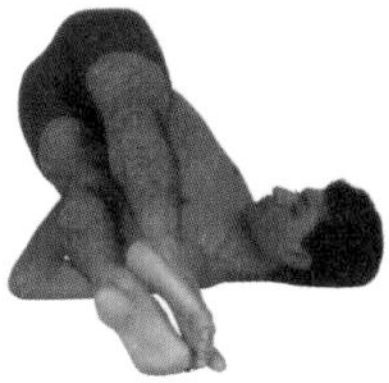 ◆◆◆   FIGURE 5-167 ◆◆◆◆

Stay in this position for an inhalation, and during the next exhalation, move your legs further in an arc, so that they are positioned at almost 90 degrees to your body *(see figure 5-167)*.

Again, stay in this position for an inhalation, and after exhalation, hold your breath, and supporting your back well, flip your waist and land on your feet, and then stretch your ankles *(see figure 5-168)*.

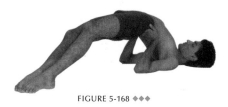

FIGURE 5-168 ◆◆◆

During the following exhalation continue with the movement until your legs are in line with your torso, to the uttana-mayurasana position (the stretched peacock pose). *(See figure 5-169.)*

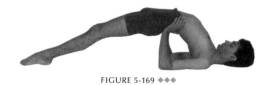

FIGURE 5-169 ◆◆◆

You may continue with the movement to the right side, step by step, until your legs are about 30 degrees to 60 degrees to your right *(see figure 5-170)*.

Then inhale and during the next exhalation, move your legs further toward the right side so that they are at about 60 degrees to your body, and stay in this position for a breath *(see figure 5-171)*.

Then during the next exhalation walk a little further to your right, flip your legs when you are halfway through the movement, and land on your toes *(see figure 5-172)*.

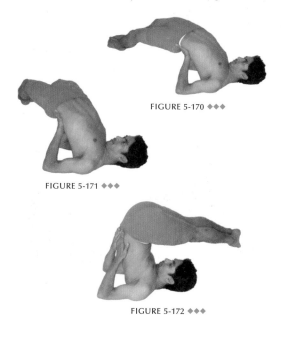

FIGURE 5-170 ◆◆◆

FIGURE 5-171 ◆◆◆

FIGURE 5-172 ◆◆◆

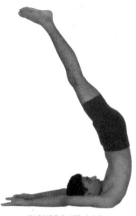

FIGURE 5-173 ◆◆◆

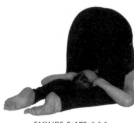

FIGURE 5-175 ◆◆◆

Stay in this position for a breath, and then while exhaling move further to finally reach the plough position from which you started *(see figure 5-173)*.

This completes the mandala, or circular ambulation in the plough pose. If you have the will, you may want to do the movement in the counterclockwise direction as well.

From the plough position, as you slowly exhale, draw up your knees and keep them beside your ears. Inhale, and during exhalation, bring your hands over your legs and cup your ears with your palms *(see figure 5-174)*.

This is known as the closed-ear pose (*karnapidasana*). Stay in this position for twelve long inhalations and exhalations. Then while you are inhaling, stretch your legs and swing your arms back to support your back.

From halasana you may now return to supta asana sthiti and rest. While in the plough pose, stretch your arms, interlock your fingers, and stretch your arms overhead. Your hands are kept beyond and outside your feet on the floor *(see figure 5-176)*.

Inhaling, straighten your arms around your legs and interlock your fingers *(see figure 5-177)*.

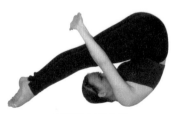

FIGURE 5-176 ◆◆◆

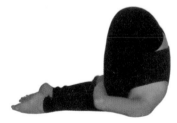

FIGURE 5-174 ◆◆◆

Another view is shown in figure 5-175.

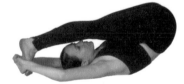

FIGURE 5-177 ◆◆◆

Then as you are inhaling, slowly, step by step, stretching each vertebra, deliberately roll back to supta asana without touching

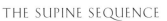

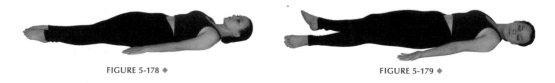

FIGURE 5-178 ◆   FIGURE 5-179 ◆

your hands. Then lower your arms as you exhale *(see figure 5-178).*

Then keep all your joints loose, turn your head to one side, and with your eyes closed watch your breath in the corpse pose for five minutes *(see figure 5-179).*

You should not go to sleep nor allow your mind to wander. When your mind starts chattering, and you recognize that fact, you should coax your mind back to your breath.

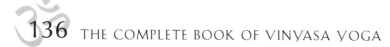

6

THE
BOW POSE
SEQUENCE

I N THE PREVIOUS chapter, we discussed several postures and vinyasas done while lying on your back. One of the important poses was the shoulder stand, which has a number of vinyasas. In this chapter, the whole sequence is done while lying prone, that is, on your stomach. Some of the simpler variations in this group can be utilized as counterposes for several poses discussed in the previous chapter.

Dhanurasana, or the bow pose, is the main posture in this sequence of movements. The vinyasa progression leading up to the hub pose follows.

LEAD SEQUENCE

Samasthiti—watch your balance, watch your breath, and do three long inhalations and exhalations (ujjayi). *(See figure 6-1.)*

Inhaling, raise your arms overhead in tadasana. Stay in this position for three breaths *(see figure 6-2)*.

Exhaling slowly, perform uttanasana, or the forward bend. Stay in this position for three breaths *(see figure 6-3)*.

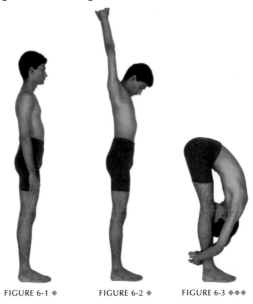

FIGURE 6-1 ◆   FIGURE 6-2 ◆   FIGURE 6-3 ◆◆◆

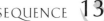

Exhaling, move to utkatasana, the hip stretch. Again, stay in this position for three breaths (*see figure 6-4*).

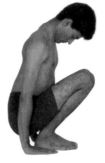

FIGURE 6-4 ◆◆◆

Inhaling, hold your breath and jump back to chaturanga-dandasana (*see figure 6-5*).

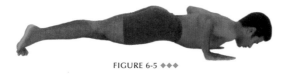

FIGURE 6-5 ◆◆◆

Stay in this position for three breaths.

Lie face down in asana sthiti. Stay in this position for three breaths.

CROCODILE POSE (Makarasana)

Exhaling, bend your elbows and place your forearms on the floor beside your chest. Then, while inhaling slowly raise your head and neck to the greatest extent possible without raising your elbows off the floor (*see figure 6-6*).

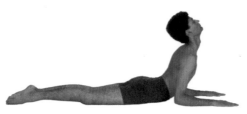

FIGURE 6-6 ◆◆

While exhaling, return to the lying-down position. Repeat this movement three to six times. This is the crocodile pose (*makarasana*).

In this group there are several poses involving back bending. These back-bending movements are generally to be done while inhaling, as you could see in the makarasana vinyasas just explained. In the introduction I discussed viloma breathing (*viloma* means "against the grain"), which should be used for back bends in certain circumstances. In some of these back bends, it may be easier and more desirable to use a smooth exhalation rather than an inhalation. People who are obese, old and therefore less supple, anxious and tense, or have some medical conditions, such as hypertension, would do well to adopt exhalation, or langhana kriya, during these back bends. Because these are belly-down positions, persons belonging to this group will be more comfortable and will achieve better results in langhana kriya.

The procedure in langhana kriya is as follows:

While in the lying-face-down (prone) position, take a short breath. As you exhale, slowly raise your head, neck, and torso to the greatest extent possible, without raising your elbows off the floor. This is makarasana performed in langhana kriya. Take a short inhalation in the position, and while exhaling lower your trunk.

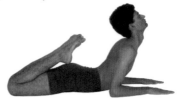

FIGURE 6-7 ◆◆

Again, as you are inhaling, raise your chest, keeping your forearms on the floor. While you are exhaling, bend both your knees to the extent you can, to draw your legs toward your thighs. It is good if you are able to touch your buttocks with your heels (*see figure 6-7*).

Inhaling, you can stretch your legs, and exhaling, lower your chest. You may repeat the movement three to six times. Return to the face-down position as you exhale. You may do the movements in langhana kriya, if need be.

FROG POSE (Manduka Asana)

Keep your legs bent as in the previous vinyasa. Exhaling, hold the dorsa of your feet (*see figure 6-8*) or the big toes of your feet with your hands.

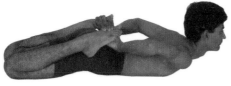

FIGURE 6-8 ◆◆

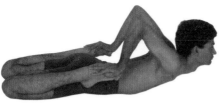

FIGURE 6-9 ◆◆

Inhale, and on the next exhalation, raise your chest while pressing your bent legs as far down as possible (*see figure 6-9*).

Stay in this posture for three to six breaths, pressing your feet down on every exhalation. This pose is called *manduka*

asana, or the frog pose. Return to asana sthiti while exhaling. Raising your trunk can be done in langhana kriya also.

COBRA POSE (Bhujangasana)

Place your palms on the floor very close to your chest. Slowly inhaling and pressing down through your palms, raise and arch your spine, keeping your pelvis on the floor. You may keep your elbows bent to avoid raising your pelvis from the floor (*see figure 6-10*).

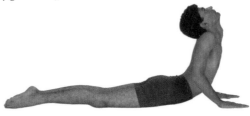

FIGURE 6-10 ◆◆◆

While exhaling, return to the starting pose. Please do the movements three to six times. This is *bhujangasana*, or the cobra pose. This can be done in langhana kriya also.

Repeat the same pose, but stretching your elbows, provided that you are able to arch your spine further (*see figure 6-11*).

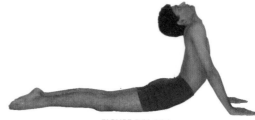

FIGURE 6-11 ◆◆◆

Repeat the movement three times, and return to the starting position while doing a long, smooth exhalation. You may, if required, use langhana breathing.

Arch your back; as you are slowly exhaling, bend your knees as well, like a cobra raising its hood, and also your tail (*see figure 6-12*).

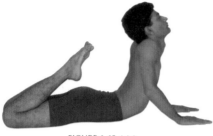

FIGURE 6-12 ◆◆◆

There will be a significant amount of pressure applied to the sacral region. Repeat the movement three times, observing the appropriate breathing.

Again inhaling, arch your back, but this time you may lift your pelvis off the floor. On exhalation, bend your knees. Anchoring your knees and pressing down through your palms, arch back to place your head on the soles of your feet (*see figure 6-13*).

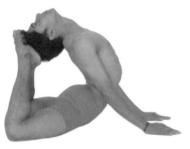

FIGURE 6-13 ◆◆◆◆

You may try the movement with langhana breathing if necessary. Keep your thighs together and do not allow your knees to spread out. This is a variation of the *rajakapotasana*, or king pigeon pose. Stay in this position for three to six breaths. Exhaling, lie down on your chest, and inhaling, stretch your legs.

Now you may do another variation to the cobra pose. Exhaling, place your palms together on your back, at the bottom of your spine. As you are slowly inhaling, open your chest, raise your torso, and arch your spine, sliding your palms further back along your spine. Your shoulder blades will touch each other (you may use langhana breathing, if warranted). Stay in this position for three long breaths (*see figure 6-14*).

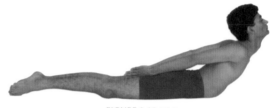

FIGURE 6-14 ◆◆◆

This is again the cobra pose. According to purists, this is the actual bhujangasana, because the use of hands is dispensed with, and the cobra has no hands. The Sanskrit name *bhujanga* means that it has only the body as its hand.

The next variation in the bhujangasana vinyasa krama will be to open the chest further. Exhaling, lower your arms, and join your palms at the bottom of your spine. Then turn your palms so that your fingers are pointing inward, and slide them along your spine until the anjali, or cupped palms, are close to your shoulder blades. As you inhale, slowly expand your chest and arch your spine (*see figure 6-15*).

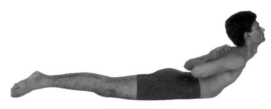

FIGURE 6-15 ◆◆◆

Certain people may find it easier to do the same movement with langhana kriya. This is very good for the entire thorax. You may move with the appropriate breath or stay in this position for three to six long inhalations and exhalations. Remember to breathe in well and expand your chest.

THE LOCUST POSE SEQUENCE

The next set of vinyasas belongs to the *salabasana* (locust) group. From the face-down lying-down position, first close your left fist. Then, inhaling, raise your right arm overhead, sweeping it along the floor. As you are slowly inhaling, raise your right arm, your head, both your shoulders, your chest, and your right leg. You should not tilt your body to the left side *(see figure 6-16)*.

(You may adopt langhana kriya breathing, if need be.) Exhaling, you may slowly lower your body to the floor. Repeat the movement three to six times. This is *dakshina-ardha-salabhasana*, the right half-locust pose.

This time as you are inhaling, slowly raise your right arm, head, shoulders, and chest. Instead of your right leg, lift your left leg, stretching it right across your body *(see figure 6-17)*.

(Langhana kriya may be used.) Exhale, and lower your trunk to the floor. Repeat the movement three to six times. This is *dakshina ardha parivritta salabhasana*, the right half-twist locust pose.

Now as you are exhaling, lower your right arm and close your right fist. During the next inhalation, slowly sweep your left arm overhead. Stay in this position for a breath. Now, while inhaling, raise your left arm, head, shoulders, and arched chest,

along with your left leg, including your thigh *(see figure 6-18)*.

(If necessary, you may use langhana kriya.) Exhaling, you may lower your trunk. You may repeat this movement three to six times. This is *vama ardha parivritta salabhasana* the left half-locust pose.

This time as you are inhaling, raise your left arm, head, shoulders, and chest, along with your right leg, stretching it from the hip *(see figure 6-19)*.

(Langhana kriya may be used.) Exhale, and return to the starting point. You may repeat the movement three to six times with the appropriate breathing. This is *vama ardha parivritta salabhasana* (left half-twist locust pose).

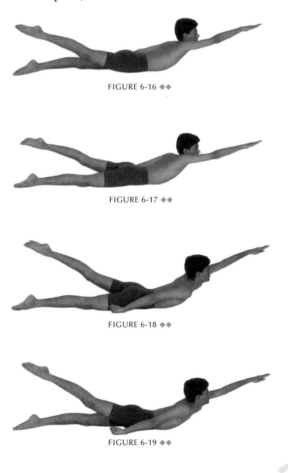

FIGURE 6-16 ◆◆

FIGURE 6-17 ◆◆

FIGURE 6-18 ◆◆

FIGURE 6-19 ◆◆

From the prone position, while inhaling stretch both arms overhead and keep both your palms together in the anjali gesture. As you slowly inhale, raise your arms, shoulders, chest, and both your feet *(see figure 6-20)*.

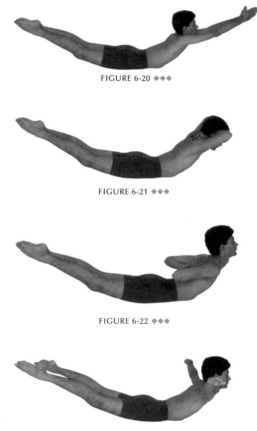

FIGURE 6-20 ◆◆◆

FIGURE 6-21 ◆◆◆

FIGURE 6-22 ◆◆◆

FIGURE 6-23 ◆◆◆

(This can be done with langhana kriya also). Try to balance on your pelvis. Exhale, and lower your trunk. You may repeat the movement three to six times. As mentioned, this is salabhasana, or the locust pose.

Keep your fingers interlocked, and as you breathe in, place your palms on the back of your neck. Slowly inhaling, raise your head and chest and push your elbows out by pressing your palms against the back of your neck. (If you are obese or tense please do the movement on exhalation). Your legs (kept together) should also be raised simultaneously *(see figure 6-21)*.

Exhaling, you may lower your trunk. Repeat the movement three to six times. Then exhaling, return to the lying-down position.

In the next variation of salabhasana, you keep your palms in anjali and slide them along your spine to a point very near your shoulder blades. Again, inhaling, lift your head and chest, and push your shoulders out. You should also raise your legs from the hips, keeping your thighs and ankles together *(see figure 6-22)*.

(Some people may prefer langhana kriya breathing here.) Exhaling, lower your trunk. Repeat the movement three to six times.

This time, inhale, and spread your arms laterally up to shoulder level. Inhaling, slowly raise your head, arms, chest, and legs, which you spread as you complete the movement *(see figure 6-23)*.

(If you find it difficult to do the movement on inhalation because of tightness of the muscles, you may resort to langhana breathing.) Exhaling, close your legs and lower your legs and your chest. Repeat the movement three to six times. Then exhale, and return to the face-down prone position. This is called *vimanasana*, or the aircraft pose.

Let us look at another variant of the locust pose. From the prone position, inhale, hold your breath, and lift your lower extremities and your pelvis off the floor by tightening your abdominal muscles. (Try the movement on exhalation if your body is tight.) *(See figure 6-24.)*

Stay in this position for five seconds, and exhaling, slowly lower your legs to the starting position.

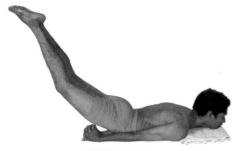

FIGURE 6-24 ♦♦♦

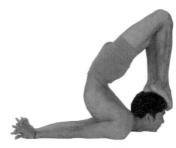

FIGURE 6-26 ♦♦♦♦♦

This time as you inhale, bend your knees slightly and raise your lower extremities and your pelvis, but swing your legs in the opposite direction, arching your spine in the process (see figure 6-25).

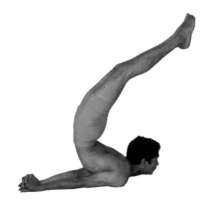

FIGURE 6-25 ♦♦♦

(Some will find it easier to do the movement on exhalation.) This posture is the bent-back locust pose (viparita salabhasana). Stay in this position for a few breaths, and on the next exhalation, slowly lower your legs to the starting position

Now, lower both your arms and close both your fists or interlock your fingers. Take a short breath, and holding your breath, lift your body up, arching your back. Stay in this position for a breath. Then slowly inhaling, lower your legs and place them on your head (see figure 6-26).

(Some experts like to do this with langhana breathing, because it helps them

relax and stretch better.) Stay in this position for six breaths. Exhaling, you can return to your supine position. This is known as Bherundasana (named after the yogi Bherunda). This is also considered a vinyasa or variation of locust pose.

THE BOW POSE SEQUENCE (DHANURASANA)

Please note that all the vinyasas in this sequence can also be done with langhana breathing if, and only if, you are tense, old, obese, or have somewhat elevated blood pressure.

We will now go into the bow posture sequence. First, inhaling, stretch your left arm overhead, moving your hand laterally. During the next exhalation, bend your right knee and catch your right ankle with your right hand. Stay in this position for a breath and get a feel for the position. Inhaling, slowly pull your leg up as you raise your left arm, chest, and head (see figure 6-27).

Exhaling, lower your trunk and your right leg. Repeat the movement three to six times. Then breathe out, lower your trunk, and stay still holding your right ankle with your right hand.

In the next vinyasa, exhaling, lower

your left hand and hold your right ankle with both your hands. Inhaling, raise your head and chest, and also pull your right leg up with both hands (see figure 6-28).

Exhaling, lower your trunk. Repeat the movement three to six times.

From the previous vinyasa, while holding your right leg with your left hand, inhale and sweep your right arm overhead. On the next inhalation, slowly raise your head and chest, and pull your right leg with your left hand, stretching it right across your body (see figure 6-29).

Repeat the movement three to six times. Then lower your trunk as you exhale.

Now catch your left leg (ankle) with your left hand. Inhaling, sweep your right arm overhead along the floor. Exhale, and then while inhaling, raise your head, and

chest, and pull your left leg up with your left hand (see figure 6-30).

Repeat the movement three to six times.

Exhaling, lower your right hand and hold your left ankle with both your hands. As you are inhaling, raise your head and chest, and pull your left leg up with both hands (see figure 6-31).

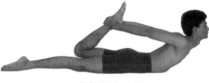

FIGURE 6-31 ◆◆

Repeat the movement three to six times.

Now hold your left leg with your right hand and keep your left hand stretched overhead. Then, as you inhale, raise your head and chest, and pull your left leg with your right hand, in the process stretching your back right across your body (see figure 6-32).

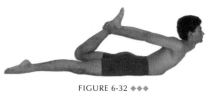

FIGURE 6-32 ◆◆◆

Repeat the movement three to six times.

For the bow pose, or dhanurasana, itself, while exhaling bend both your knees and catch your ankles with the respective hands. Then while inhaling raise your head and chest, and pull both your legs up with your hands (see figure 6-33).

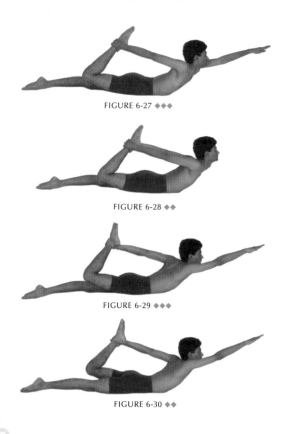

FIGURE 6-27 ◆◆◆

FIGURE 6-28 ◆◆

FIGURE 6-29 ◆◆◆

FIGURE 6-30 ◆◆

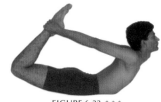

FIGURE 6-33 ◆◆◆

You may repeat the movement three to six times. This is the classical dhanurasana, or bow pose.

As an additional vinyasa, while exhaling bend both your knees; catch your left ankle with your right hand and your right ankle with your left hand. While you are inhaling, raise your head and chest, and pull your legs up with both hands (*see figure 6-34*).

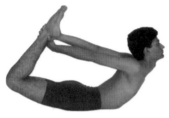

FIGURE 6-34 ◆◆◆

You may repeat the movement six times.

Again, hold your ankles with the respective hands; inhaling, arch your body into the bow pose. Now, exhaling, roll over to the right side (*see figure 6-35*).

Then inhaling, roll back to the bow pose. Once again as you breathe out, roll over to the left side (*see figure 6-36*).

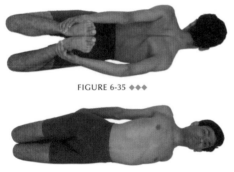

FIGURE 6-35 ◆◆◆

FIGURE 6-36 ◆◆◆

Then return to asana sthiti as you breathe in. Now inhaling, stretch both your legs. You are back to the prone position, the starting point of this vinyasa krama.

You may rest for a while and return to samasthiti.

THE RETURN SEQUENCE

You are now in the prone position. Exhale, and place your palms close to your chest. Exhale, hold your breath, and pressing down through your palms and anchoring your big toes, lift your body to chaturanga-dandasana (*see figure 6-37*).

Stay in this position for three breaths.

On the next exhalation, press down with your palms and your big toes, and bend back, lifting your torso up to the upward-facing-dog position (*see figure 6-38*).

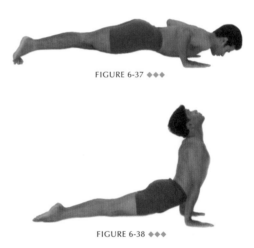

FIGURE 6-37 ◆◆◆

FIGURE 6-38 ◆◆◆

Stay in this position for three breaths.

Exhaling, lower your torso and raise your waist; now flex the dorsa of your feet to get to the downward-facing-dog pose (*see figure 6-39*).

Stay in this position for three breaths.

Exhale, hold your breath, and jump forward to land gently between your palms. This is utkatasana (*see figure 6-40*).

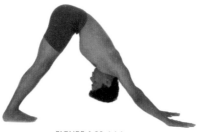

FIGURE 6-39 ◆◆◆

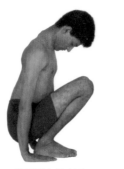

FIGURE 6-40 ◆◆◆

The back-bending movements in this "lying-prone" sequence can be strenuous. You may want to practice a few vinyasas each day and slowly master all the exercises in the sequence. Though the default breathing in all the back-bending movements in this sequence is inhalation, because of the pressure this places on the abdomen, some find it easier to use the langhana mode of breathing. Each method of breathing confers different benefits.

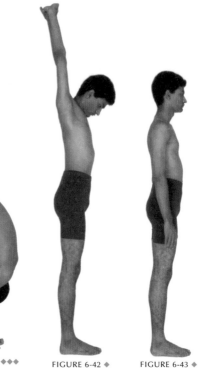

FIGURE 6-41 ◆◆◆   FIGURE 6-42 ◆   FIGURE 6-43 ◆

Stay in this position for three breaths.

Inhaling, straighten your knees, and lift your buttocks up while keeping your palms on the floor. This is uttanasana *(See figure 6-41).*

Stay in this position for three breaths.

Inhaling, raise your body, keeping your arms overhead. This is tadasana *(see figure 6-42).*

Exhale, and lower your arms to samasthiti *(see figure 6-43).*

THE
TRIANGLE POSE
SEQUENCE

ONE OF THE more popular asanas among younger practitioners is *trikonasana*, or the triangle pose. In this sequence, a number of vinyasas centered on and progressing from the triangle position will be described.

SIMPLE STRETCHING IN TRIANGLE POSE (UTTITA TRIKONASANA)

Start from samasthiti *(see figure 7-1)*.

Stay in this position for a minute, watching your balance and your breath. Do six long ujjayi inhalations and exhalations, keeping your chin down *(see figure 7-2)*.

Inhaling, raise your arms laterally to shoulder level. Then exhale, and holding your breath, gently jump and spread your legs about three feet apart, landing gently on the floor *(see figure 7-3)*.

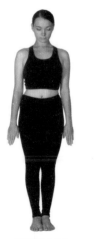

FIGURE 7-1 ◆

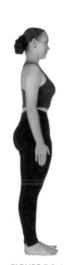

FIGURE 7-2 ◆

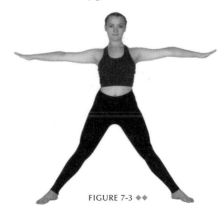

FIGURE 7-3 ◆◆

Your feet should be turned slightly outward to allow for the slight turn of your hip joints from the spreading of your legs. Stay in this position for three long inhalations and exhalations. This is the *trikonasana sthiti* (position of triangle pose).

Inhale, and as you are breathing out, slowly bend to your right, and place your right palm beside your right foot and look up *(see figure 7-4)*.

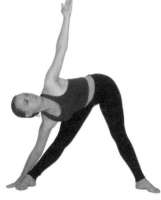

FIGURE 7-4 ◆◆◆

Inhaling, return to trikonasana sthiti. Repeat the movement three times. Then stay in the posture for three breaths. And then, return to the trikonasana position on inhalation.

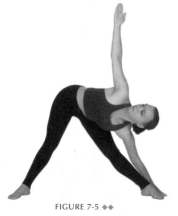

FIGURE 7-5 ◆◆

From the asana sthiti, while exhaling bend to the left this time, place your left palm beside your left foot. Your right arm should be held up, and you should also turn your head and look up *(see figure 7-5)*.

Repeat the movement three times, and then stay in the posture for three breaths before returning to asana sthiti while you are inhaling slowly.

TWISTING MOVEMENTS
(PARIVRITTA TRIKONASANA)

This time, as you breathe out slowly turn to the left, keeping your feet in their original position *(see figure 7-6)*.

Stay in this position for a breath. Then on exhalation, slowly bend down, keeping your body horizontal *(see figure 7-7)*.

Stay in this position for a breath. Then press down and anchor your feet well. While you are exhaling, twist your body, lower your trunk, and place your right palm beside your left foot *(see figure 7-8)*.

Stay in this position for three to six long inhalations and exhalations. On every exhalation, slowly twist more and look up. The side view is shown figure 7-9.

This is known as *parivritta trikonasana* (triangle pose with a twist) The rear view is shown in figure 7-10.

To return to asana sthiti, first, from the asana pose, slowly inhaling, raise your trunk, unwind it, and bring it to the horizontal position. Stay in this position for a breath *(see figure 7-11)*.

During the following slow inhalation, straighten your back, but keep it still turned to the left side *(see figure 7-12)*.

Stay in this position for a breath. While you are inhaling, return to trikonasana sthiti *(see figure 7-13)*.

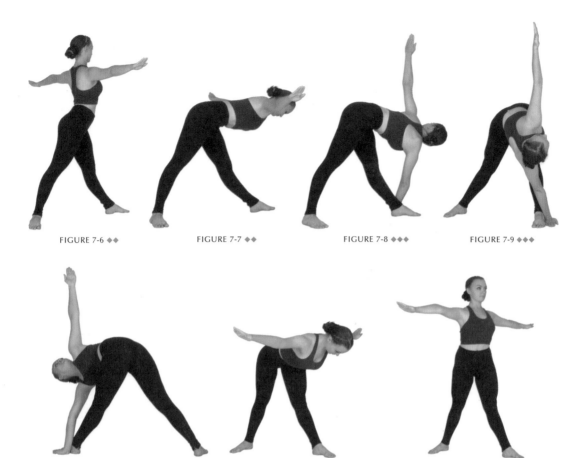

FIGURE 7-6 ◆◆   FIGURE 7-7 ◆◆   FIGURE 7-8 ◆◆◆   FIGURE 7-9 ◆◆◆

FIGURE 7-10 ◆◆◆   FIGURE 7-11 ◆◆   FIGURE 7-12 ◆◆

This sequence can then be done on the other side. As you breathe out, slowly turn to the right side, keeping your feet in the same position (*see figure 7-14*).

Stay in this position for a breath. Then on the next exhalation, slowly bend forward and down, keeping your body horizontal (*see figure 7-15*).

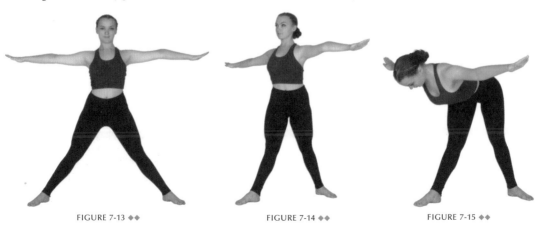

FIGURE 7-13 ◆◆   FIGURE 7-14 ◆◆   FIGURE 7-15 ◆◆

Stay in this position for a breath. Then press down and anchor your feet well; while you are exhaling, twist, lower your trunk, and place your left palm beside your right foot (see figure 7-16).

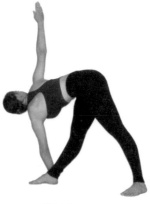

FIGURE 7-16 ◆◆◆

The rear view is shown in figure 7-17.

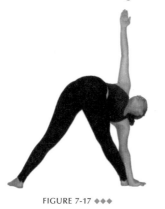

FIGURE 7-17 ◆◆◆

Stay in this position for three to six long inhalations and exhalations. On every exhalation, slowly twist and look up. You can return to the asana sthiti in three steps, as explained previously. You can see that the movement from the trikonasana position and the final posture is made in three distinct steps.

SIDE STRETCH TRIANGLE POSE (UTTITA PARSVA KONASANA)

From the trikonasana position, while exhaling turn your right foot out sideways, keeping your left foot straight. Slowly exhaling, bend your right knee, push your body sideways to the right, and lower your trunk. Place your right palm by the side of your turned right foot. You may also swing your left arm overhead; do not look up; look straight in front of you (see figure 7-18).

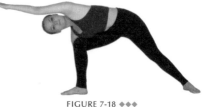

FIGURE 7-18 ◆◆◆

While inhaling, return to asana sthiti. Repeat the movement three times. On the fourth occasion, stay in this position for six long breaths, moving your knee out and lowering your body as much as you can, and in the process stretching your hip and the gluetial and thigh muscles of your left leg. Inhaling, you may return to trikonasana sthiti. This pose is known as *uttita parsva konasana* (the side stretch triangle pose).

From trikonasana position, once again do uttita parsva konasana. Now, balancing well, stretch your right arm up and keep both your palms together (see figure 7-19).

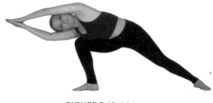

FIGURE 7-19 ◆◆◆

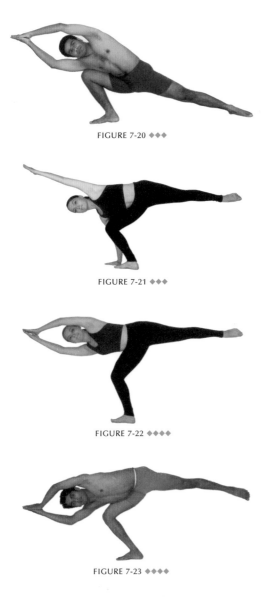

FIGURE 7-20 ◆◆◆

FIGURE 7-21 ◆◆◆

FIGURE 7-22 ◆◆◆◆

FIGURE 7-23 ◆◆◆◆

Stay in this position for six breaths. With every exhalation, try to lower your trunk and slide your body further to the right. Then as you inhale, return to the asana sthiti. Another view is shown in figure 7-20, in which you can see that the yogi has lowered his body by moving his right knee out.

Now exhale, lower your right hand, and place your palm on the floor beside your right foot. Then balancing on your right foot and pressing down with your right hand, slowly raise your left leg as you exhale (see figure 7-21).

Stay in this position for three breaths, and during the next exhalation, lower your leg to the floor. This is a good preparation for balancing on your right leg.

Balancing on your bent right leg, and holding your breath after exhalation, slowly raise your left leg laterally, lifting it from your hip (see figure 7-22).

Stay in this position for three long inhalations and exhalations. Once you are able to balance well, slowly lower your body further down, bending your right knee (see figure 7-23).

This should be done while smoothly exhaling and maintaining good balance. Stay in this position for a few breaths. Inhale lower your left leg and return to trikonasana sthiti.

Yoga demands that one's practice be balanced. All postures should be done on both sides to maintain symmetry. Many books provide an explanation of how to perform exercises only on one side, and the reader is left to practice it on the other side. But if the instructions are available for both sides, this makes it much easier, and one can be sure that practice will be done bilaterally. So, the preceding uttita parsva konasana should be practiced on the other side as well.

From trikonasana sthiti, while exhaling bend your left knee and place your left palm on the floor beside your left foot. Also bring your right hand overhead. Look straight ahead, not up. Stay in this position for three to six breaths (see figure 7-24).

Inhale, lower your right leg and return to trikonasana sthiti.

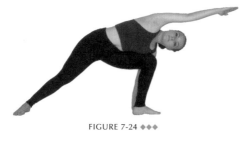

FIGURE 7-24 ◆◆◆

This time as you inhale, raise your left hand and keep both your palms together. Stay in this position for six breaths (*see figure 7-25*).

From the previously practiced position, exhale and hold your breath. Then slowly raise your right leg, balancing on your bent left leg (*see figure 7-26*).

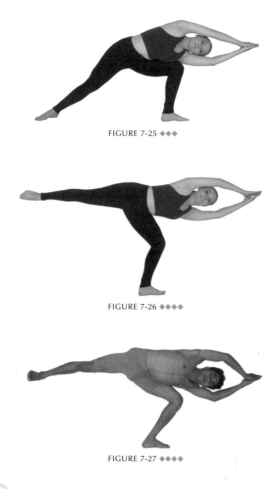

FIGURE 7-25 ◆◆◆

FIGURE 7-26 ◆◆◆◆

FIGURE 7-27 ◆◆◆◆

Once you are able to balance well, slowly lower your body further down, bending your left knee (*see figure 7-27*).

This should be done while smoothly exhaling and maintaining good balance. Stay in this position for three breaths. Inhaling, lower your right leg and return to trikonasana sthiti.

SIDE STRETCH MOVEMENTS (PARSVA KONASANA VINYASAS)

From trikonasana sthiti, you can move on to another group of vinyasas centered on side stretch asana, or *parsva konasana*. From the trikonasana sthiti, while inhaling raise both arms overhead. While exhaling, turn to the right and also turn your right foot. Stay in this position for three breaths.

Next, as you inhale lift your chest and bend back (*see figure 7-28*).

Then as you are breathing out, stretch your torso from your left hip, bend forward, and place your palms on the floor, and your forehead on your right knee or your shin (*see figure 7-29*).

Repeat the movement three times, and then stay in the forward-bend position another three to six breaths. Then as you are inhaling, lift your arms and your trunk to come back to parsva konasan sthiti.

From the asana sthiti, while slowly exhaling turn to the left side this time, turning your left foot out. Stay in this position for three breaths. Inhaling, bend back, lifting your heart (*see figure 7-30*).

As on the other side, while exhaling deeply, stretch your spine and your right hip, and bend forward. Place your palms

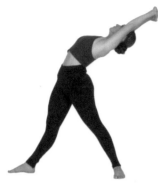

FIGURE 7-28 ♦♦

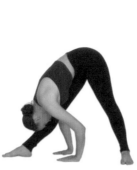

FIGURE 7-29 ♦♦♦

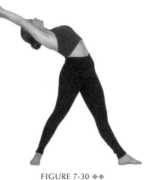

FIGURE 7-30 ♦♦

on the floor and your face on your left knee (*see figure 7-31*).

Repeat the movement three times, and then stay in the pose for another three to six breaths. Finally, while inhaling slowly return to asana sthiti.

In the asana sthiti, while exhaling, lower your arms and hold your elbows behind your back. Inhaling, bend back, and while you are exhaling, stretch your back and bend forward, placing your forehead on your right knee or your shin (*see figure 7-32*).

Stay in this position for three long inhalations and exhalations. Return to asana sthiti while inhaling.

In a similar fashion, inhale, and as you are exhaling, bend forward and place your forehead on your left knee or shin (*see figure 7-33*).

Stay in this position for three long inhalations and exhalations. Then, as you are breathing in, return to asana sthiti to the right.

Again, in the parsva konasana position, while inhaling raise both arms overhead, and while exhaling, lower your arms and swing your arms behind your back. Join your palms in anjali and slide your hands along your spine close to your shoulder blades (in prishtanjali, or the back salute). Inhaling, bend back, and with the next exhalation stretch well and bend forward to place your face on your right knee or your shin. Stay in this position for three long inhalations and exhalations. Return

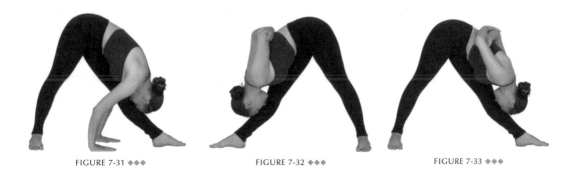

FIGURE 7-31 ♦♦♦   FIGURE 7-32 ♦♦♦   FIGURE 7-33 ♦♦♦

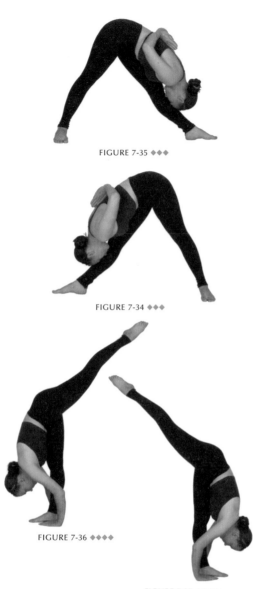

FIGURE 7-35 ◆◆◆

FIGURE 7-34 ◆◆◆

FIGURE 7-36 ◆◆◆◆

FIGURE 7-37 ◆◆◆◆

sthiti. Then breathing out slowly, bend forward, and place your palms on the floor. Now as you inhale, lift your left leg as high as you can, still keeping your face down (*see figure 7-36*).

Stay balanced for three breaths. Exhaling, you may lower your left leg. Then during your inhalation, return to asana sthiti.

This vinyasa should be done on the left side as well (*see figure 7-37*).

Now return to trikonasana sthiti as you are inhaling.

VIRABHADRASANA SEQUENCE (THE WARRIOR POSE)

From here we go to the next group, popularly known as virabhadrasana. From the triangle pose position, while exhaling turn to the right. Turn your right foot as well. Inhale, raise your arms overhead, and bend back (*see figure 7-38*).

As you are exhaling, bend your right knee, lower your trunk, rotate your shoulders, and bring your arms in front of you in a circular motion. Keep your upper body straight (*see figure 7-39*).

to asana sthiti while you are inhaling (*see figure 7-34*).

Following the same procedure, do the vinyasa on the left side as well (*see figure 7-35*).

As you are inhaling, return to your starting position.

Again from the trikonasana sthiti, while inhaling, raise your arms overhead and interlock your fingers. Exhale, and turn to your right side for the parsva konasana

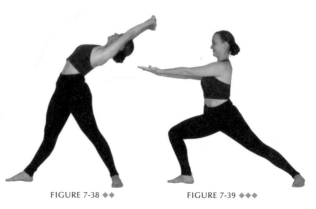

FIGURE 7-38 ◆◆

FIGURE 7-39 ◆◆◆

Stay in this position for six long inhalations and exhalations. This is virabhadrasana.

Stay in virabhadrasana; inhaling slowly, expand and lift your chest and bend back (see figure 7-40).

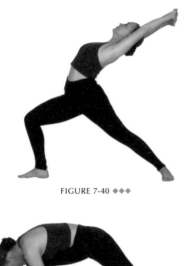

FIGURE 7-40 ◆◆◆

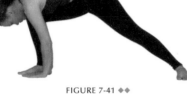

FIGURE 7-41 ◆◆

Stay in this position for six long inhalations and exhalations.

Now from this position, exhale smoothly and completely, and bend forward to place your face on your bent right knee. Keep your palms on the floor beside/behind your right leg. Stay in this position for three to six inhalations and exhalations (see figure 7-41).

Keeping your right knee bent and your hands on the floor, slowly inhale and lift your left leg, straighten your left knee, and keep your left leg horizontal. Exhale, and during the next inhalation, raise your upper body and stretch your arms over-

head. Now your whole body is horizontal, your right knee bent, and you are balancing on your right leg (see figure 7-42).

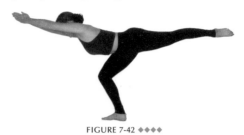

FIGURE 7-42 ◆◆◆◆

This is another variation of virabhadrasana. Stay in this position for three breaths. When you are able to maintain good balance, slowly exhale, bend your right knee a little more, and lower your whole body, which is still horizontal (see figure 7-43).

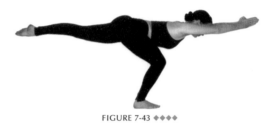

FIGURE 7-43 ◆◆◆◆

Stay in this position for another three breaths. This gives a tremendous stretch to your hip joint and also stretches your thigh muscle. Lower your body as far down as possible; the low center of gravity gives lot more stability to this posture. It also helps to stretch the gluteal muscles and the hip joint (see figure 7-44).

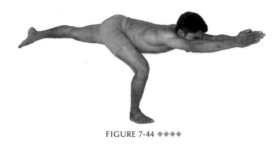

FIGURE 7-44 ◆◆◆◆

Your knee must be kept relaxed.

Now balancing on your right leg, and slowly inhaling, straighten your right knee, so that both your knees are stretched (*see figure 7-45*).

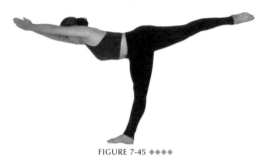

FIGURE 7-45 ◆◆◆◆

This is another vinyasa of virabhadrasana. Stay in this position for three breaths. Exhaling, lower your leg and return to the starting position, the triangle pose, while you are inhaling.

Here is yet another variation. From the triangle position, while exhaling keep your arms behind you and clasp your hands. Inhale, and while you are exhaling, bend your right knee, lower your upper body, twist it to the right side, and place your head on your right foot (*see figure 7-46*).

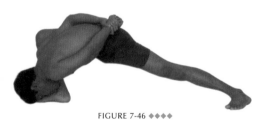

FIGURE 7-46 ◆◆◆◆

Stay in this position for six long inhalations and exhalations.

Now do virabhadrasana on the left side. From the triangle pose, while exhaling turn to the left. Turn your left foot as well. Inhale, raise your arms overhead, and bend back (*see figure 7-47*).

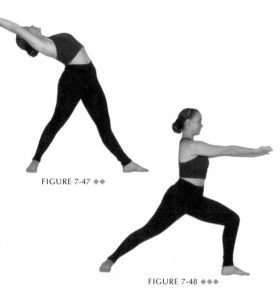

FIGURE 7-47 ◆◆

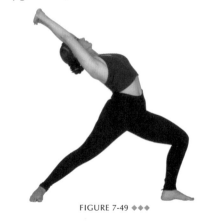

FIGURE 7-48 ◆◆◆

As you exhale, bend your left knee, lower your trunk, rotate your shoulders, and bring your arms in front of you in a circular motion. Keep your upper body straight (*see figure 7-48*).

Stay in this position for six long inhalations and exhalations.

Stay in virabhadrasana; inhaling slowly, expand and lift your heart, and bend back (*see figure 7-49*).

FIGURE 7-49 ◆◆◆

Stay in this position for six long inhalations and exhalations.

Now from this position, exhale smoothly and completely, and bend forward to place your face on your bent left knee and your palms on the floor. Stay in this position for three to six inhalations and exhalations *(see figure 7-50)*.

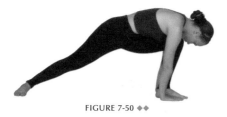

FIGURE 7-50 ◆◆

Keeping your left knee bent and your hands on the floor, while slowly inhaling raise your right leg, straighten your knee, and keep your right leg horizontal. Exhale, and during the following inhalation, raise your upper body and stretch your arms overhead. Now your whole body is horizontal, your left knee is bent, and you are balancing on your left leg *(see figure 7-51)*.

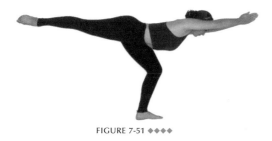

FIGURE 7-51 ◆◆◆◆

Stay in this position for three breaths. When you are able to maintain good balance, slowly exhale, bend your left knee a little more, and lower your whole body, which is still horizontal *(see figure 7-52)*.

Stay in this position for another three breaths. It gives a tremendous stretch to your hip joint and also stretches your thigh muscle. Lower your body as far down as possible; the low center of gravity gives lot more stability to the posture. It also helps

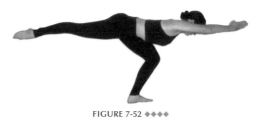

FIGURE 7-52 ◆◆◆◆

to stretch the gluteal muscles and the hip joint *(see figure 7-53)*.

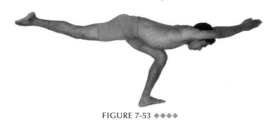

FIGURE 7-53 ◆◆◆◆

Your knee must be kept relaxed.

Now, balancing on your left leg and slowly inhaling, straighten your left knee so that both your knees are stretched *(see figure 7-54)*.

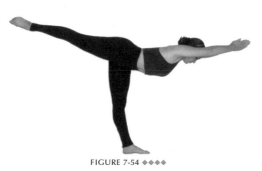

FIGURE 7-54 ◆◆◆◆

This is another vinyasa of virabhadrasana. Stay in this position for three breaths. Exhaling, lower your leg and return to the triangle pose while inhaling.

Here is yet another variation. From the triangle position, while exhaling keep your arms behind and clasp your hands. Inhale, and while you are exhaling, bend your left knee, lower your upper body, twist it to the left side, and place your head on your left foot (*see figure 7-55*).

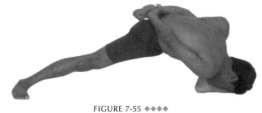

FIGURE 7-55 ◆◆◆◆

Stay in this position for six long inhalations and exhalations.

EXAGGERATED SPREAD-FEET STRETCH POSE
(PRASARITA PADOTTANASANA)

All the groups of vinyasas done so far in this sequence have required you to keep your feet about three to four feet apart, depending mainly upon your height and the condition of your hips. Now we go on to the next group in which the spreading of the feet is more exaggerated—about six to seven feet. You can reach this position by spreading your legs further from trikonasana.

Inhale, and stretch your arms overhead. Now exhaling, bend forward and place your palms on the floor and the crown of your head on the floor in line with your feet (*see figure 7-56*).

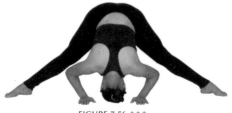

FIGURE 7-56 ◆◆◆

Stay in this position for three long inhalations and exhalations. While you are inhaling, return to the asana sthiti.

This time, keeping your arms overhead, stay in the position for a breath. Now as you are slowly exhaling, again bend forward, but spread your arms and clasp the big toes of your feet. Place your crown on the floor in line with your feet. Stay in this position for six long inhalations and exhalations (*see figure 7-57*).

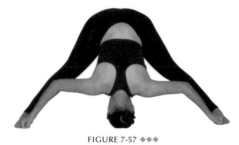

FIGURE 7-57 ◆◆◆

Now as you breathe in, still holding your toes, arch your back and raise your head before raising your trunk. Return to the asana sthiti.

Now you will do forward bending without support. Exhaling, move your arms back and do prishtanjali, or the back salute. Inhale well, and expand your chest. Now as you are breathing out slowly, stretch your back and bend forward to place the crown of your head on the floor in line with your feet (*see figure 7-58*).

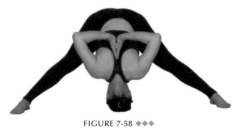

FIGURE 7-58 ◆◆◆

Stay in this position for six long inhalations and exhalations. Another figure with a broader base is shown in figure 7-59).

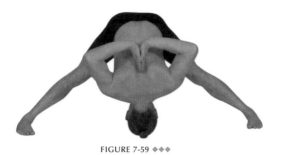

FIGURE 7-59 ◆◆◆

Return to asana sthiti while you are inhaling.

This time from asana sthiti, while exhaling twist to the right side, lower your upper body, and hold your right foot with both your hands (see figure 7-60).

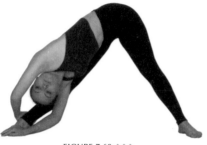

FIGURE 7-60 ◆◆◆

Stay in this position for three long inhalations and exhalations. Return to the starting position while you are inhaling.

Now do the same movement on the left side as you slowly breathe out (see figure 7-61).

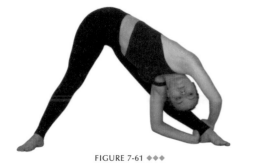

FIGURE 7-61 ◆◆◆

Stay in this position for three breaths, and return to the starting point while you are slowly inhaling.

With this group completed, the logical next step is to spread your legs fully to sit on the floor, which is known as samakonasana, or the straight angle posture. From *prasarita padottanasana*, bend forward and place your palms on the floor a little in front of you. Then as you are exhaling, slide your legs along the floor until you are able to sit on the floor with your legs pointing in opposite directions (see figure 7-62).

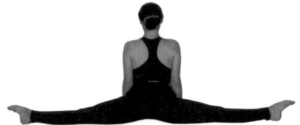

FIGURE 7-62 ◆◆◆◆◆

The front view is shown in figure 7-63, and forward bending on exhalation is shown in figure 7-64).

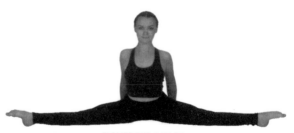

FIGURE 7-63 ◆◆◆◆◆

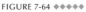

FIGURE 7-64 ◆◆◆◆◆

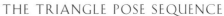

Now exhaling swing your hands back and do a back salute. This is *niralamba samakonasana*, or the straight-angle pose, without support *(see figure 7-65)*.

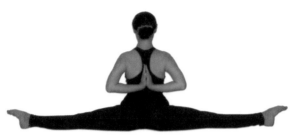

FIGURE 7-65 ◆◆◆◆◆

Stay in this position for three breaths. Lower your arms on exhalation. Place your palms on the floor in front of you, and pressing down with your palms and holding your breath, return to prasarita pada uttanasana, then to trikonasana, and finally to samasthiti. Stay in each position for a breath.

We have seen a number of postures emanating from the triangle pose position. These vinyasas give considerable power to your legs, and athletes, especially runners, will find that these vinyasas work very well on the lower extremities.

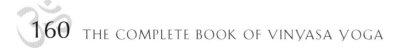

8

THE
INVERTED POSTURE
SEQUENCE

INVERTED POSTURES (*viparita karani*) have a very important place in yoga asana practice. They are unique innovations of ancient yogis. All antigravity poses have a tonic effect on the internal organs, if done properly. The yogis have a very definite view about the efficacy of these postures. Because of the constant downward pull of gravity, our muscles are dragged down as we stand or sit. We also know that the muscles lose their tone as we get older. Like the external muscles, the muscle tissues inside the body also slowly lose their tone.

The internal organs—they are called *kosas*, or sacs—are kept in place by various groups of muscles, tendons, and other tissues. The kosas are *hridaya kosa* (heart), *swasa kosa* (lungs), *anna kosa* (stomach), *garbha kosa* (uterus), *mutra kosa* (bladder), *bindu kosa* (prostate), and *mala kosa* (the large intestines). When they start losing their tone from the constant downward pull, the internal organs also tend to sag, like the facial muscles. We do not see this, however.

The yogis say that this process displaces the internal organs from their original positions because the space inside the body is not packed tightly. This, according to yogis, is the cause, or one of the causes, of ailments. The organs tend to lose their efficiency, to say the least. The yogis invented a simple procedure to try to correct this natural process as much as possible: inverted poses.

By staying in such poses as the shoulder stand and headstand, you can get the organs to move back to their correct positions. Of course, you must stay upside down for a sufficiently long time for the postures to have any effect. In these poses, if you can also breathe out very well, you may even be able to hold your breath out for a healthy ten to fifteen seconds or more. During that time, if you have good control over your rectal, gluteal, and abdominal muscles, you can use these muscles along with the pelvic diaphragm and the thoracic diaphragm to gently, but effectively access the internal organs and press or massage them. Further, by manipulating the body in the inverted poses through various vinyasas or movements, you may be able to reach a specific group of muscles or internal organs.

That is the theory. The problem is that these are difficult asanas to practice and master. But to the earnest practitioner, such as a yogi, it is possible. Of course, you have to be very careful about your neck and your spine. One cannot practice yoga without attention. With coordinated breathing, as in vinyasa krama, maintaining the required attention becomes much easier. And sirsasana is thus an important innovation in the arsenal of the yogi.

PROCEDURE FOR THE HEADSTAND

The starting point for *sirsasana* is *vajrasana* (the bolt pose), which itself is reached by a series of vinyasas starting from samasthiti (see page 176). Another starting point for sirsasana or its unsupported form, *mukta hasta*

sirsasana (also known as *kapala asana*, or the skull pose) is the hub pose of the downward-facing-dog pose.

From vajrasana, slowly bend forward while exhaling, and place your forearms on the floor with your fingers interlaced and cupped (*see figure 8-1*).

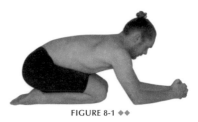

FIGURE 8-1 ◆◆

As you inhale, slowly raise your haunches while still kneeling (*see figure 8-2*).

While inhaling, straighten your knees (*see figure 8-3*).

Stay in this position for a breath.

As you exhale, pressing down with your elbows, bend your knees, lift your feet off the floor, and draw your legs close to your body, balancing on your head and your forearms (*see figure 8-4*).

Stay in this position for three long inhalations and exhalations.

Now as you are inhaling, straighten your waist, still keeping your knees bent (*see figure 8-5*).

Again stay in this position for three long inhalations and exhalations.

Now as you are inhaling, straighten your knees so that your body is straight (see figure 8-6).

You are in the headstand. Stay in this position for three to six breaths. This is a pose where you can stay in this position for a long time. Adepts stay in this position for a half-hour to an hour. Here your breath should be very smooth and very long. Your breathing rate is the key to the success in

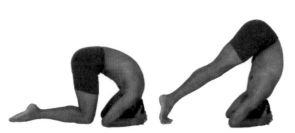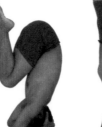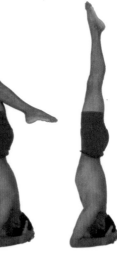

FIGURE 8-2 ◆◆   FIGURE 8-3 ◆◆   FIGURE 8-4 ◆◆◆   FIGURE 8-5 ◆◆◆   FIGURE 8-6 ◆◆◆◆

this pose. Six breaths per minute is acceptable, but slowly you can reduce this to three or even two per minute. The straight view is shown figure 8-7. The rear view, in figure 8-8, shows the position of the hands.

The front view in figure 8-9 shows the legs close to and touching each other.

This position helps one to remain relaxed and affords better balance.

Knee Bends (Akunchanasana)

Now for some vinyasas performed in the headstand position. Exhaling slowly, bend your right knee and lower it, rounding your back. Keep your left leg straight *(see figure 8-10)*.

Inhaling, raise your right leg. Repeat the movement very slowly, synchronizing it with your breath. This is *dakshina pada akunchanasana*. Inhaling, you may return to the headstand.

See whether you are balancing on your head correctly. You have to make frequent adjustments of your head position to maintain your balance, because your head tends to become displaced during when moving your body while in the headstand. Exhaling, slowly bend your left knee and lower your left leg close to your chest, rounding your back a little *(see figure 8-11)*.

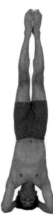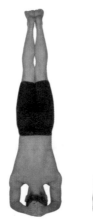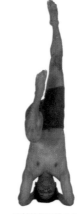   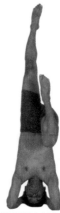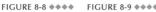

FIGURE 8-7 ◆◆◆◆   FIGURE 8-8 ◆◆◆◆   FIGURE 8-9 ◆◆◆◆   FIGURE 8-10 ◆◆◆   FIGURE 8-11 ◆◆◆

Inhaling, raise your left leg. Repeat the movement three times. This is *vama pada akunchanasana.*

Now, as you are exhaling, bend both your knees and lower both your legs in front of your chest (*see figures 8-12 and 8-13*).

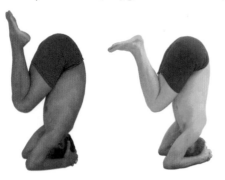

FIGURE 8-12 ◆◆◆   FIGURE 8-13 ◆◆◆

While you are inhaling, return to the headstand. Repeat the movement three times. Then return to headstand while inhaling. This is akunchanasana, or the contraction posture. In this vinyasa, the back is very well rounded to maintain balance. There will be a tendency to straighten your back. With your legs coming down, your body will have to be balanced by pushing your torso back, that is, by rounding your back.

This time as you are exhaling, bend your left knee and keep your left foot on your right thigh close to your groin, in half-lotus position. Stay in this position for three breaths. Then as you are exhaling, slowly bend your right knee and lower your right leg (with both your knees bent) close to your body (*see figure 8-14*).

Inhale, and straighten your right leg. Repeat the movement three times. Then on the next inhalation, straighten your left and right legs. This is *ardha padma akunchanasana* (half-lotus contraction pose).

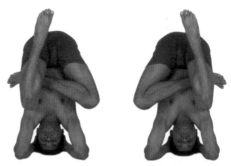

FIGURE 8-14 ◆◆◆◆   FIGURE 8-15 ◆◆◆◆

Now, repeat the movement with your right leg bent in half-lotus position, while you are exhaling. Inhale, and during exhalation bend your left knee and lower your left leg close to your chest (*see figure 8-15*).

Inhale, and straighten your left leg. Repeat the movement three times. During the next inhalation, straighten both your legs to return to the headstand position.

As you are exhaling, slowly lower your right leg all the way down to the floor (*see figure 8-16*).

Inhaling and pressing down through your elbows, slowly raise your leg back to the headstand. Repeat the movement three times, then raise your right leg back to the headstand on inhalation. This is *dakshina-(eka) pada-sirsasana.*

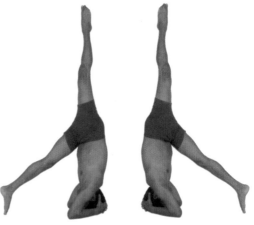

FIGURE 8-16 ◆◆◆   FIGURE 8-17 ◆◆◆

This may be done on the left side as well. Exhaling, from headstand position, slowly lower your left leg all the way down to touch the floor (*see figure 8-17*).

Inhaling, slowly return to the headstand. Repeat the movement three times. Then return your left leg to the headstand, while doing a slow inhalation.

From the headstand position again, slowly exhaling, lower your right leg to the right side until it touches the floor. Inhaling, raise your leg back to the headstand (*see figure 8-18*).

Repeat the movement three times, carefully maintaining your balance. Return to the headstand as you are inhaling.

This may also be done on the left side. Exhaling, slowly lower your left leg all the way down to your left side (*see figure 8-19*).

Inhaling, return to the headstand. Repeat the movement three times, and then return to the headstand by raising your left leg while you are inhaling.

From the headstand position, while you are exhaling and balancing well, entwine your right leg around your left—as a snake

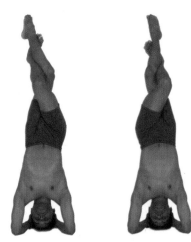

FIGURE 8-20 ◆◆◆　　　FIGURE 8-21 ◆◆◆

would do around the trunk of a tree (*see figure 8-20*).

Stay in this position for three long inhalations and exhalations. This is known as *viparita garudasana*, or the inverted eagle pose. The twisted leg resembles a snake around the leg of an eagle, the king of birds. The eagle (*garuda*) is deified in epics and is considered the vehicle of Lord Vishnu.

Return to the headstand pose while inhaling. This time as you are exhaling, wrap your left leg around your right leg (*see figure 8-21*).

Stay in this position for three breaths, and return on inhalation.

Slowly exhaling, turn your body to the right side and also bend back, twisting your torso well, by anchoring your head and your elbows (*see figure 8-22*).

Stay in this position for three breaths, twisting a little more on each exhalation. Return to the headstand as you slowly inhale.

Again as you are exhaling, anchoring your head and elbows, slowly twist to the left side and bend back as much as you can (*see figure 8-23*).

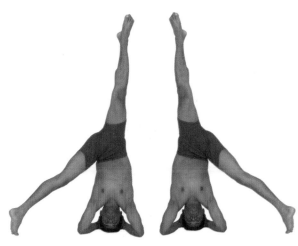

FIGURE 8-18 ◆◆◆　　　FIGURE 8-19 ◆◆◆

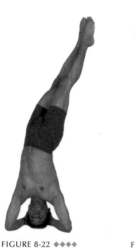

FIGURE 8-22 ◆◆◆◆

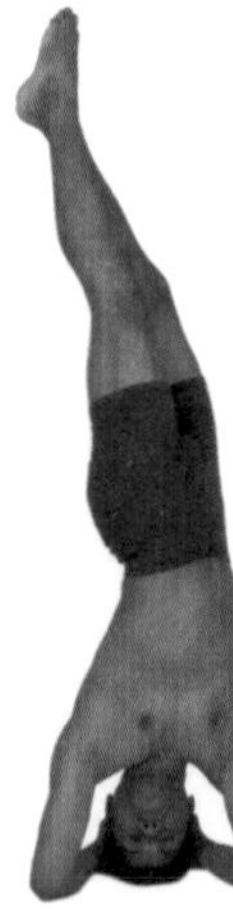

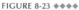

FIGURE 8-23 ◆◆◆◆

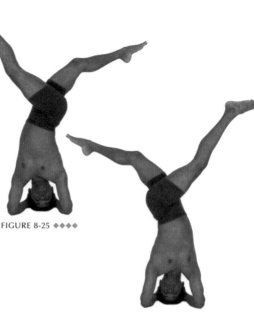

FIGURE 8-25 ◆◆◆◆

FIGURE 8-26 ◆◆◆◆

Stay in this position for three long inhalations and exhalations. While you are inhaling, return to the asana sthiti.

This time, while inhaling, slowly spread your legs evenly, maintaining good balance (*see figure 8-24*).

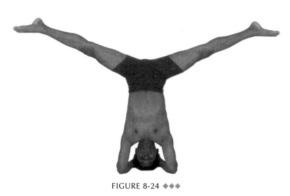

FIGURE 8-24 ◆◆◆

Stay in this position for six long inhalations and exhalations. Exhaling, return to asana sthiti. This is urdhwa konasana, or the upward triangle pose.

Remaining in urdhwa konasana and slowly exhaling, twist your trunk to the right side (*see figure 8-25*).

Stay in this position for three breaths, twisting a little more on each exhalation. Return to asana sthiti while you are inhaling.

The movement should be done on the other side as well. Exhaling, slowly twist your trunk to the left side, maintaining good balance (*see figure 8-26*).

Stay in this position for three breaths, and during every exhalation try to twist a little more. After three breaths, you may return to asana sthiti.

This time while exhaling, from the asana sthiti, bend your knees and bring your soles together, pushing your bent knees out laterally (*see figure 8-27*).

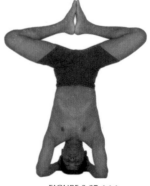

FIGURE 8-27 ◆◆◆

Stay in this position for six long breaths. This is urdhwa baddha konasana. Now inhaling, return to the headstand position.

Remaining in the headstand position, while inhaling spread your legs to to urdhwa konasana position. Then as you are exhaling, bend your right knee and place it on your left thigh, near your groin. Inhale, and during the following exhalation, while pushing your right knee back slightly, bend your left knee and place your left foot on your right thigh close to your groin. During the next exhalation, manipulate your feet carefully and reach the lotus position (*see figure 8-28*).

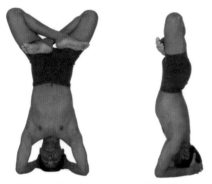

FIGURE 8-28 ♦♦♦♦   FIGURE 8-29 ♦♦♦♦

Stay in this position for six long inhalations and exhalations. This is urdhwa padmasana. The side view is shown in figure 8-29.

From the upward lotus position, while you are slowly exhaling, twist your spine and your hips to the right side, anchoring your head and elbows (*see figure 8-30*).

Stay in this position for three breaths, twisting a little more to the right each time you exhale. Inhaling, return to the starting point.

This time as you are exhaling, anchoring your elbows and your head well, turn your spine and twist your hips to the left side;

maintain good balance and remain relaxed (*see figure 8-31*).

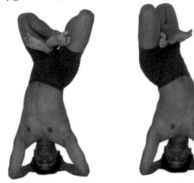

FIGURE 8-30 ♦♦♦♦   FIGURE 8-31 ♦♦♦♦

Stay in this position for three breaths, twisting a little more each time you exhale. Return to the starting point as you are inhaling.

From the upward lotus position, while exhaling slowly fold your waist and lower your lower extremities still locked in lotus position. Bring your legs up to your chest (*see figure 8-32*).

Inhaling, return to the starting point. Repeat the movement slowly with long, slow inhalations and exhalations. This is akunchita urdhwa padmasana.

From the previous position, while exhaling, further round your back and lower your legs until your feet almost touch your chin. The whole lower half of your body should be hanging from your absolutely relaxed hip joints (*see figure 8-33*).

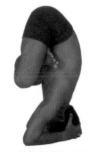 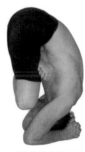

FIGURE 8-32 ♦♦♦   FIGURE 8-33 ♦♦♦

This is known as *viparita yoga mudra* (upside-down yoga seal).

Your legs can be brought further down to touch the floor, all the time maintaining good control and balance. Exhaling, slowly bring your legs down, first with your knees close to your armpits or your biceps *(see figure 8-34)*, and then to the floor *(see figure 8-35)*.

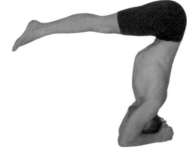

FIGURE 8-36 ◆◆◆

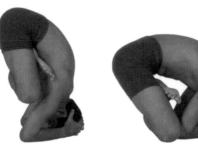

FIGURE 8-34 ◆◆◆   FIGURE 8-35 ◆◆◆

In each of the stages, you may stay in this position for a breath. Do not rush through the movements. Then inhaling, return to the starting pose, urdhwa padmasana. This return journey should be done while you are inhaling. You may also stop at each position where you stopped during the downward movement, and breath once. Stretch your legs to the headstand position, while you are inhaling.

Now as you are exhaling, slowly lower your legs and keep them horizontal, in the process pushing your hips back and also curving your back *(see figure 8-36)*.

Stay in this position for six long inhalations and exhalations. During the next inhalation, slowly bring your legs up, pulling your back forward, to get to the headstand. This pose is called *urdhwa dandasana*, or the raised-stick pose (your legs are straight, horizontal).

From the headstand position, press

down through your elbows, bring your shoulder blades together, and push out your upper chest up inhaling. Stay in this position for a breath. During the next inhalation, push your chest further forward, bend your knees, and drop or hang your legs behind your back *(see figure 8-37)*.

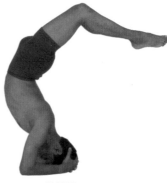

FIGURE 8-37 ◆◆◆

Stay in this position for a breath and check how well you are balancing. Inhaling again, slowly lower your legs to the floor—your toes first, and then your feet. Your knees should still be bent. Stay in this position for a breath. Now inhaling, you may stretch your legs completely, keeping your head and your elbows on the floor *(see figure 8-38)*.

This is known as *viparita dandasana*, or the crooked staff pose. Stay in this position for six breaths. During every inhalation,

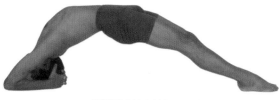

FIGURE 8-38 ◆◆◆◆

open your chest well and lift your chest up. After six breaths, while exhaling bend your knees and draw your legs closer to your body. Exhale again; hold your breath, and slowly kick your legs up, back to the headstand.

From the headstand, lower your legs straight to the floor in front of you while you are exhaling (*see figure 8-39*).

Inhale, and on exhalation, while anchoring your head and pressing down

through your elbows, slowly walk around on the right side until your legs are at an angle of about 30 degrees (*see figure 8-40*).

Walk further on your toes, to your right, twisting your waist to almost 90 degrees (*see figure 8-41*).

Stay in this position for a breath. Now exhale; hold your breath, flip your legs over, and then walk with your feet on the floor beyond your head position (*see figure 8-42*).

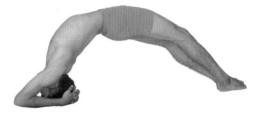

FIGURE 8-42 ◆◆◆◆

Inhale, and stay in this position for a breath. Again while exhaling, walk further until your feet are exactly behind your legs, as in viparita dandasana (*see figure 8-43*).

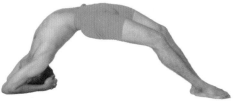

FIGURE 8-43 ◆◆◆◆

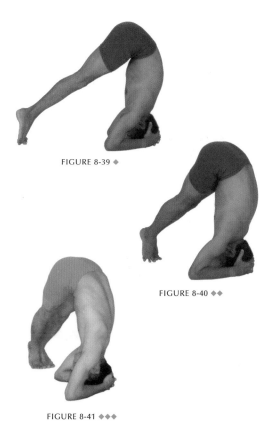

FIGURE 8-39 ◆

FIGURE 8-40 ◆◆

FIGURE 8-41 ◆◆◆

Take a breather. Then as you are exhaling, move your legs step by step to the other side, and when your legs are at an angle of about 90 degrees, flip over and land on your toes (*see figure 8-44*).

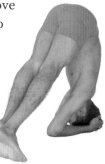

FIGURE 8-44 ◆◆◆

Stay in this position for a breath. Then as you exhale, continue the journey until your legs are about 30 degrees off-center (*see figure 8-45*).

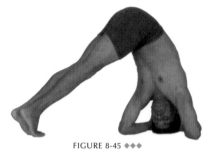

FIGURE 8-45 ◆◆◆

Stay in this position for another breath. Finally as you exhale, move your legs until you reach the starting point. Now as you are exhaling, complete the circle (mandala) to return to the starting position (*see figure 8-46*).

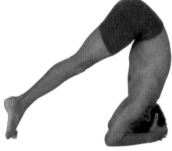

FIGURE 8-46 ◆◆◆

Inhaling, raise your trunk back to the headstand. Some yogis would do this circular ambulation counterclockwise also.

The mandala in both the shoulder stand and the headstand is a very powerful exercise. It strengthens your arms, shoulders, and torso, while making your waist and hips lighter. Your hip joints and your knees also get good flexion. This subsequence should be done slowly without violating the method of breathing. Fast movements and heavy breathing are tiring and clumsy.

Now let us look at the procedure for returning from the headstand. From the asana sthiti, while exhaling slowly, bend your knees to akunanasana. Inhale, and then exhaling lower your legs, land on your toes, and place your knees on the floor. Stay in this position for three breaths. Now raise your head and sit in vajrasana, from which position you started the headstand sequence.

Headstand with Straight Knees

We have seen the headstand being reached through akunchanasana, or bending your knees. Exercises can also be done from this position without bending your knees. In this krama, or procedure, from vajrasana (*see figure 8-47*), while inhaling, push your body up, still on your knees (*see figure 8-48*).

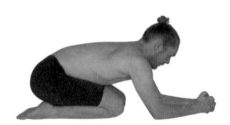

FIGURE 8-47 ◆◆

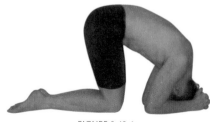

FIGURE 8-48 ◆

Straighten your knees as you inhale (*see figure 8-49*).

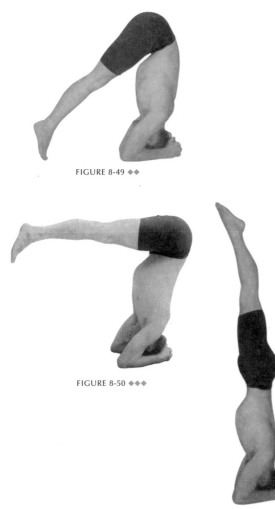

FIGURE 8-49 ◆◆

FIGURE 8-50 ◆◆◆

FIGURE 8-51 ◆◆◆◆

During the next inhalation, slowly raise your legs straight until they are halfway up (*see figure 8-50*).

Stay in this position for a breath. Now during the following inhalation, raise your legs all the way up to the headstand (*see figure 8-51*).

Stay in this position for several minutes, while doing slow inhalations and exhalations. To return to vajrasana, the starting position, you may follow the reverse route and also maintain the appropriate breathing.

Headstand, without Support (Niralamba Sirsasana)

So far we have seen the headstand variations practiced with your fingers interlocked and supporting your head. After some practice with the vinyasa krama, many practitioners are able to stand on their heads without their hands close to their head. This is known as *niralamba sirsasana*, or the headstand without support (to your head). Sometimes this is referred to as mukta hasta sirsasana, or headstand with the hands released. These headstand variations help to lift your body off the floor (utpluti) and include several balancing poses.

In the first of these variations, you will place your forearms on the floor and do the headstand. From vajrasana, place your forearms on the floor and your head in between your hands, while you are slowly exhaling. Now lift your knees, and during the following inhalation, while balancing on your forearms, lift your legs to the headstand (*see figure 8-52*).

You may stay in the pose for twelve long inhalations and exhalations. While exhaling, lower your legs back to vajrasana.

By pressing your forearms and relaxing your whole body, it is possible to lift your body (utpluti) off the ground and balance. Exhale completely; hold your breath, press down through your forearms, and lift your body off the floor, while arching

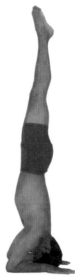

FIGURE 8-52 ◆◆◆◆

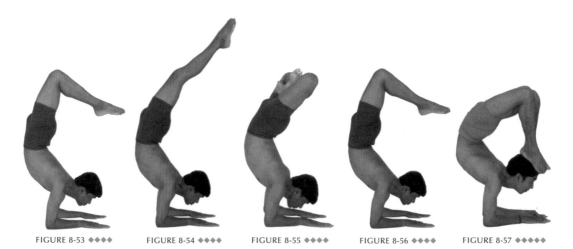

FIGURE 8-53 ◆◆◆◆   FIGURE 8-54 ◆◆◆◆   FIGURE 8-55 ◆◆◆◆   FIGURE 8-56 ◆◆◆◆   FIGURE 8-57 ◆◆◆◆◆

your back and stretching your legs back-ward *(see figure 8-53)*.

Stay in this position for three long inhalations and exhalations. As you are inhaling, stretch your knees and keep your whole body arched uniformly *(see figure 8-54)*. This is pinchamayurasana, or the peacock with lifted feathers pose.

Remaining in the previous pose, balance yourself well; carefully place your right foot on your left thigh close to your groin. This is done as you are exhaling. Now wait for one inhalation, and on the next exhalation place your left foot on your right thigh near your groin. Now relaxing your hip joints, push your feet closer to your groin *(see figure 8-55)*.

This is *padma pincamayurasana* (feathers-up lotus peacock pose). Stay in this position for three to six breaths. Inhaling, stretch your legs back to pinchamayurasana.

There is another exquisite pose that is an extension of this pinchamayurasana. From pinchamayurasana, inhale, lift your chest up slightly by arching your back a little more, and lower your legs by bending them. The halfway stage is shown in figure 8-56.

Then, while inhaling, slowly lower your legs and gently place your feet on your head, still balancing on your forearms and keeping your legs and feet together *(see figure 8-57)*.

Stay in this position for three to six breaths. This is *vrischikasana*, or the scorpion pose. Exhaling, quickly round your back (moving your pelvis toward the floor) and land on your toes. This will look similar to figure 8-46 (on page 170) except that your head will be off of the floor and your forearms will still be flush with it.

So far we have seen one position of hands in the unsupported headstand—there are other hand positions as well. First go to the supported headstand. Then as you are inhaling, spread your arms laterally to the sides of your body, and anchor your palms to the floor. Now you will be balancing with your crown and your two palms, with all three in line *(see figure 8-58)*.

Stay in this position for three breaths; exhaling, bring your arms close to your head, interlock your fingers, and support your head. During the next exhalation, you may lower your trunk. (With some practice, from vajrasana, you may also be able to place your head on the floor and spread your arms laterally with your palms placed

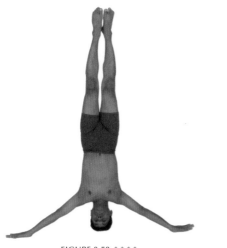

FIGURE 8-58 ♦♦♦♦

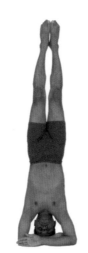

FIGURE 8-59 ♦♦♦♦

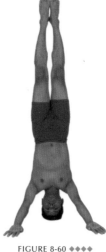

FIGURE 8-60 ♦♦♦♦

on the floor.) Now, balancing carefully, slowly raise your legs in stages to the headstand, stopping in akunchanasana and then straightening your legs. You may return in steps, while you are exhaling.

In the next vinyasas, as before, reach the salamba headstand. Then exhaling, keep your arms bent in front of your face on the floor. You will be keeping your hands folded in front of your head on the floor (see figure 8-59).

Stay balanced for three breaths. Inhaling return to the headstand, and then while exhaling return to vajrasana sthiti in stages. As in the previous asana vinyasa, you may proceed by first placing your arms in asana sthiti and then going up to the headstand, carefully balancing.

Another variation of arm position is to keep your arms spread at about 45 degrees in front of you, with your palms turned upward (see figure 8-60).

We have so far seen the headstand started from vajrasana. Let us consider another procedural variation leading to the headstand.

Headstand from the Downward-Facing-Dog Position

You may start the headstand from the downward-facing-dog pose. Because your palms are on the floor, this particular headstand becomes the hub pose for several of the poses requiring you to lift your body (utpluti). Now from the downward-facing-dog position (see figure 8-61), while exhaling, stretch your body forward, and lower your head and place your crown on the floor (see figure 8-62).

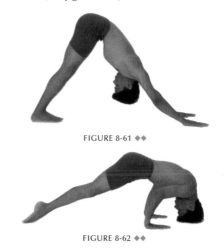

FIGURE 8-61 ♦♦

FIGURE 8-62 ♦♦

The next step will be to move your body forward, by walking your toes up toward your body: your upper body will be almost straight while your big toes help move your body almost vertical (see figure 8-63).

Stay in this position for a breath.

From this vinyasa, while inhaling, slowly lift your legs to the intermediate level; keep your legs horizontal, while balancing on your head and both your palms (see figure 8-64).

This is a vinyasa of urdhwa dandasana.

Inhaling, lift your legs further up until your body is straight (see figure 8-65).

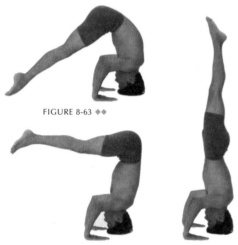

FIGURE 8-63 ♦♦

FIGURE 8-64 ♦♦   FIGURE 8-65 ♦♦♦

You will be balancing on both your palms and your crown. This pose is called mukta hasta sirsasana, or the headstand with the hands released. It is also known as kapala asana, or the skull pose. Stay in this position for twelve long inhalations and exhalations, and get a good feel for the posture.

Because of the position of your hands (which remains the same from the stage of the dog pose), this becomes the posture for several handstand postures. We can practice a few of them. Pressing your palms,

raise your head and arch your back to lift your head. Simultaneously, push your legs a little by bending your waist. Now your whole body is nicely arched back, as you balance on your hands (see figure 8-66).

This is a vinyasa of handstand also known as viparita vrikshasana, or the inverted tree pose. It is also considered a vinyasa of pinchamayurasana. Stay in this position for three breaths, and slowly lower your legs back to the floor for asana sthiti.

Remaining in kapalasana, while slowly exhaling, bend your knees, round your back, and lower your legs. Place your knees against the sides of your upper arms, but keep your feet close to each other. During the following inhalation, slowly raise your heads while still balancing on your hands (see figure 8-67).

This handstand variation is a vinyasa of bhuja peedasana, or the shoulder-pressure pose. Return to kapalasana while you inhale.

As in the previous pose, while exhaling, come to bhuja peedasana. Now inhaling and balancing on your hands, stretch your

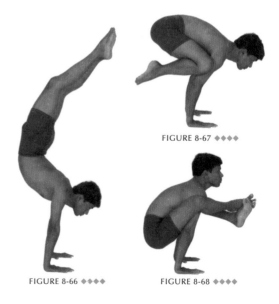

FIGURE 8-67 ♦♦♦♦

FIGURE 8-66 ♦♦♦♦   FIGURE 8-68 ♦♦♦♦

legs forward past your shoulders and cross your ankles as well (see figure 8-68).

Stay in this position for three to six breaths. This is another vinyasa of bhuja peedasana.

This time, while in kapalasana, and exhaling, bend your right knee and place it on your left thigh close to your groin. During the next exhalation, slowly bend your left knee and place your left foot on your right thigh near your right groin. Stay in this position for three breaths, adjusting the lotus position of your legs. Now as you are smoothly exhaling, round your back, and lower your legs. As you raise your upper body during the next inhalation, lift your legs up to a horizontal position to abut your shoulders (see figure 8-69).

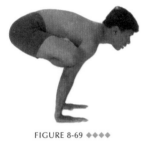

FIGURE 8-69 ♦♦♦♦

This is *urdhwa kukkutasana*. Stay in this position for three long inhalations and exhalations. Inhale, and return to asana sthiti.

From the kapalasana position, bend your knees and lower your legs, while rounding your back and exhaling. Lower your leg as in akunanasana; exhaling, this time move your legs to the right side and place your left knee abutting your right shoulder. Now inhaling, while anchoring your left knee on your right shoulder, stretch your legs to the right side as you raise your head and upper body, balancing on your hands. This is *Ashtavakrasana*, which was named after the sage Ashtavakra (see figure 8-70).

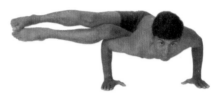

FIGURE 8-70 ♦♦♦♦

Stay in this position for three breaths. Exhaling, bend your knees and lower your head. On the next inhalation, raise your legs back to kapalasana.

Following the same procedure do this variation on the left side (see figure 8-71).

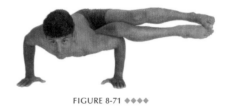

FIGURE 8-71 ♦♦♦♦

9

MEDITATIVE POSE
SEQUENCE

OTHER THAN THE lotus pose (which is discussed in the next chapter), there are a few yoga postures that are used for such practices as pranayama and meditation. Some of these are important poses, especially the vajrasana, around which a number of asana vinyasas are practiced.

Vajrasana, or the bolt pose, is the hub for several vinyasas and asanas. The vinyasa krama for vajrasana is described in this chapter. Vajrasana is a compact and relatively easy pose. With some practice you may be able to stay in the position for a long time. Many yogis who are not comfortable with the lotus pose choose vajrasana for their yoga sadhanas (meditative practices).

LEAD SEQUENCE (SIMPLE)

Start from samasthiti (*see figure 9-1*).

Watch your breath. Watch your balance. Do three inhalations and exhalations, using throat breathing (ujjayi breathing).

Inhaling, raise both arms overhead, interlacing your fingers (*see figure 9-2*).

As you are exhaling slowly and extensively, bend forward to the forward stretch pose known as uttanasana (*see figure 9-3*).

Stay in this position for three long inhalations and exhalations.

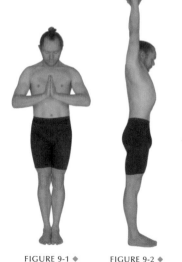
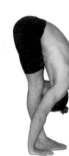

FIGURE 9-1 ◆   FIGURE 9-2 ◆   FIGURE 9-3 ◆◆◆

176 THE COMPLETE BOOK OF VINYASA YOGA

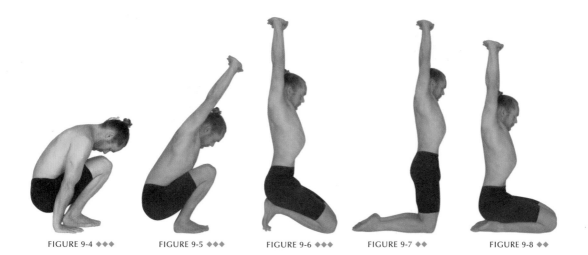

FIGURE 9-4 ◆◆◆   FIGURE 9-5 ◆◆◆   FIGURE 9-6 ◆◆◆   FIGURE 9-7 ◆◆   FIGURE 9-8 ◆◆

Inhale, and on the next exhalation, sit on your haunches, in utkatasana *(see figure 9-4).*

Stay in this position for three long inhalations and exhalations.

Now as you are inhaling, while still in utkatasana raise both your arms up and interlock your fingers *(see figure 9-5).*

Stay in this position for three long inhalations and exhalations.

While you are on the next exhalation, lean forward slightly and land on your knees and your toes on the floor *(see figure 9-6).*

Inhaling, raise your trunk and stand on your knees in the kneeling position, and stretch out your ankles keeping the dorsum of your feet on the floor *(see figure 9-7).*

Exhale slowly and sit on your legs *(see figure 9-8).*

Now as you are exhaling, lower your arms and place your palms on your knees *(see figure 9-9).*

Stay in this position for six long inhalations and exhalations. This is vajrasana.

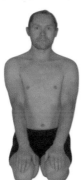

FIGURE 9-9 ◆◆

LEAD SEQUENCE (CLASSICAL)

We have seen a krama, or flow, of vinyasas leading to vajrasana. A more classical approach is described now. From samasthiti to utkatasana, the approach is the same. From utkatasana, inhale; hold your breath and jump (or pump) back to chaturanga-dandasana *(see figure 9-10).*

The next vinyasa will be the upward-facing-dog pose, which is done while inhaling *(see figure 9-11).*

The next vinyasa in the flow is the downward-facing-dog pose, which is done while doing a long, smooth ujjayi exhalation *(see figure 9-12).*

Keeping your chin down, exhale. Then holding your breath, bend your knees slightly, press down through your palms, and swing your bent legs to a position between your arms. Balance yourself in the position *(see figure 9-13).*

A variation of this is shown in figure 9-14.

Stay in this position for a breath, and slowly ease your whole body onto the floor with your legs still bent *(see figure 9-15).*

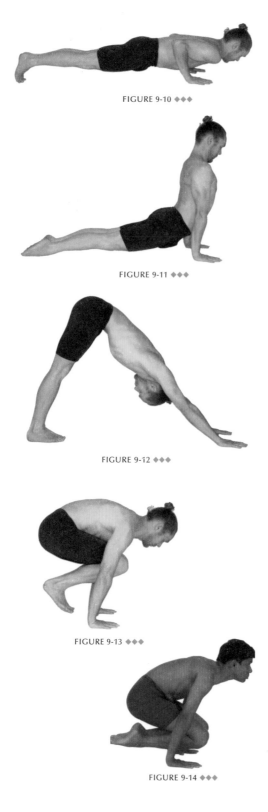

FIGURE 9-10 ◆◆◆

FIGURE 9-11 ◆◆◆

FIGURE 9-12 ◆◆◆

FIGURE 9-13 ◆◆◆

FIGURE 9-14 ◆◆◆

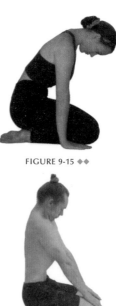

FIGURE 9-15 ◆◆

FIGURE 9-16 ◆◆

Now straighten your back as you inhale. Figure 9-16 shows all the three bandhas being done in this classic pose.

This is the more classical progression to vajrasana, by means of the vinyasa karma approach.

VAJRASANA VINYASAS

Now let us try to do vinyasas in vajrasana. First, as you are inhaling, raise your arms and interlock your fingers, turning them outward. Exhale, and again while inhaling, raise your trunk and remain kneeling (*see figure 9-17*).

As you breathe out, slowly return to vajrasana sthiti, while bending your elbows and placing your interlaced hands on the back of your neck (*see figure 9-18*).

Repeat the movement three to six times. The side view is shown in figure 9-19 with all the three bandhas in operation.

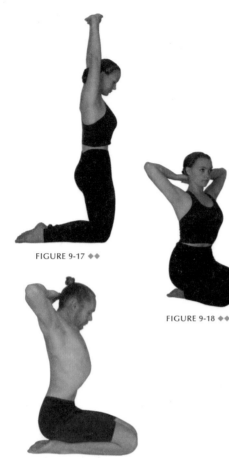

FIGURE 9-17 ◆◆

FIGURE 9-18 ◆◆

FIGURE 9-19 ◆◆

three times, then stay in the bent forward position for another three breaths. Inhaling, return to vajrasana sthiti, and then exhaling lower your arms and place your palms on your knees.

This time as you are inhaling, raise your arms laterally to shoulder level (*see figure 9-21*).

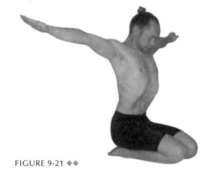

FIGURE 9-21 ◆◆

Stay in this position for a breath. Then during the following exhalation, stretch your back thoroughly and bend forward, placing your forehead on the floor (*see figure 9-22*).

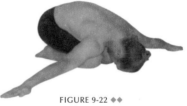

FIGURE 9-22 ◆◆

Keep your buttocks on your heels. Stay in this position for three long, smooth, relaxed breaths. Remain in the bent forward position; exhaling, lower your arms along the floor and place your hands behind your buttocks (*see figure 9-23*).

While coming down for the last time in this vinyasa, keep your arms overhead with your fingers interlaced and return to vajrasana, but with your arms still stretched up. Now inhale, and during the long smooth exhalation, stretch your back, and fold smoothly forward and place your forehead on the floor in front of you (*see figure 9-20*).

You are not supposed to lift your buttocks off your heels. Repeat the movement

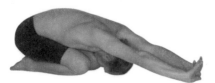

FIGURE 9-20 ◆◆

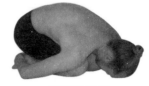

FIGURE 9-23 ◆◆

Stay in this position for another three breaths, then bring you hands to shoulder level on inhalation. Exhale, and while you slowly inhale again, return to the starting position. Exhaling, you may lower your arms to asana sthiti.

While you are exhaling, interlock your fingers and place your palms so that they are covering your lower abdomen, just above the pelvic bone. You may dig your hands a little into your lower abdomen (see figure 9-24).

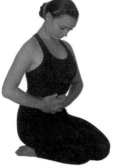

FIGURE 9-24 ◆◆

Inhale, and slowly exhaling, bend forward and place your forehead on the floor. In the process, do not allow your lower abdomen to bulge, but try to contain it within the grasp of your palms (see figure 9-25).

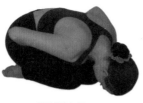

FIGURE 9-25 ◆◆◆

This will be facilitated to an extent by a deeper and more complete exhalation. This will also provide a gentle massage to your abdominal and pelvic organs. Practitioners of kundalini yoga experience some positive benefits from this pose. The side view is shown in figure 9-26).

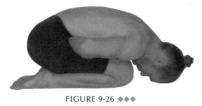

FIGURE 9-26 ◆◆◆

Inhaling, raise you arms overhead. Exhaling slowly, swing your arms behind you and keep your palms together in prishtanjali, or the back salute. Exhaling slowly and very deeply, bend forward and place your forehead on the floor (see figure 9-27).

Stay in this position for three long inhalations and exhalations. Inhaling, push your arms and shoulders out, lift your chest, and raise your head (see figure 9-28).

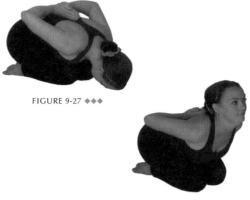

FIGURE 9-27 ◆◆◆

FIGURE 9-28 ◆◆

Expanding your chest, return to vajrasana sthiti.

We have seen many variations of the forward bend in vajrasana. Now let us look at the counterpose, or pratikriya, and other advanced back-bending vinyasas. Inhaling, raise your arms overhead. Slowly exhaling, lean back your body a bit on your heels, on which you are sitting, and place your palms on the floor behind you about a foot away (see figure 9-29). Your palms should be turned inward. Stay in this position for a breath, keeping your chin down.

While you are slowly inhaling, raise your waist/hips, arch your spine, and drop your head back. Lift your chest and expand your chest well (*see figure 9-30*).

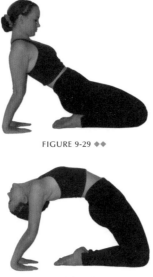

FIGURE 9-29 ♦♦

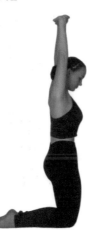

FIGURE 9-30 ♦♦

Exhaling, return to asana sthiti. Repeat the movement three to six times. Then, inhaling, raise your arms and pull yourself back to vajrasana sthiti.

THE CAMEL SUBROUTINE
(USHTRASANA)

From vajrasana sthiti, while inhaling, you lift your arms, interlace your fingers, and raise your trunk (*see figure 9-31*).

Stay in this position for a breath, then inhaling, place your hands on your hips and slightly bend back your neck. During the next inhalation, slowly

arch your spine, and balancing on your knees (pressing down with your stretched ankles), lower your upper body and place your cupped palms so that they cover your heels. Your fingers will be pointing downward, and your hands will be in a supine position (*see figure 9-32*).

Stay in this position for six long inhalations and exhalations. During every inhalation, while pressing your palms against your heels, you can elevate your chest up and arch your spine a little more. This posture is called *ushtrasana*, or the camel pose. It is also known as *ushtra nishada*, or a position resembling a camel, because your torso looks like the hump of a camel. As you are exhaling, return vajrasana sthiti.

Again from vajrasana sthiti, inhaling, raise your trunk to the kneeling position. Exhale, and as you are inhaling, bend back, keeping your arms in the overhead position. Arching your back, place your cupped palms on your heels, with your fingers turned inward; your hands will now be in prone position (*see figure 9-33*).

This advanced vinyasa of ushtrasana involves more bending of your spine, and your shoulders also come into play. Stay in this position for three to six long inhalations

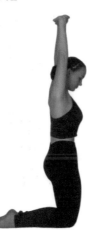

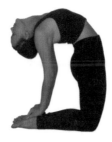

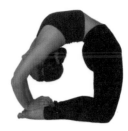

FIGURE 9-31 ♦♦   FIGURE 9-32 ♦♦♦   FIGURE 9-33 ♦♦♦♦

and exhalations, arching your torso on every and inhalation. Stay in this position for a few breaths. As you are slowly inhaling, try to straighten your elbows, accentuating the curvature of the posture. Stay in this position for three breaths (*see figure 9-34*).

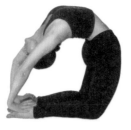

FIGURE 9-34 ◆◆◆◆

Camel to Pigeon

From this advanced camel pose vinyasa, let us try one more vinyasa. As you are slowly inhaling, press your palms, tighten your gluteal muscles, and lower your head and place it on your heels. Stay in this position for a breath. During the next exhalation, stretch your arms along your legs and hold your thighs close to your knees (*see figure 9-35*).

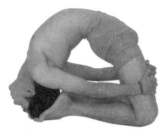

FIGURE 9-35 ◆◆◆◆◆

Stay in this position for six breaths, taking care to see that the entire stretching is controlled from your gluteal muscles. This pose is called *kapotasana*, or the pigeon pose. The chest curvature is very prominent in this pose, hence the name. Bring your arms back to your heels on inhalation,

and as you breath out, return to the starting position and then to vajrasana sthiti.

The Camel Walk Sequence

Once again from vajrasana, as you are breathing in, raise your trunk to the kneeling position (*see figure 9-36*).

Inhale, and on the next exhalation, bend your right knee and place your right leg in front of you by about a foot (*see figure 9-37*).

Once again, inhale and on the following exhalation, bend forward and place your palms on either side of your right foot and your face/chin on your right knee (*see figure 9-38*).

Stay in this position for three long inhalations and exhalations. Inhaling, straighten your trunk.

While you are inhaling, slowly bend back and clasp your left heel with both cupped palms (*see figure 9-39*).

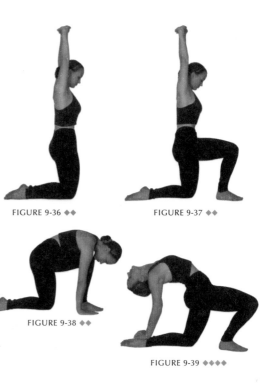

FIGURE 9-36 ◆◆   FIGURE 9-37 ◆◆

FIGURE 9-38 ◆◆

FIGURE 9-39 ◆◆◆◆

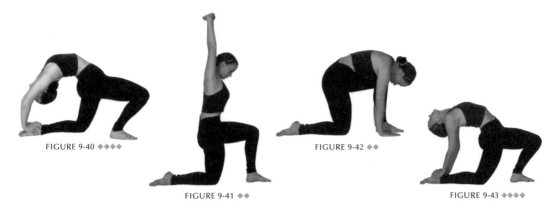

FIGURE 9-40 ♦♦♦♦

FIGURE 9-41 ♦♦

FIGURE 9-42 ♦♦

FIGURE 9-43 ♦♦♦♦

Stay in this position for six long inhalations and exhalations, while also lifting your chest (facilitated by the breathing in). This is a variation of camel pose. Some experts call this variation alone the camel pose, because it gives the impression of a camel walking leisurely.

Here is an advanced vinyasa. From asana sthiti inhale, and arching your back, place your cupped palms on your left heel, with your fingers turned inward and your hands in a prone position (see figure 9-40).

Stay in this position for three breaths, arching your back each time to a greater degree on every inhalation. Exhaling, return to the starting position. Inhaling, bring your right leg back to the vajrasana position.

Once again from vajrasana, as you are breathing in, lift your trunk to the kneeling position. Inhale, and on the next exhalation, place your left leg forward by about a foot, bending your left knee (see figure 9-41).

Once again inhale, and on the following exhalation, bend forward and place your palms on either side of your left foot and your face/chin on your left knee (see figure 9-42).

Stay in this position for three long inhalations and exhalations. Inhaling, straighten your trunk.

While you are inhaling, slowly bend

back and clasp your right heel with both cupped palms (see figure 9-43).

Stay in this position for six long inhalations and exhalations and also lift your chest (facilitated by the breathing in). This is a variation of camel pose.

Here is another advanced vinyasa. From asana sthiti inhale, and arching your back, place your cupped palms on your right heel, with your fingers turned inward and your hands in a prone position (see figure 9-44).

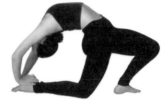

FIGURE 9-44 ♦♦♦♦

Exhaling, you may return to the starting position. Inhaling bring your right leg back to the starting position.

Vajrasana is a classical pose. It is used by many yogis for pranayama, or yogic breathing exercises; for the mudras, or internal exercises; and for meditation. Hence even though here we are considering only the vinyasa krama, this does not preclude us from remaining static for such specific exercises. Figure 9-45 is vajrasana with all the bandhas, which are done after a very long and complete exhalation.

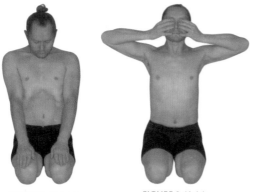

FIGURE 9-45 ◆◆◆   FIGURE 9-46 ◆◆

Figure 9-46 is *shanmukhi mudra* in vajrasana.

Shanmukhi mudra, or closing of all the ports (of senses), with a mudra called shanmukhi. *Shanmukhi* means the six ports, which are the two eyes, two ears, the nose, and the mouth. In the vinyasas krama system this is resorted to as a rest procedure. During the period when you are in this mudra, you will closely watch your breath (but not regulate it) unlike in vinyasa krama or in pranayama.

HERO'S POSE AND MOVEMENTS (VIRASANA)

Next will be vinyasas involving *virasana*, or the hero's pose. This again is a classical posture, mention of it is found in texts like the *Ramayana*. The invocation verse of the great epic Valmiki's *Ramayana* mentions Lord Rama being seated comfortably in virasana.

From the vajrasana position, while inhaling, raise your trunk to the kneeling position. On the next exhalation you may spread your feet, but keep both your knees together (*see figure 9-47*).

Stay in this position for a breath. The rear view is shown in figure 9-48.

Now exhaling slowly, lower your trunk and sit between your feet (*see figure 9-49*).

The rear view is shown in figure 9-50.

During the next exhalation, slowly lower your arms as well, and place your palms on your knees or thighs (*see figure 9-51*).

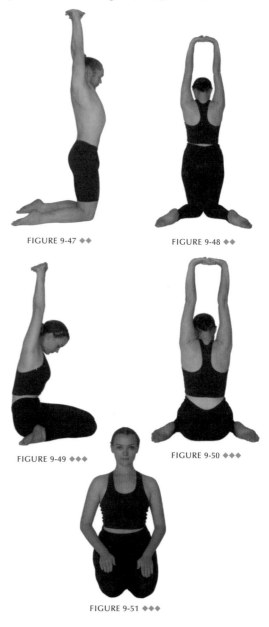

FIGURE 9-47 ◆◆   FIGURE 9-48 ◆◆

FIGURE 9-49 ◆◆◆   FIGURE 9-50 ◆◆◆

FIGURE 9-51 ◆◆◆

This is virasana, or the hero's pose. Stay in this position for six to twelve breaths, keeping your chin in jalandhara bandha *(see figure 9-52)* and doing all the bandhas at the end of each exhalation at least for five seconds. The side view with bandhas is shown in figure 9-53).

Remaining in virasana, while inhaling, extend your arms and interlock your fingers. While you are exhaling, slowly bend forward to place your forehead and your arms on the floor in front of you *(see figure 9-54).*

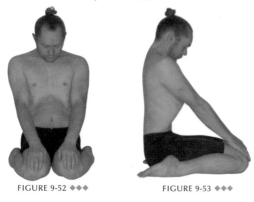

FIGURE 9-52 ◆◆◆   FIGURE 9-53 ◆◆◆

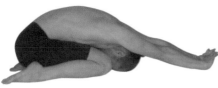

FIGURE 9-54 ◆◆◆

Do not raise your buttocks off the floor. Stay in this position for six breaths. Inhaling, you may return to virasana sthiti.

Stay with your arms still overhead in virasana; as you slowly inhale, round your back slightly and lie down. As you breathe out, lower your arms and place your hands on your thighs. Stay in this position for six long inhalations and exhalations *(see figure 9-55).* Or you may keep your hands on your heels to straighten your back a little more *(see figure 9-56).*

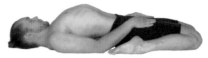

FIGURE 9-55 ◆◆◆

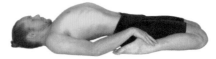

FIGURE 9-56 ◆◆◆

This posture is called *paryankasana,* or the couch pose. Now, holding your breath out, come up to sit in virasana.

It may be easier to go down to or come up from the couch pose by either holding your heels *(see figure 9-57)* or asking someone to hold your hands *(see figure 9-58).*

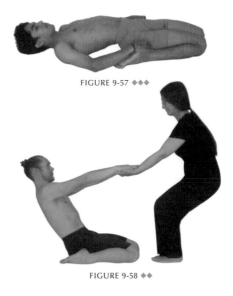

FIGURE 9-57 ◆◆◆

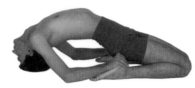

FIGURE 9-58 ◆◆

Holding your heels, while inhaling, arch your back and place your head on the floor *(see figure 9-59).*

FIGURE 9-59 ◆◆◆

This is called *laghu vajrasana* (simple bolt pose). Stay in this position for three to six breaths, and return to paryanksana, or the couch pose. Then return to virasana sthiti on exhalation.

LION POSE (Simhasana)

Inhaling, raise your trunk. While exhaling, cross your legs at your ankles so that your right foot is on the left side and your left foot is on the right side *(see figure 9-60)*.

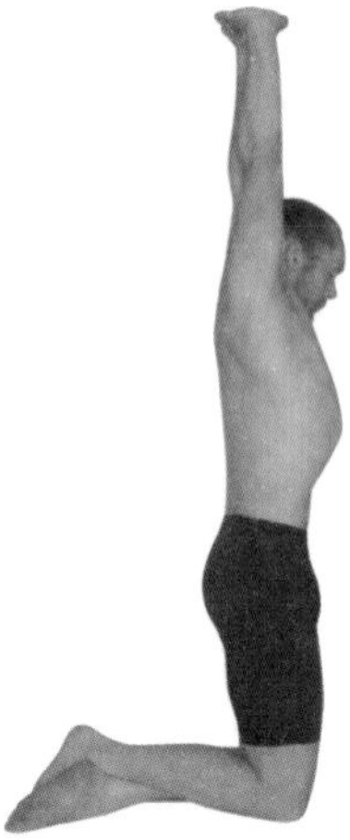

Then as you are exhaling, ease into the posture by sitting right on your heels. Stick your tongue out, look at the middle of your eyebrows, and spread your fingers *(see figure 9-61)*.

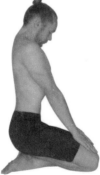

FIGURE 9-60 ◆◆

This is a vinyasa of *simhasana*, or the lion posture. The side view is shown in figure 9-62.

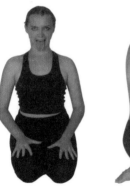

FIGURE 9-61 ◆◆◆   FIGURE 9-62 ◆◆◆

In this pose you may inhale by the ujjayi method, but when you breathe out, stick your tongue out and exhale with a throaty roar—the way that a lion roars. (*A close-up of the face is shown in figure 9-63*). The side view is shown in figure 9-64.

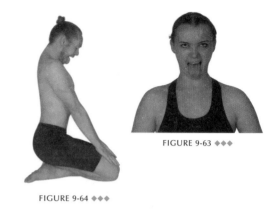

FIGURE 9-63 ◆◆◆

FIGURE 9-64 ◆◆◆

Inhaling, raise your trunk and repeat the pose, switching first your left foot and then your right. After doing the vinyasa, while inhaling, raise your trunk, bring your legs together, and sit down on your heels for vajrasana.

RETURN SEQUENCE

Remaining in vajrasana, lean forward slightly and place your palms by the sides of your bent legs.

Exhale, and hold your breath; pressing down through your palms, lift your body and balance on your hands *(see figure 9-65)*.

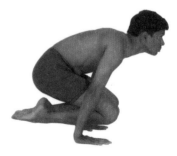

FIGURE 9-65 ◆◆◆

Inhale; hold your breath, and jump back to gently land on your big toes in chaturanga-dandasana (*see figure 9-66*).

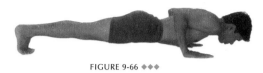

FIGURE 9-66 ◆◆◆

Stay in this position for three breaths.

The next inhalation should be synchronized with the upward, arching movement of your torso, as you press down through your palms (*see figure 9-67*).

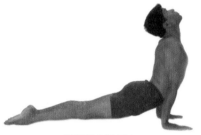

FIGURE 9-67 ◆◆◆

As you know, this is the upward-facing-dog position. With a chin lock, stay in this position for three ujjayi breaths. During the next exhalation, lift your waist, stretch your legs, and flex the dorsa of your feet to reach the downward-facing-dog pose (*see figure 9-68*).

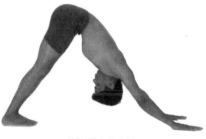

FIGURE 9-68 ◆◆◆

Stay in this position for three breaths.

Exhale, and hold your breath; pressing down through your palms, jump forward to land between your palms. You are now in utkatasana (*see figure 9-69*).

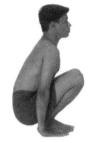

FIGURE 9-69 ◆◆◆

Stay in this position for a few breaths. Inhale; straighten your knees, pressing down through your palms kept close to your feet (*see figure 9-70*).

Stay in this uttanasana position for three breaths. Inhale, and stand up to tadasana (*see figure 9-71*).

On the next exhalation, lower your arms to return to samasthiti (*see figure 9-72*).

FIGURE 9-70 ◆◆◆   FIGURE 9-71 ◆   FIGURE 9-72 ◆

Many yogis, especially women yogis, prefer vajrasana to other seated poses. It is a compact and very effective pose. Your stretched ankles help to act as a nice arch to support your spine. Once your knees and ankles become supple by practicing these past several vinyasas, it will become easy to stay in vajrasana for a long time. Every yogi must try to master a seated pose, vajrasana, virasana, padmasana, or siddhasana, so that other advanced yoga angas (limbs) such as *dhyana*, pranayama, and chanting, can be practiced without the body distracting the mind.

10

THE
LOTUS POSE
SEQUENCE

THE LOTUS POSTURE (padmasana) is considered by conventional yogis to be the most important seated posture. Mention of this posture can be found not merely in old yoga texts but also in epics and other very ancient Indian religious and cultural books. However, many people who do contemporary yoga do not like this posture. Many consider it boring and static and even a pain. Without much emphasis these days on the practice of breathing exercises or meditation, this posture appears unimportant to most people. But if this pose is done according to vinyasa krama, where movements that progressively lead to the posture are done, followed by various elaborations, subsequent counterposes, and the return sequence, it can be a lot more fun. Further, by going through the process of vinyasa krama, the chances of performing the posture without pain for a long period of time are increased considerably. It is a great posture to be in as a yogi and practice some of the subtler aspects of yoga, such as pranayama and meditation. Please pay attention to your breathing, which should be synchronized with the movements. Take at least five seconds each for inhalation and exhalation unless otherwise specified.

THE LEAD SEQUENCE

Per the general procedure adopted in vinyasa krama, start from samasthiti *(see figure 10-1).*

As you inhale, slowly raise your arms overhead and interlock your fingers in tadasana *(see figure 10-2).*

Then exhaling slowly and completely, bend forward to the forward stretch pose (uttanasana). Place your palms beside your feet *(see figure 10-3).*

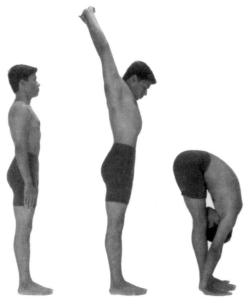

FIGURE 10-1 ◆   FIGURE 10-2 ◆   FIGURE 10-3 ◆◆◆

Breathe out slowly and smoothly and sit on your haunches, with your palms beside your feet. This is the hip stretch, or utkatasana *(see figure 10-4).*

After one or two inhalations and long exhalations, inhale, then hold your breath and jump back gently to land on your toes, stretching your legs in the process *(see figure 10-5).*

Stay in this position for three long, smooth breaths. It is the four-legged staff posture (chaturanga-dandasana).

While inhaling, stretch and lift your torso up to the upward-facing-dog position (urdhwa-mukha-swanasana). *(See figure 10-6.)*

Again stay in this position for three long, smooth breaths.

Now while exhaling long and smoothly, raise your waist and drop your head to do the downward-facing-dog pose (adhomukha swanasana). *(See figure 10-7.)*

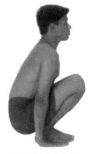

FIGURE 10-4 ◆◆◆

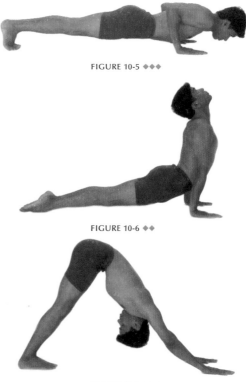

FIGURE 10-5 ◆◆◆

FIGURE 10-6 ◆◆

FIGURE 10-7 ◆◆◆

Again stay in this position for three long inhalations and exhalations. Now exhale, hold your breath, bend your knees slightly, press down through your palms, and jump through the space between your hands. Stay balanced on your palms while keeping your legs stretched. This is *dandasana utpluti* (meaning to lift the body up in staff pose). *(See figure 10-8).*

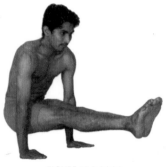

FIGURE 10-8 ◆◆◆◆

Stay in this position for a breath.

Inhale, hold your breath, and ease your body onto the floor. This is the staff pose, or dandasana *(see figure 10-9)*.

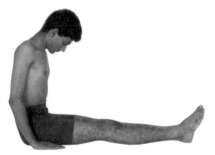

FIGURE 10-9 ◆◆

Stay in dandasana for three to six long inhalations and exhalations.

HALF-LOTUS SUBROUTINE
(ARDHA PADMASANA VINYASAS)

As you exhale, bend your right knee and place your right foot on your left thigh near your groin. Keep your back erect, and stay in this position for three long inhalations and exhalations. This is the first vinyasa in the right half-lotus (*dakshina-ardha-padmasana*) subsequence. Inhaling, raise your arms and stay in this position for another three breaths *(see figure 10-10)*.

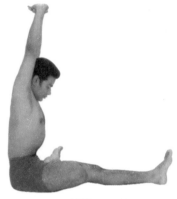

FIGURE 10-10 ◆◆

Slowly (while exhaling), bend forward and place your forehead on your stretched left knee, and stay in the position for three long, smooth breaths *(see figure 10-11)*.

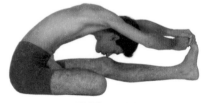

FIGURE 10-11 ◆◆

Inhaling, return to half-lotus position.

As you inhale, raise both arms overhead. During the next exhalation, swing your right arm around your waist and behind your back. Clasp the big toe of your right foot with your right hand (*see figure 10-12*).

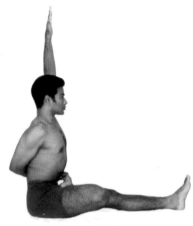

FIGURE 10-12 ◆◆

Stay in this position for three long inhalations and exhalations, stretching your spine on every inhalation. This position is known as locked half-lotus pose (*ardha-baddha-padmasana*).

After three breaths, while slowly exhaling, stretch your back and bend forward, placing your forehead on your left knee (*see figure 10-13*).

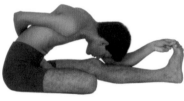

FIGURE 10-13 ◆◆◆

Stay in this position for three to six breaths. During every exhalation, try to stretch your back. Hold your breath for five seconds after exhalation, and do rectal and abdominal locks (mula bandha and uddiyana bandha).

Now exhaling, lean back slightly and place your left palm (turned out by 90 degrees) on the floor about a foot behind

you. Your right hand should still be holding the big toe of your right foot, placed on your left thigh. As you inhale, press down through your left hand, anchor the outside of your left foot, tilt your body to the left side, and lift your body, especially raising your hips. As you reach the posture, turn your head and look up (*see figure 10-14*).

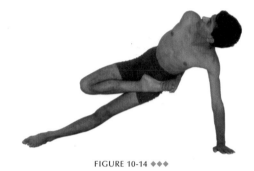

FIGURE 10-14 ◆◆◆

This posture is known as Kashyapasana, or ardha-baddha-padma Vasishtasana. This is a very effective posture, enabling a lateral movement and stretch of your hip. Stay in this position for six breaths, nudging your tailbone laterally up a little bit more on every inhalation. Return to the starting position on exhalation.

Stay in the same ardha-baddha-padmasana position. Exhaling, lean forward and clasp the inside of your left foot with your left hand. Holding your left foot firmly, and slowly inhaling, turn or twist your body to the right and look over your right shoulder. Stay in this position for a few breaths. Return to the starting position on exhalation. This is another a variant of half-kingfish pose (ardha Matsyendrasana). (*See figure 10-15*).

Next is another variant of ardha Matsyendrasana. Inhaling, raise both arms overhead as in the ardha padmasana position. Keep exhaling, lean forward, and clasp the outside of your left foot with your right hand. Then inhale; as you exhale, twist to the left side and clasp your right thigh with your left hand, swung from behind your back *(see figure 10-16).*

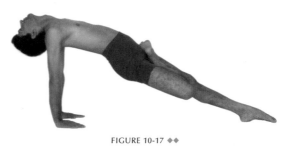

FIGURE 10-17 ◆◆

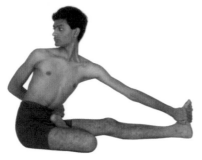

FIGURE 10-15 ◆◆

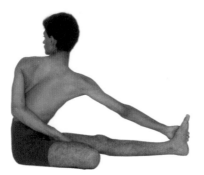

FIGURE 10-16 ◆◆

Stay in this position for three breaths, turning even more on every exhalation. Inhale and return to the half-lotus position.

Now for the counterpose, or prathikriya, in half-lotus. Inhaling, raise both arms overhead. As you keep breathing out, lean back a little and place both your hands behind your back, about a foot away, on the floor. Your fingers should be pointing toward you, with your palms turned inward. As you inhale, slowly press down through your palms. Raise your hip while stretching your left ankle to place your left foot on the floor *(see figure 10-17).*

Exhaling, return to the starting point and repeat the movement three times. Stretch your right leg straight to return to the dandasana position.

This time, while you exhale, slowly, bend your left knee, stretch your left ankle fully, and place the outer edge of your left foot on your right thigh close to your groin. Inhaling, raise both arms overhead. This position is *vama-ardha-padmasana* (left half-lotus pose) *(see figure 10-18).*

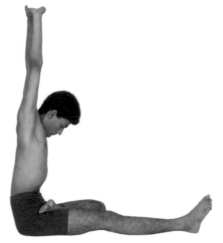

FIGURE 10-18 ◆◆

Stay in this position for a few breaths; adjust your left leg in the posture so that you feel comfortable and well anchored. Your buttock bones should be firmly placed. As you exhale slowly and smoothly, stretch your back and bend forward, hold your right foot with your left hand and place your right hand on top of it. Place your head on your stretched right knee. Stay in this position for three to six breaths, making the exhalation as complete as possible. During every exhalation try to stretch forward and bring your body down lower. You may use the bandhas, or locks, after exhalation and when holding your breath out. This is *vama-ardha-padma paschmatanasana* (left half-lotus posterior-stretch posture). *(See figure 10-19.)*

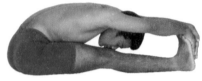

FIGURE 10-19 ◆◆

As you slowly inhale, stretch your arms overhead. Then during the next slow exhalation, swing your left arm behind your back and firmly clasp the big toe of your left foot. Keep your back straight, and stay in this position for three long breaths. *(see figure 10-20).*

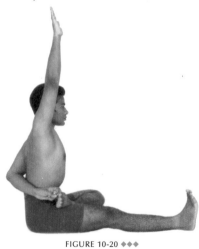

FIGURE 10-20 ◆◆◆

This posture is left-tied-half-lotus posture (vama-ardha-baddha-padmasana).

Then, inhale and while exhaling smoothly and slowly, stretch your back and bend forward. Place your forehead on your stretched left knee or beyond it. You may stay in this position for a few breaths, concentrating on making the exhalation long, smooth, and as complete as possible. After some practice, you may attempt to do rectal and abdominal locks after exhalation and while holding your breath out. This has a long name, vama-ardha-baddha-padma-paschima-uttanasana. Translated, it is left-side-tied, half-lotus posterior stretch posture *(see figure 10-21).*

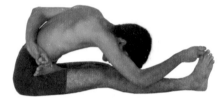

FIGURE 10-21 ◆◆◆

Exhaling, place your right palm, (turned out 90 degrees) on the floor at about a foot behind you. Your left hand should be holding your big toe of your left foot, placed on your right thigh. As you inhale, press down through your right hand and the outside of your right foot, tilt your body to the right side, and raise your body, especially lifting your hips. As you achieve the posture, turn your head and look up *(see figures 10-22 and 10-23).*

This posture is known as Kashyapasana, or ardha-baddha-padma Vasishtasana. This is a very useful posture effecting lateral movement of and stretching your hip. Stay in this position for a few breaths, pushing your body up a little bit on every inhalation. Return to the starting position on exhalation.

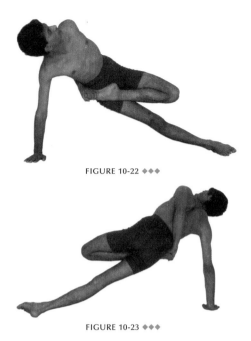

FIGURE 10-22 ◆◆◆

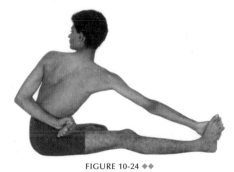

FIGURE 10-23 ◆◆◆

Now in the ardha baddha padmasana position, while exhaling, lean forward and clasp the inside of your right foot with your right hand. Holding your right foot firmly and inhaling slowly, turn or twist your body to the left side and look over your left shoulder. Stay in this position for a few breaths. Return to the starting position on exhalation. This is also a variant of ardha Matsyendrasana or the half-kingfish pose (*see figure 10-24*).

FIGURE 10-24 ◆◆

Inhaling, raise both arms overhead. During the exhalation, slowly turn to your right side; swinging your right from behind your back, clasp your left thigh. Inhale, and as you slowly exhale, lean forward slightly and clasp the outside of your outstretched right foot with your left hand. Turn and look over your right shoulder (*see figure 10-25*).

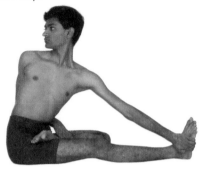

FIGURE 10-25 ◆◆

Stay in this position for three breaths, twisting your trunk a little more on each exhalation. This is another vinyasa of half-Matsyendrasana. Inhaling, return to asana sthiti.

Now for the counterpose. Exhaling, place both your palms (turned inward) behind your back on the floor about a foot away from your body. While you are inhaling slowly, press down through your palms and lift your body up as much as you can. As you complete the movement during inhalation, stretch your right ankle and place your right foot on the floor. Of course, your right knee should remain outstretched and straight (*see figure 10-26*).

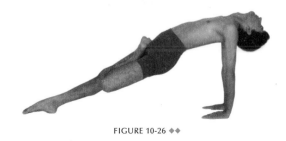

FIGURE 10-26 ◆◆

There are a number of postures done with the half-lotus position while standing, lying down, in a headstand, in a shoulder stand, and so on. To prepare for the lotus pose, these vinyasas should be practiced so that your legs are in better condition to proceed. All the vinyasas discussed up to now are preparatory vinyasas for the lotus posture. They also form part of the asymmetric seated pose sequence.

THE LOTUS POSE (PADMASANA)

The next vinyasa is the lotus pose. Keep your legs outstretched in the staff pose. Exhaling, lean forward, grab your right foot, bend your right knee, and place your right foot on your left thigh near your groin. Stay in this position for one or two breaths and then once again as you exhale, slightly lean forward clasp your left foot, bend your left leg, and place your left foot on your right thigh (*see figure 10-27*).

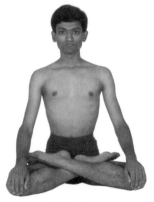

FIGURE 10-27 ◆◆

Try to stay in this position for a few breaths. Repeat the procedure at least six times. Over time, you may develop the ability to stay in this position for a considerable amount of time.

Now the vinyasas in padmasana can be practiced. The first one is a nice stretch to the spine called *parvatasana*, or the hill pose. Inhaling in lotus pose, lift your arms overhead and interlock your fingers. Keep your chin locked (*see figure 10-28*).

Stay in this position for a long time, doing long ujjayi inhalations and exhalations. Exhaling, lower your arms, returning to the lotus position.

From parvatasana, while exhaling, lower your arms, turning your palms inward, and place your palms on your thigh close to your groin. Press your palms against your thighs and stretch your back while you are inhaling. Stay in this position for three to six breaths. This posture known as *bhadrasana* (peaceful pose or auspicious pose) helps to stretch your spine still more (*see figure 10-29*).

In a slightly different vinyasa, bhadrasana is done with the hands on the thighs but closer to the knees (*see figure 10-30*).

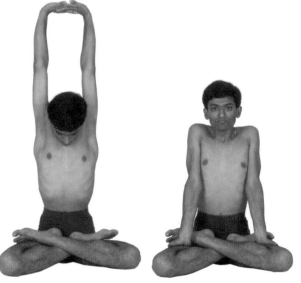

FIGURE 10-28 ◆◆   FIGURE 10-29 ◆◆◆

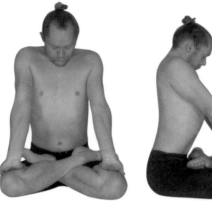

FIGURE 10-30 ◆◆◆   FIGURE 10-31 ◆◆◆

Stay in this position for three to six breaths. The side view is shown in figure 10-31.

Because there is space available for the abdomen to move as a result of the stretching of the spine, this pose is ideal for doing the three bandhas effectively. At the end of every exhalation, hold your breath out and draw in your rectal and abdominal muscles (mula and uddiyana bandhas). Maintain the bandhas for the duration of your external breath holding (*bahya kumbhaka*). Maintain the chin lock as well (jalandhara bandha). The posture with the bandhas, or locks, is shown in figure 10-32, and the side view is shown in figure 10-33.

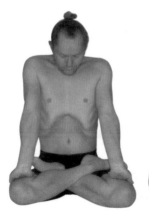

FIGURE 10-32 ◆◆◆   FIGURE 10-33 ◆◆◆

Return to parvatasana, or the hill pose, on inhalation. Then as you very slowly and smoothly exhale, with a rubbing sensation in your throat (ujjayi), stretch your back, bend forward, and place your face on the floor (*see figure 10-34*).

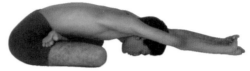

FIGURE 10-34 ◆◆◆

Stay in this position for three to six breaths. During every exhalation try to stretch a little more. Also practice rectal and abdominal locks during bahya kumbhaka. This is known as the simple yoga seal (*laghu yoga mudra*). Because the heels press against the lower abdomen, along with the stomach lock, this massages the internal abdominal area. It is an effective procedure to tone up the pelvic and abdominal organs. As you are inhaling, return to the hill pose.

Remaining in the hill pose, make one or two long inhalations and exhalations. Exhaling, slowly lower your arms and place your palms on the floor by your sides. Exhale completely, and hold your breath out. Pressing down with your hands, lift your body, and while doing so, bend forward by folding the pelvic joint (*see figure 10-35*).

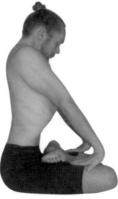

FIGURE 10-34 ◆◆◆◆

This is yoga mudra, but with your body in air. The lifting procedure is called utpluti.

Inhaling, return to starting position, which in this case, is the hill pose. Now do three long inhalations and exhalations. While you are very slowly exhaling, turn to your right by about 45 degrees, and bend down, placing your head on the floor (see figure 10-36).

Stay in this position for three long inhalations and exhalations, being especially careful that your exhalations are long. Again do the locks after exhalation. This is again a good exercise for the abdominal organs, especially those on the right side. This is a right-side simple yoga seal (*dakshina-parsva laghu yoga mudra*).

Inhaling, return to the hill pose. Then as you exhale smoothly, stretch, turn to the left, and bend down and forward. Place your forehead on the floor, and stay in this position for three to six long breaths (see figure 10-37).

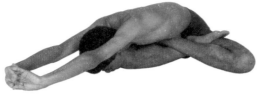

FIGURE 10-36 ◆◆

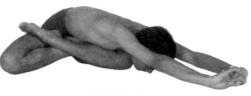

FIGURE 10-37 ◆◆

This is *vama-parsva laghu yoga mudra*, or the left-side simple yoga seal.

Next you may consider doing the classical padmasana, which is also known as *baddha padmasana*, or the locked lotus

pose. Some texts assert that only this position should be called the lotus pose. From the hill pose, while exhaling, swing your arms behind your back one at a time, cross your hands, and clasp the big toes of the opposite feet. Open your chest cavity, lift your heart, and do three to six long inhalations and exhalations (see figure 10-38).

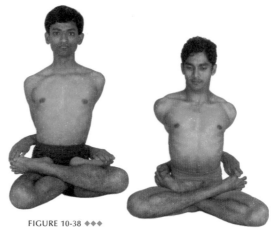

FIGURE 10-38 ◆◆◆

FIGURE 10-39 ◆◆◆

The same pose with right leg on top is shown in figure 10-39.

Concentrate on slow smooth inhalations, doing ujjayi with a chin lock. You may practice all the locks in this posture. The side view is shown in figure 10-40.

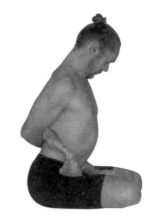

FIGURE 10-40 ◆◆◆

The rear view of this important pose is shown in figure 10-41 so that you will know how to correctly position your hands.

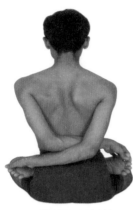

FIGURE 10-41 ◆◆◆

Stay in baddha padmasana. Slowly exhaling, bend forward and place your head or forehead on the floor. Stay in this position for three to six breaths (*see figure 10-42*).

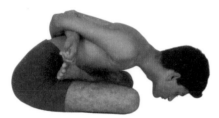

FIGURE 10-42 ◆◆◆

While you are inhaling, return to the starting point. This is yoga mudra, or the seal of yoga (yoga mudra).

Remain seated in baddha padmasana. As you very slowly and smoothly exhale, turn your torso to the right side by about 45 degrees, and continuing your exhalation stretch your back and bend down and place your face on the floor (*see figure 10-43*).

This is *dakshina-parsva yoga mudra*—the right-side yoga seal. Stay in this position for several inhalations and exhalations. You

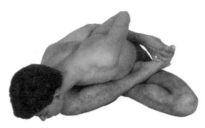

FIGURE 10-43 ◆◆◆

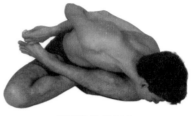

FIGURE 10-44 ◆◆◆

may practice the locks after exhalation. Return to the starting position on a slow, smooth inhalation.

This may be repeated on the left side now. From the baddha pamasana position, while deeply exhaling, turn your torso to left side by about 45 degrees, and continuing your exhalation, bend down to touch the floor with your head (*see figure 10-44*).

Stay in this position for several breaths, concentrating on comprehensive exhalation. These yoga mudras help you to achieve complete exhalation (*recaka bala*) and practice of the three bandhas; your heels help to gently massage your abdomen. All these factors are very useful to stimulate the pelvic organs.

You have done a number of postures bending forward. Now it may be good to do a back-bending vinyasa, while still in lotus pose. Inhaling, slowly lift your arms overhead laterally and interlock you fingers as in the hill pose. Then while you are exhaling, lower your arms to place your palms on the floor about a foot behind you. As you inhale slowly, press down through your palms, and anchoring your knees, slowly lift your body especially your hip as high as you can, arching your spine in the process *(see figure 10-45)*.

Exhaling, you may return to the starting point. Repeat the movement three to six times. This is the upward-facing-lotus pose (*urdhwa-mukha padmasana*). This counterpose can be used whenever you have done a number of forward bends in padmasana sthiti, and you think a counterpose movement is needed.

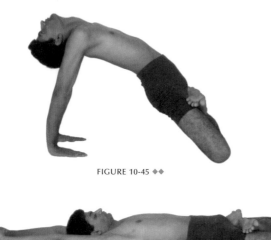

FIGURE 10-45 ◆◆

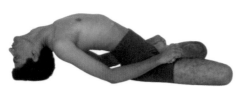

FIGURE 10-46 ◆◆

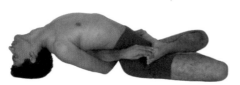

FIGURE 10-47 ◆◆◆

FIGURE 10-48 ◆◆◆

Some rest? Okay. From the hill pose position, as you inhale, slowly round your back. Slowly lie down, curving your back, and keeping your legs still in the lotus position *(see figure 10-46)*.

Stay in this position for six long inhalations and exhalation. This is the reclining lotus pose (*supta padmasana*).

Then you can practice the well-known fish pose. As you are in the reclining lotus pose, exhale, place your palms on the floor (fingers facing downward) below your shoulder blades. While you are inhaling, press down through your palms, lift your torso, arch your spine, and place your crown on the floor, with your upper body forming a nice arch between your head and your anchored buttock bones. The top of your head and your buttocks bones act as pivots. Place your hands on your thighs or, better yet, hold your toes *(see figure 10-47)*.

Stay in this position for six long inhalations and exhalations. This is a good opportunity to open up your thorax, so you should concentrate on very relaxed smooth inhalation. Support your back by placing your palms once again on the floor, and while exhaling return to the reclining lotus position.

The same posture can be done holding your toes from behind your back, as in baddha padmasana. This is more difficult, but helps to open your chest even more *(see figure 10-48)*.

The procedure is the same as for the king-fish pose explained in the preceding vinyasa. Another method of reaching the posture is to start from baddha padmasana and while inhaling arch your back and place your head on the floor. This is definitely a very involved procedure. Some people use the fish pose as a counterpose for the shoulder stand. But the general rule is that the counterpose should be a relatively simple pose, and the fish pose is a very involved pose. There are other postures and vinyasas that will do the job of relieving the strain in the neck from shoulder stand practice.

From supta padmasana, inhale, and after completing a very long exhalation, hold your breath, press through your arms, and lift your body to a shoulder stand. This posture is also known as urdhwa padmasana, or the lifted-up lotus pose (see figure 10-49).

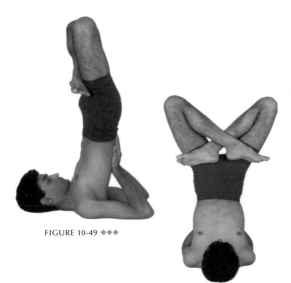

FIGURE 10-49 ◆◆◆

FIGURE 10-50 ◆◆◆

Stay in this position for a very long time, concentrating on long, smooth exhalations, at the end of which all the three locks can be very effectively employed. The front view is shown in figure 10-50.

You may have wondered why this leg position is called the lotus. The position of the legs looks like a lotus flower, and the two feet resemble two petals hanging.

From urdhwa padmasana position, as you slowly exhale, bend your waist and bring your legs in lotus position close to your chest; stay in this position for three long inhalations and exhalations (see figure 10-51).

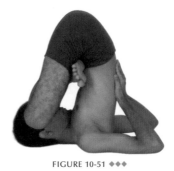

FIGURE 10-51 ◆◆◆

This is *akunchita urdhwa padmasana* (the drooping lotus pose).

Remaining in the same pose, exhale, hold your breath, lower your legs in the lotus position further down by rounding your back, embrace your legs with both hands, and clasp your hands (see figure 10-52).

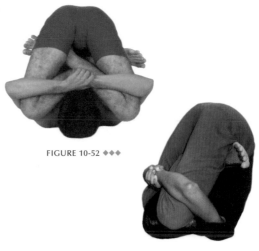

FIGURE 10-52 ◆◆◆

FIGURE 10-53 ◆◆◆

Figure 10-53 shows another view, indicating how close your thighs can get to your upper body.

Stay in this position for six breaths, tightening the noose on every exhalation. This pose is the fetus pose (pindasana). The side view is shown in figure 10-54.

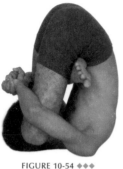

FIGURE 10-54 ◆◆◆

While you are inhaling, return to upward lotus position.

Remaining in urdhwa padmasana, while slowly exhaling, twist your body to the right. Stay in this position for three long inhalations and exhalations (see figure 10-55).

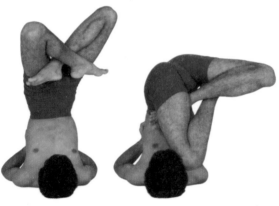

FIGURE 10-55 ◆◆◆   FIGURE 10-56 ◆◆◆

Inhale, and as you exhale slowly lower your lower extremities to the left side. Again stay in this position for three long, smooth breaths (see figure 10-56).

Inhaling, return to urdhwa padmasana. Then while you are exhaling, twist your waist, and turn as much as possible to the

left side. Stay in this position for three long breaths (see figure 10-57).

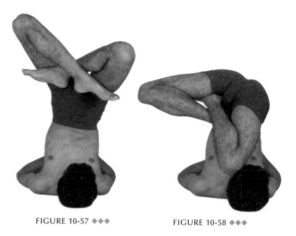

FIGURE 10-57 ◆◆◆   FIGURE 10-58 ◆◆◆

Inhale, and on the next exhalation lower your lower extremities to the left side (see figure 10-58).

Stay in this position for six long inhalations and exhalations. Then as you inhale return to urdhwa padmasana.

Because you have done a lot of forward bending by now, a simple back bend in urdhwa padmasana can be performed as a counterposition. Stay in the posture and as you are inhaling and supporting your low back, bend back from your waist, maintaining the lotus position (see figure 10-59).

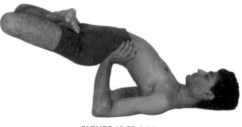

FIGURE 10-59 ◆◆◆

Stay in this position for three breaths. Alternately, you may bring your legs down to akunchita padmasana, and then on the following inhalation move to this counter-pose (pratikriya).

In the next move, while exhaling, lower your trunk to akunchita urdhwa pad-masana (*see figure 10-60*).

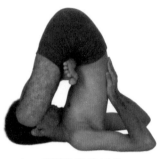

FIGURE 10-60 ◆◆◆\

Now as you are inhaling, stretch your arms overhead on the floor—you are still in the shoulder stand but with your legs in the lotus position (*see figure 10-61*).

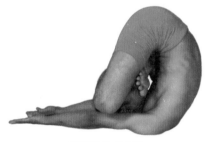

FIGURE 10-61 ◆◆◆

Completely exhaling, hold your breath. Roll down to the floor, to the reclining lotus position, then sit up in a mountain pose in lotus. In the same continuous movement, lean forward, and supported by your hands, lie down prone on the floor, with your legs still in the lotus position (*see figure 10-62*).

This is known as *adho mukha pad-masana*, or the downward-facing-lotus position.

Inhaling, stretch your arms overhead and keep your hands in anjali, or prayer position (*see figure 10-63*).

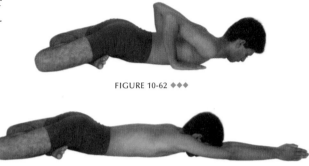

FIGURE 10-62 ◆◆◆

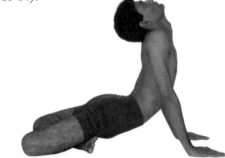

FIGURE 10-63 ◆◆

This pose is known as *padma danda namaskara*, or the surrender (sticklike) salutation in lotus.

Now bring your arms down, place your palms close to your chest. Then inhaling, arch your back by pressing down through your palms and anchoring your knees (*see figure 10-64*).

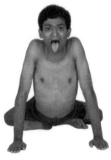

FIGURE 10-64 ◆◆◆

This is the lotus-cobra posture (*padma bhujangasana*).

Remaining in the same position, keep your back straight. Exhaling, stick your tongue out (*see figure 10-65*).

FIGURE 10-65 ◆◆◆

Inhale, and on the next exhalation, breathe out hoarsely through your throat like a lion roaring. This is a variation of lion pose, or simhasana. You may focus your attention on the middle of your eyebrows, squinting like the lion's eyes. Exhaling, return to the simple yoga mudra position by pressing down with your palms, pulling back, and lowering your body to the floor. As you are inhaling, return to the lotus position.

This time, while inhaling, raise your arms overhead and interlock your fingers as in the hill pose. Stay in this position for one breath. Then as you smoothly exhale, slowly turn to the right side. Stay in this position for a breath. On the next exhalation, lower your arms and place your intertwined palms on the floor next to your right thigh (see figure 10-66).

Stay in this position for three long inhalations and exhalations. This posture is known as Bharadwajasana, named after an ancient Vedic sage. During every exhalation—which should be long and smooth—bearing your body down and anchoring your palms, twist to the left side. After three breaths, return to the hill pose as you are slowly inhaling.

Again from the hill pose with your fingers interlocked, while you are exhaling, turn to left side. Stay in this position for a breath, and during the following exhalation, lower your arms and place your hands on the floor close to your left thigh. Exhaling, twist your trunk and your head to the right, anchoring your palms and your buttock bones well (see figure 10-67).

Stay in this position for three breaths, then return to the hill pose on inhalation. This is Bharadwajasana.

Now for some fun vinyasas. In the lotus position, keep your palms by your sides. Keep your back straight, and stay in this position for three long inhalations and exhalations. Then, after a very complete smooth exhalation, hold your breath out, and pressing down through your palms (without pushing your shoulders up), lift your trunk and balance on both hands. If you can, you may stay in this position for three breaths (see figure 10-68).

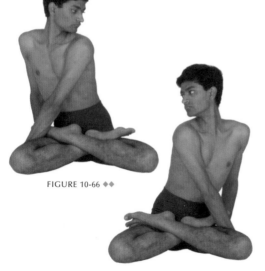

FIGURE 10-66 ◆◆

FIGURE 10-67 ◆◆

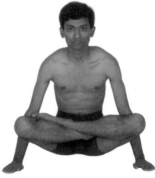

FIGURE 10-68 ◆◆◆

This is *tolangulasana*, or the balance pose in lotus. This is also called utpluti, or the pumping (lifting) vinyasa in lotus pose. The side view is shown in figure 10-69 and the view with all the bandhas in the posture is shown in figure 10-70.

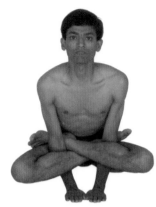

FIGURE 10-71 ◆◆◆◆

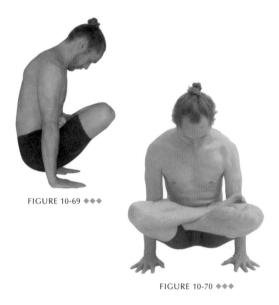

FIGURE 10-69 ◆◆◆

FIGURE 10-70 ◆◆◆

Spread your arms wider. You may choose to swing forward and backward with your body in the air—this is the swing pose (*lolasana*).

Next is another pumping or lifting pose. While in lotus, as you exhale slowly, insert your hands between the thigh and calf muscles of each leg, and place your palms on the floor. Stay in this position for a long breath. Then after a long exhalation, hold your breath, and by pressing your hands, lift your body up and stay in this position for a few breaths, balancing on your hands with your body lifted up (*see figure 10-71*).

This is the rooster pose (*kukkutasana*).

The next pose is a bit more involved. From the previous pose, sit back, balancing on the bones of your buttocks. As you keep

exhaling, stick your arms further out, until your elbows are pushed outside your legs. Slowly bend your elbows, hold your chin, and look forward (*see figure 10-72*).

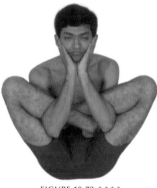

FIGURE 10-72 ◆◆◆◆

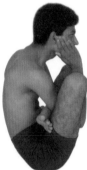

FIGURE 10-72 ◆◆◆◆

Stay in this position for a few breaths. The inhalations will be brief, but you should try to exhale as completely as possible. During every exhalation, you should try to narrow the gap between your upper body and your lower extremities. This is the fetus-in-the-womb pose (*garbha pindasana*). The side view is shown in figure 10-73.

While slowly exhaling, try to close the gap between your torso and your lower extremities by holding the back of your head. Again, stay in this position for three to six breaths, closing the gap between the upper and lower parts of your body on every exhalation (see figure 10-74).

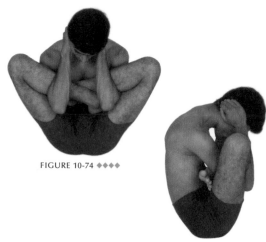

FIGURE 10-74 ♦♦♦♦

FIGURE 10-75 ♦♦♦♦

The side view is shown in figure 10-75.

When there is virtually no gap then, this is *purna garbha pindasana* (complete fetus pose). Further, the position of the hands around the neck resembles the chord around the neck of a fetus (see figure 10-76).

The side view is shown in figure 10-77).

You can see in figure 10-78 that there is no gap between the torso and the legs and that the flexion of the whole spine is complete, with the neck also bent and forming a smooth curve with the rest of the spine.

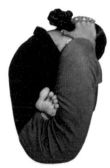

FIGURE 10-78 ♦♦♦♦♦

This posture, among a few other poses, is said to be an effective contraceptive. It could be practiced once a day.

Now from the previous fetus pose, without taking your hands off your neck, exhale, hold your breath, gently rock back, and lie on your back. You will rock once or twice on the floor and will settle to another posture, the upturned-turtle pose (*uttana-kurmasana*). (See figure 10-79.)

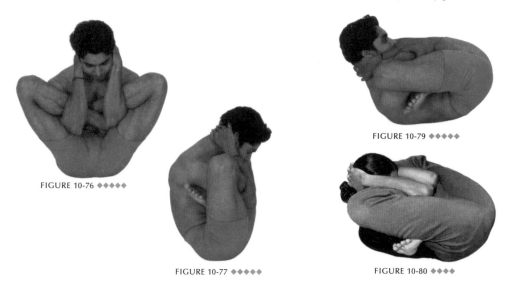

FIGURE 10-76 ♦♦♦♦♦

FIGURE 10-77 ♦♦♦♦♦

FIGURE 10-79 ♦♦♦♦♦

FIGURE 10-80 ♦♦♦♦

The posture looks like a "turned turtle." A well-compacted version of the posture is shown in figure 10-80.

Stay in this position for a few breaths. Then slowly release your head and pull your hands out of the tangle and stretch them overhead, as you inhale deeply, while stretching your waist to supta padmasana. Now raise your arms and interlock your fingers as you inhale *(see figure 10-81)*.

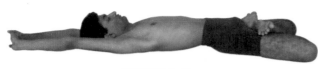

FIGURE 10-81 ♦♦

Bend your waist, exhale, hold your breath, and sit up to the hill pose *(see figure 10-82)*.

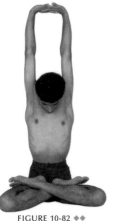

FIGURE 10-82 ♦♦

So far we have seen a number of vinyasas leading to the lotus pose and a number of others in which the integrity of the lotus pose is maintained while the body is manipulated (of course with the appropriate breathing). Some other well-known postures, such as the shoulder stand, were also demonstrated. Now we will see a few more

of the vinyasas of lotus in another classic posture, the headstand. These hybrid vinyasas, such as urdhwa padmasana, can be considered vinyasas of both the lotus pose and the headstand. However, they are determined to belong to one group or the other according to the approach used to enter them. Thus, when you move from the lotus pose to the headstand, it is a vinyasa of the lotus pose and included in the lotus sequence (vinyasas krama). However, as you could surmise, if the lotus position is entered while in the headstand, it would form part of the headstand sequence. Thus the postures may look the same, but the approaches could vary.

LOTUS SPECIAL BALANCING POSES

First, we will look at some special balancing poses that evolved from the lotus position.

From the lotus pose, keep your hands in front of you. While holding your breath after exhalation and pressing down with your palms, lift your body up and bring it close or abutting to your shoulders *(see figure 10-83)*.

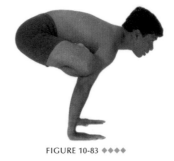

FIGURE 10-83 ♦♦♦♦

This is the jumping rooster pose (urdhwa-kukkutasana).

Again from lotus position, place your palms on the floor about a foot in front of you. Your palms should be turned inward with your fingers facing toward you. Press down through your palms, raise your buttocks, and stand on your knees with your palms still on the floor. Exhale completely, hold your breath out, and slowly lift the lower portion of your body and balance on your hands. Look straight ahead (*see figure 10-84*).

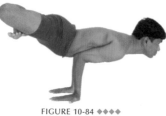

FIGURE 10-84 ◆◆◆◆

Stay in this position for three to six breaths. This is known as the lotus-peacock pose (*padma-mayurasana*). Exhaling, you may return to the lotus position.

In this variation, instead of keeping your palms flat on the ground, place only your fingers on the floor, but keep your thumb bent and pressed against the floor. Some prefer this variation because they get a better grip on the floor (*see figure 10-85*).

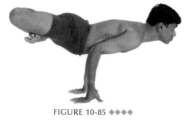

FIGURE 10-85 ◆◆◆◆

Stay in this position for three to six breaths, then return to the lotus position while slowly exhaling.

LOTUS IN HEADSTAND
(URDHWA PADMA SIRSASANA)

Now for a brief subroutine in *padma sirsasana*, or lotus-headstand. From the lotus position, while you are exhaling, lean forward and place your interlaced hands on the floor about a foot in front of you. Then exhaling and rounding your back well, move the lower portion of your body close to the rest of your body. This is the starting position for padma sirsasana, also known as *urdhwa padmasana* (*see figure 10-86*).

The next step is the important one. Do three long inhalations and exhalations. Now after exhalation is over, hold your breath out, then anchoring your elbows and tightening your rectal and abdominal muscles or doing a mild version of the two bandhas, gently shift your weight to your arms, especially your elbows. Your legs in the lotus position will be very close to your body and your knees barely off the ground (*see figure 10-87*).

Observe how you balance in this position. Stay in this position for three long inhalations and exhalations. This position is called the contracted upward lotus pose (*akunchita urdhwa padmasana*).

Now inhaling slowly, lift the lower portion of your body halfway up, keeping it

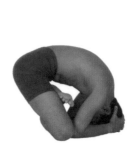

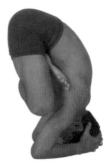

FIGURE 10-86 ◆◆◆   FIGURE 10-87 ◆◆◆◆

very close to the rest of your body (*see figure 10-88*).

Stay in this position for three inhalations. This pose is the inverted yoga seal (*viparita yoga mudra*). We have already seen the normal yoga mudra, which is a seated vinyasa, not vertical as in this case. Stay in this position for three long inhalations and exhalations. Be fully aware of the posture, observe the "feeling" of balance and smooth breathing.

This time, as you slowly inhale, stretch and straighten your waist and bring your lower extremities in the lotus position straight up (*see figure 10-89*).

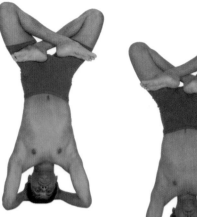

FIGURE 10-90 ◆◆◆

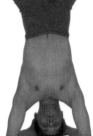

FIGURE 10-91 ◆◆◆

While in urdhwa padmasana, slowly twist to the right as you exhale (*see figure 10-92*).

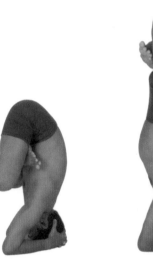

FIGURE 10-88 ◆◆◆   FIGURE 10-89 ◆◆◆

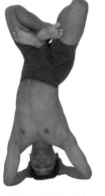

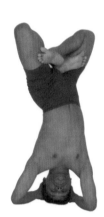

FIGURE 10-92 ◆◆◆

FIGURE 10-93 ◆◆◆

This is urdhwa padmasana, or the upright lotus pose. Stay in this position for six to twelve breaths, or even more. This is a pose in which one should stay for a considerable length of time. The front view is shown in figure 10-90).

Figure 10-91 shows the same pose but with the position of the leg changed.

Stay in this position for three breaths, turning a little more on every exhalation.

You may repeat the same movement on the left side (*see figure 10-93*).

Return to urdhwa padmasana as you slowly inhale.

HANDSTANDS AND BALANCING VINYASAS WITH LOTUS

One more variation. Here you change the way you keep your forearms. Instead of keeping your hands around your head, now, release the interlock and place both forearms on the floor parallel to each other. Now as you inhale, press through your forearms. Lift your body, arch your spine, and also bend back your waist (*see figure 10-94*).

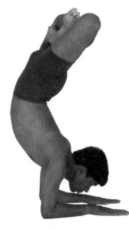

FIGURE 10-94 ◆◆◆◆

The posture is the stretched (feathers) lotus-peacock pose (padma pinchamayurasana). Stay in this position for three breaths and return to urdhwa padmasana, and revert your hand position.

To return to padmasana, step by step lower your trunk by rounding your back, while on exhalation. Then lower your body and place your knees on the floor. Then anchoring your knees and forearms, return to padmasana, while simultaneously inhaling.

At the completion of this sequence, stretch your legs as you inhale and sit in the staff pose (dandasana). (*See figure 10-95.*)

Stay in this position for six long inhalations and exhalations, and then lie down and rest in savasana.

After rest get back to the staff pose (dandasana) to return to samasthiti.

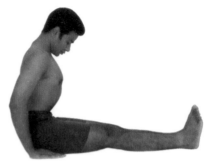

FIGURE 10-95 ◆◆

While in dandasana, slightly, bend forward and place your palms on the floor beside your thighs. Hold your breath after a short inhalation, and lift your body off the floor by pressing dow through your palms (*see figure 10-96*).

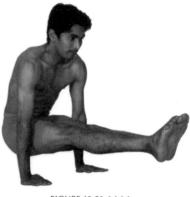

FIGURE 10-96 ◆◆◆◆

Balance yourself carefully for a moment. Exhale, hold your breath, and bend your knees back (*see figure 10-97*).

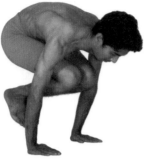

FIGURE 10-97 ◆◆◆◆

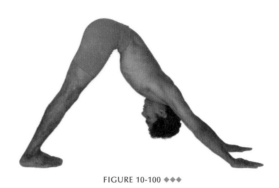

FIGURE 10-100 ◆◆◆

Inhale hold your breath and kick your legs back in the air to land gently on your toes. This is four-legged the staff pose *(see figure 10-98)*.

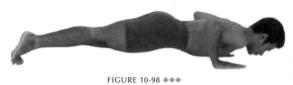

FIGURE 10-98 ◆◆◆

Stay in this position for a breath. Inhaling, arch your back and press your pelvis down. You are now in upward-facing-dog position *(see figure 10-99)*.

Stay in this position for three breaths, doing the bandhas at the end of each exhalation. Exhale, hold your breath, and gently hop so that you land between your planted palms. You are now in utkatasana *(see figure 10-101)*.

Keep your chin down and do three ujjayi breaths. During the next inhalation, straighten your knees as you press down through your palms and feet to get to uttanasana *(see figure 10-102)*.

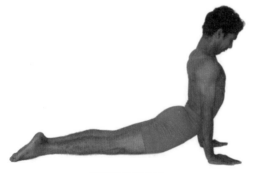

FIGURE 10-99 ◆◆◆

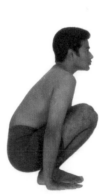

· FIGURE 10-101 ◆◆◆

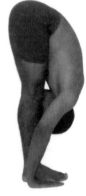

FIGURE 10-102 ◆◆◆

With the chin lock you may do three ujjayi breaths. On the next exhalation, raise your hips to get to the downward-facing-dog pose *(see figure 10-100)*.

Stay in this position for three breaths. Next inhalation, raise your arms, interlock your fingers and stand up to tadasana vinyasa *(see figure 10-103)*.

Exhaling, lower your arms to samasthiti *(see figure 10-104)*.

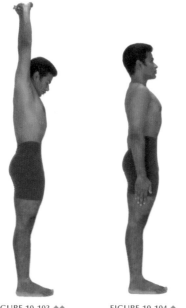

FIGURE 10-103 ◆◆   FIGURE 10-104 ◆

The lotus series is a beautiful sequence. With your lower extremities completely locked, the other parts of your body are exercised in several positions. Bending forward, twisting, bending back, jumping, and inversions are all included in the series. With good, controlled coordinated breathing, your mind will be totally engrossed in the exercise routine, making your mind ever more calm and focused.

11

VISESHA VINYASA KRAMAS

THERE ARE SEVERAL subroutines in the overall vinyasa methodology. These subroutines, which are more commonly practiced, include the sun salutation and several sequences stemming from the downward-facing-dog position, an important hub pose. We will look at some of the important sequences in this chapter. They can be practiced independently.

SUN SALUTATION

This is a very popular exercise. But different schools practice it with some variations. In vinyasa krama:

- There are twelve vinyasas.
- Each movement should be done with the correct breathing.
- Normally mantras are used. They are to be chanted, heard, or mentally recited while holding one's breath in or out as the case may be. You may do the exercise without the mantras, but during the time allotted for the mantra, you must hold your breath preferably for the time needed to chant the mantra. When you do the mantra for the sun salutation (*samantraka-suryanamaskara*), it is chanted at the end of a particular movement and when holding your breath (*kumbhaka*). So, at the time the mantra is recited, there is no movement of the body and no movement of the breath. The mind focuses on the mantra and its import. The mantra consists of three parts. Part 1 of the mantra is called *bijakshara mantra*, or a one-syllable basic mantra. Part 2 is the mantra taken from the Veda. And part 3 is called *laukika mantra*, or the commonly chanted name of the deity, which here, is the sun.

This sun salutation is best done facing east and at dawn.

The sequence follows.

Start in samasthiti/tadasana. Stand erect with your back straight, and your palms in anjali. Stay in this position for a few breaths. Hold your breath after an inhalation and focus on the first mantra. This is the first vinyasa (*see figure 11-1*).

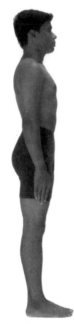

FIGURE 11-1 ◆

The mantra, consisting of three parts, will be:
1. *Om Hram.*
2. *Uddannadya mitramahah,*
3. *mitraya namah.*

The meaning of the mantra is:
1. Om Hram.
2. (You,) the One rising now and daily, (are) the great friend,
3. salutations to the great friend.

Inhaling smoothly, raise your arms. Interlock your fingers and pull your arms back (*see figure 11-2*).

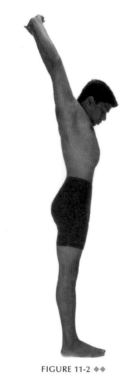

FIGURE 11-2 ◆◆

As you hold your breath in, mentally chant the mantra (or stay quiet without the mantra):
1. *Om Hrim.*
2. *Arohannuttaram divam.*
3. *Ravaye namah.*

The meaning is:
1. Om Hrim.
2. Climbing, the great one, up the sky.
3. Oh the fast mover, salutation to you.

Exhaling smoothly, stretch and bend forward, place your forehead on your knees or your shins (*see figure 11-3*), and as you hold your breath out, chant and meditate on the following mantra:

Inhale and while you are exhaling, bend your knees and sit on your haunches to utkatasana or the hip stretch pose (*see figure 11-4*).

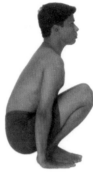

FIGURE 11-4 ◆◆◆

As you hold your breath out, meditate on the following mantra:

1. *Om Hraim.*
2. *Harimanancha nasaya.*
3. *Bhanave namah.*

This means:
1. Om Hraim.
2. And the green patches (on my skin) you do destroy.
3. Salutations to you, the provider of light to the world.

Note: the greenish or dark blue patches in the skin are due to heart ailment.

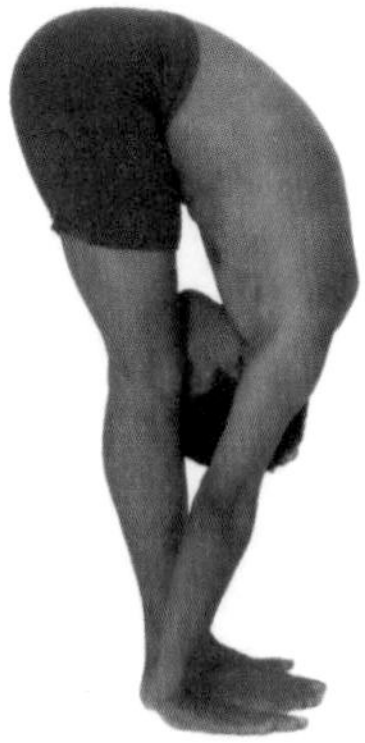

FIGURE 11-3 ◆◆◆

1. *Om Hrum.*
2. *Hrudrogam mama surya.*
3. *Suryaya namah.*

This means:
1. Om Hrum.
2. My heart ailment, O the divine guide.
3. My salutations to the divine (Surya).

Inhaling, hold your breath. Lean slightly forward, raise your heels (see figure 11-5), and gently jump back landing smoothly on your big toes.

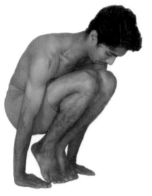

FIGURE 11-5 ◆◆◆

Keep both your feet and ankles together as you push yourself back. This pose is chaturanga-dandasana or four-legged-staff pose (see figure 11-6).

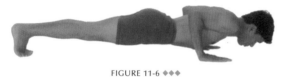

FIGURE 11-6 ◆◆◆

Breathe out, and as you hold your breath, meditate on the following mantra:
1. *Om Hraum.*
2. *Sukeshu mey harimanam.*
3. *Khagaya namah.*

This means:
1. Om Hraum.
2. Give away the green color to the parrots.
3. Salutations to Thee, the mover in space.

The next vinyasa is the actual surya namaskara, and the pose is known as *danda samarpana*, or surrendering oneself to the deity which is the sun itself (see figure 11-7).

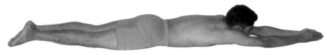

FIGURE 11-7 ◆

From the previous pose, slowly exhale and lie prostrate. Meditate on the following mantra:
1. *Om Hrah.*
2. *Ropanakasu dadhmasi.*
3. *Pushne namah.*

This means:
1. Om Hrah.
2. And give to the herbs used for healing paste.
3. Salutations to thee, the great Nourisher.

Perform chaturanga-dandasana (see figure 11-8).

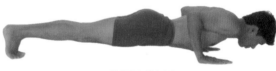

FIGURE 11-8 ◆◆

Chant the following mantra:
1. *Om Hram.*
2. *Atho Haaridraveshu mey.*
3. *Hiranyagarbhaaya namah.*

This means:
1. Om Hram.
2. Or to the green trees.
3. My salutations are to the Golden Creator (womb).

Perform urdhwa-mukha swanasana, the upward-facing-dog pose *(see figure 11-9)*.

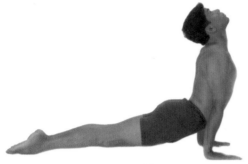

FIGURE 11-9 ◆◆

Chant the following mantra:
1. *Om Hrim.*
2. *Harimanannidaddhmasi.*
3. *Marichaye namah.*

This means:
1. Om Hrim.
2. Deposit the green patches.
3. Salutations to the radiant one.

Perform the downward-facing-dog pose *(see figure 11-10)*.

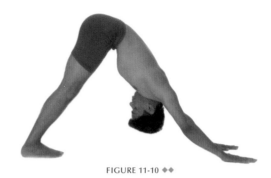

FIGURE 11-10 ◆◆

Chant the following mantra:
1. *Om Hrum.*
2. *Udagadayamadityah.*
3. *Adityaya namah.*

This means:
1. Om Hrum.
2. This Sun rising in the sky.
3. Salutations to Aditya.

Perform utkatasana (*see figure 11-11*).

Perform uttanasana (*see figure 11-12*).

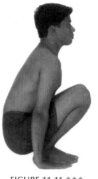

FIGURE 11-11 ◆◆◆

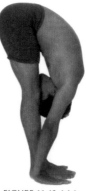

FIGURE 11-12 ◆◆◆

Chant the following mantra:
1. *Om Hrom.*
2. *Viswena sahasa saha.*
3. *Savitre namah.*

This means:
1. Om Hrom.
2. Energize the world to effort and work.
3. Salutations to the luminous one.

Chant the following mantra:
1. *Om Hraum.*
2. *Dwishantam mama randhayan.*
3. *Arkaya namah.*

This means:
1. Om Hraum.
2. Remove all my obstacles.
3. To the venerable one, my salutations.

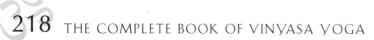

Perform samasthiti *(see figure 11-13).*

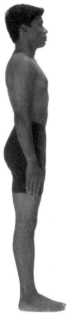

FIGURE 11-13 ◆

Chant the following mantra:
1. *Om Hrah.*
2. *Mo aham dwishato radham.*
3. *Bhaskaraya namah.*

This means:
1. Om Hrah.
2. May I stop all inimical forces [With the energy you give, may I be able to overcome all inimical forces].
3. Salutations to the great illuminator.

You may do few surya namaskaras at a time, always taking care to see that your breathing does not get hurried. Doing too many surya nakmaskaras in succession is not recommended in yoga. In the *Hathayogapradipika*, the bible of all hatha yogis, the author, Swatmarama, gives a list of dos that are helpful for progress in yoga and don'ts that are detrimental to yoga. Quoting another great yogi, Gorakhanatha, Swatmara forbids yogis from doing activities that are painful and injurious (*kayaklesa*). Brahmananda, the commentator to the great yoga treatise, gives examples of what constitutes kayaklesa. He warns against weightlifting and too many sun salutations. Sun salutations done in moderation, however, are excellent exercises for the body, breath, and mind.

VASISHTASANA SEQUENCE

The next group we will consider is Vasishtasana. This asana is named after a great sage known for his wisdom. A well-known work of his is *Yoga Vasishta*, which is a yoga classic. He was an important character in the great epic *Ramayana*, being the guru of Lord Rama, an incarnation of Vishnu.

This is a simple sequence. As described earlier, you should get to the downward-facing-dog vinyasa *(see figure 11-14)*.

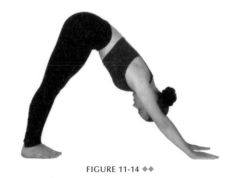

FIGURE 11-14 ◆◆

In that pose, exhale, and turn your right palm outward. During the next inhalation, pressing down through your right palm and anchoring your right foot, tilt your body, raise your free arm straight up, and look up (see figure 11-15).

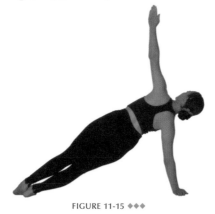

FIGURE 11-15 ◆◆◆

This is Vasishtasana with your left arm up. Stay in this position for a breath.

Anchor your right palm and press down through your right leg. Exhaling, bend your knee and draw your left foot toward your chest. Now clasp your big toe with your left hand. Inhaling, stretch your leg along with the hand holding your big toe; you may also look up as you complete the inhalation (see figure 11-16).

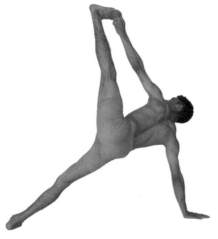

FIGURE 11-16 ◆◆◆

Stay in this position for three breaths; on every exhalation, lift your pelvis up (laterally).

Again as you exhale, draw your left foot toward you, and place it on your right thigh near your groin for the half-lotus position. Stay in this position for a breath, and during the following inhalation, lift your hip laterally up, stretch your left arm, and look up. Stay in this position for three breaths. Now slightly relax your pelvic joints. As you inhale, swing your left arm around your back and (if possible—only if possible) clasp the big toe of your left foot (see figure 11-17).

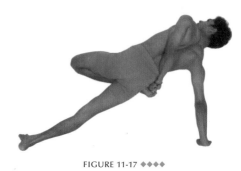

FIGURE 11-17 ◆◆◆◆

Inhaling, lift your pelvis laterally, and look up and stay in this position for three breaths in this Kashyapasana pose.

Lower your left leg to Vasishtasana sthiti as you inhale.

During the next exhalation, turn your palm by 90 degrees and inward. Then as you inhale, tilt your body by further 90 degrees, land on your left hand and push your body up. Now both your palms are on the floor, so are your feet, stretched and planted on the floor (see figure 11-18).

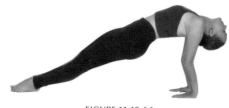

FIGURE 11-18 ◆◆

Stay in this position for one breath. This is purvatanasana.

From purvatanasana, while exhaling turn your left palm outward. During the next inhalation, tilt your body up, pressing down with your left palm and your left foot, and look up. You are again in Vasishtasana, but with your right hand up (see figure 11-19).

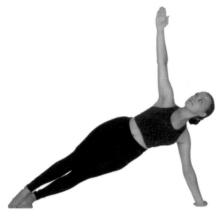

FIGURE 11-19 ◆◆◆

lm and anchor your left leg. Exhaling, bend your knee, and draw your left foot toward your chest. Now clasp your big toe with your right hand. Inhaling, stretch your right leg upward along with the hand holding your big toe; you may also look up as you complete the inhalation (see figure 11-20).

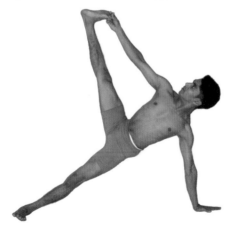

FIGURE 11-20 ◆◆◆

Stay in this position for three breaths; on every exhalation, lift your pelvis up (laterally). This is another vinyasa of Vasishtasana.

Again as you exhale, draw your right foot toward you, and place your right foot on your left thigh near your groin for the half-lotus position. Stay in this position for a breath and during the following inhalation, lift your hip laterally up, stretch your right arm, and look up. Stay in this position for three breaths. Now if possible, do the next movement. Slightly relax your pelvic joints. As you inhale, swing your right arm around your back and clasp the big toe of your right foot (see figure 11-21).

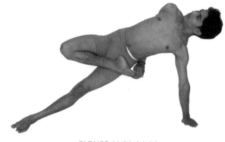

FIGURE 11-21 ◆◆◆◆

Inhaling, lift your pelvis laterally, and look up. Stay in this kashyapasana pose for three breaths.

Lower your right leg on exhalation to return to Vasishtansana sthiti.

From the Vasishtasana position, tilt downward and place your right palm on the floor, keeping both your palms on the floor, fingers forward. Now you have reached the adho-mukha swanasana position (see figure 11-22).

Exhaling, turn your left palm outward, and inhaling, tilt your body up, pressing down with your left palm and your left foot. While you are inhaling, you may tilt your

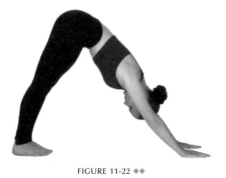

FIGURE 11-22 ◆◆

body to the right side, raising your right arm up and looking up (*see figure 11-23*).

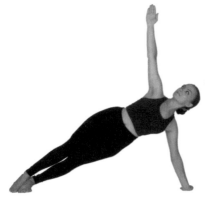

FIGURE 11-23 ◆◆◆

You are now in Vasishtasana.

From the Vasishtasana pose, turn your palm inward by 90 degrees, and tilting your body up, land on your right palm. Now inhaling, lift your body (*see figure 11-24*).

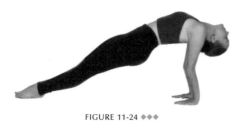

FIGURE 11-24 ◆◆◆

This is purvatsnasana.

From purvatanasana, pressing down with your right palm, tilt to the right side

and raise your left arm up and look up. You are again in Vasishtasana (*see figure 11-25*).

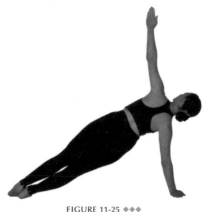

FIGURE 11-25 ◆◆◆

From Vasishtasana, tilt your body downward on exhalation, placing your left palm to the floor. You are now in the downward-facing-dog pose, from which you started the sequence (*see figure 11-26*).

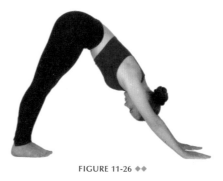

FIGURE 11-26 ◆◆

This sequence is very good for the shoulders and also the hip because the rotation takes place freely in space, rather than being restricted when you are seated or lying down. This sequence is invigorating. The next time, you may start by raising your right arm instead of your left. This sequence is calorie-consuming. So, please watch your breath. As it quickens, rest in between positions.

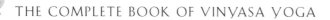

Vasishtasana is done following a simpler sequence. You start from the staff pose—the sequence used to reach the staff pose has been discussed earlier.

From dandasana, or the staff pose (*see figure 11-27*), exhale, place your right palm on the floor by your right side.

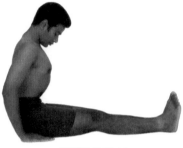

FIGURE 11-27 ◆◆

Then as you are inhaling, slowly press down with your right palm and your right foot, and pushing up your body, reach Vasishhtasana. In the pose, you will be looking up and your left hand will be stretched up (*see figure 11-28*).

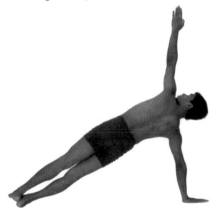

FIGURE 11-28 ◆◆◆

From here there are two alternatives. You may continue the cycle as explained earlier. Or you may return to the staff pose on a slow exhalation and repeat the movement on the other side (*see figure 11-29*).

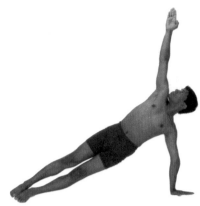

FIGURE 11-29 ◆◆◆

VISESHA VINYASA— ANJANEYASANA

We have seen that Anjaneyasana can be approached as an extension of tiryang-mukha-ekapada-asana, which is an asymmetric seated pose. In this sequence it is approached from the hub pose, the downward-facing-dog posture.

Start from the downward-facing-dog. The approach to it has been described earlier. Basically it will involve the following vinyasas in sequence:

1. SAMASTHITI
2. TADASANA (arms raised during inhalation)
3. UTTANASANA (forward bend, while exhaling)
4. UTKATASANA (hip stretch sitting on haunches)
5. CHATURANGA-DANDASANA (Inhale, hold breath)
6. UPWARD-FACING-DOG POSE (inhaling)
7. DOWNWARD-FACING-DOG POSE (exhaling) (*see figure 11-30*)

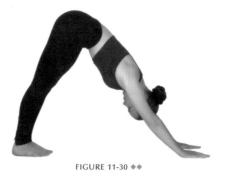

FIGURE 11-30 ◆◆

Stay in downward-facing-dog position for three long breaths.

From this pose, while slowly exhaling, bend your right knee, move your right leg forward, and place it between your palms. Bend forward to place your belly on your right thigh. This is *godhasana*, or the iguana pose (*see figure 11-31*).

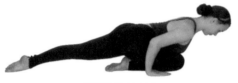

FIGURE 11-31 ◆◆◆

Inhaling, raise your arms overhead (*see figure 11-32*).

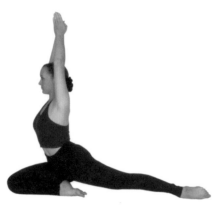

FIGURE 11-32) ◆◆◆

This posture is a variation of godhasana. Stay in this position for three long inhalations and exhalation. Then slowly lower

your body to the floor, stretching your thighs (*see figure 11-33*).

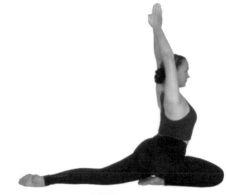

FIGURE 11-33 ◆◆◆

Stay in this position for another three breaths.

From godhasana, as you are exhaling, step out with your right foot. Inhaling, rotate your shoulder and stretch your arms in front of you. Stay in this position for six long inhalations and exhalations. This is a vinyasa of Anjaneyasana (*see figure 11-34*).

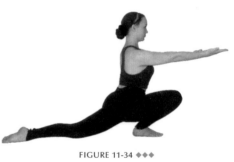

FIGURE 11-34 ◆◆◆

Some call it *Hanumanasana*. It gives the impression of Hanuman—the monkey-god, devotee of Rama in the epic *Ramayana*—flying and carrying the herbal mountain from Himalayas to Lanka.

Here is another variation of Hanumanasana. Inhaling, bend back and stay in this position for three breaths (*see figure 11-35*).

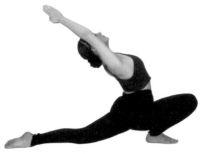

FIGURE 11-35 ◆◆◆◆

You may adjust the position of your left foot to anchor it well so that you may maintain perfect balance while bending back (*see figure 11-36*).

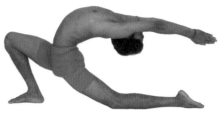

FIGURE 11-36 ◆◆◆◆

Exhaling, you may return to the asana sthiti.

In Hanumanasana sthiti, while exhaling, lower your arms and place your palms on the floor. Stay in this position for a breath. Then holding your breath after exhalation and anchoring your hands, slowly stretch your right leg forward, until you "split your legs" fully and sit. Making

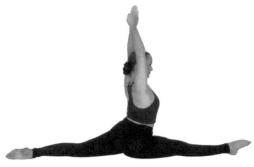

FIGURE 11-37 ◆◆◆◆◆

sure that your legs are not tight and inhaling slowly, raise your arms up and hold your hands in anjali, or the salutation position. This is Anjaneyasana (*see figure 11-37*).

Another popular position of your hands in prayer is also shown as another vinyasa of Anjaneyasana (*see figure 11-38*).

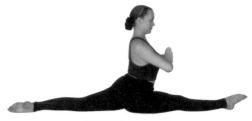

FIGURE 11-38 ◆◆◆◆◆

While in Anjaneyasana, inhale and once again raise your arms. While exhaling, slowly bend forward to place your head on your right knee or your shin. Stay in this position for six long inhalations and exhalations (*see figure 11-39*).

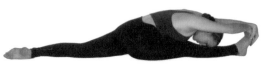

FIGURE 11-39 ◆◆◆◆◆

Inhaling, return to the asana sthiti.

The next variation will involve a very good control over the hips. In the asana sthiti, while exhaling, bring your hands down and back for the back salute (*see figure 11-40*).

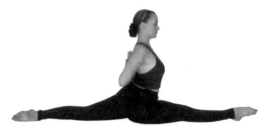

FIGURE 11-40 ◆◆◆◆◆

Stay in this position for three breaths, opening your chest on every inhalation.

Keeping your hands in back salute, exhale very slowly and completely bend forward and place your head on your right knee or your shin (*see figure 11-41*).

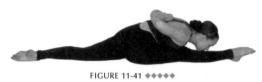

FIGURE 11-41 ◆◆◆◆◆

Inhaling, return to asana sthiti. Then exhale and lower your arms, placing your hands on the floor for support. Slowly, lift your hip and bring your right leg to Hanumanasana. Stay in this position for a breath. On the next exhalation, bring your right leg to godhasana. Stay in this position for a breath. Finally inhale, raise your hips, and push your right leg back to reach the downward-facing-dog pose.

From the downward-facing-dog pose, slowly exhaling, bend your left knee, move your left leg forward and place it between your palms, and bend forward to place your belly on your right thigh. This is godasana, or the iguana pose (*see figure 11-42*).

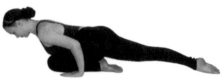

FIGURE 11-42 ◆◆◆

Inhaling, raise your arms overhead (*see figure 11-43*).

This posture is a variation of godasana, or the iguana pose. Stay in this position for three long inhalations and exhalations. Then slowly lower your body further to the floor, stretching your thighs (*see figure 11-44*).

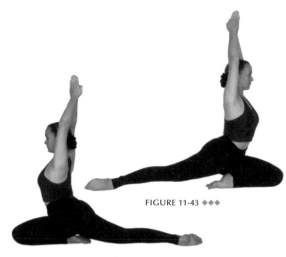

FIGURE 11-43 ◆◆◆

FIGURE 11-44 ◆◆◆

Stay in this position for another three breaths.

From godasana, as you are exhaling, step in front with your left foot. Inhaling, rotate your shoulder (first backward and then forward in one circular motion) with your arms in front of you. Stay in this position for six long inhalations and exhalations. This is a vinyasa of Anjaneyasana (*see figure 11-45*). Some call this Hanumanasana.

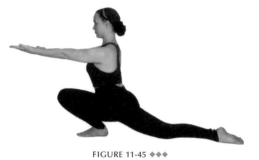

FIGURE 11-45 ◆◆◆

Another variation of Hanumanasana is seen here. Inhaling, bend back and stay in this position for three breaths (*see figure 11-46*).

You may adjust the position of your left foot to anchor it well so that you can maintain perfect balance while bending back (*see figure 11-47*).

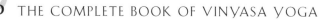

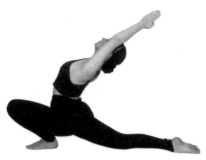

FIGURE 11-46 ◆◆◆◆

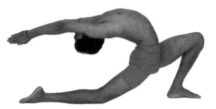

FIGURE 11-47 ◆◆◆◆

Exhaling, return to the asana sthiti.

In Hanumanasana sthiti, while exhaling, lower your arms and place your palms on the floor. Stay in this position for a breath. Then holding your breath after exhalation and pressing down through your palms, slowly stretch your left leg forward, until you split your legs fully and sit. Making sure that your legs are not tight and inhaling, slowly raise your arms up and hold your hands in anjali, or the salutation position. This is Anjaneyasana (see with figure 11-48).

Another popular position of your hands in prayer is also shown as another vinyasa of Anjaneyasana in figure 11-49.

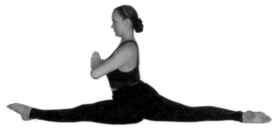

FIGURE 11-49 ◆◆◆◆◆

While you are in Anjaneyasana, inhale once again, and raise your arms. While exhaling, slowly bend forward to place your head on your left knee or your shin. Stay in this position for six long inhalations and exhalations (see figure 11-50).

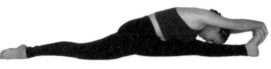

FIGURE 11-50 ◆◆◆◆◆

Inhaling, return to the asana sthiti.

The next variation will involve maintaining very good control over your hips. In asana sthiti, while exhaling, bring your hands down and back for the back salute (see figure 11-51).

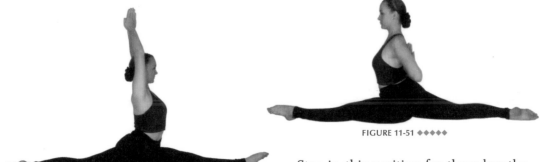

FIGURE 11-48 ◆◆◆◆◆

FIGURE 11-51 ◆◆◆◆◆

Stay in this position for three breaths, opening your chest on every inhalation.

Keeping your hands in the back salute, exhale very slowly and completely bend forward and place your head on your left knee or your shin (*see figure 11-52*).

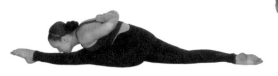

FIGURE 11-52 ◆◆◆◆◆

Inhaling, return to asana sthiti. Then, exhale lower your arms, and place your hands on the floor for support. Slowly, lift your hip and bring your left leg to Hanumanasana. Stay in this position for a breath. On the next exhalation, bring your left leg to godasana. Stay in this position for a breath. And finally inhale, raise your hips, and push your left leg back to reach the downward-facing-dog pose.

HALASANA-PASCHIMATANASANA

Start from dandasana, or the staff pose. The procedure to arrive at this pose has been discussed earlier. From dandasana, raise your arms while inhaling and interlock your fingers. During the next exhalation, roll back and lie down on your back with your arms stretched overhead. Exhale and lower your arms. You are in supta asana sthiti (*see figure 11-53*).

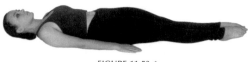

FIGURE 11-53 ◆

Stay in this position for three long inhalations and exhalations. Now inhaling, stretch your arms overhead and stay in this position for thee breaths (*see figure 11-54*).

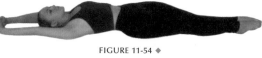

FIGURE 11-54 ◆

Exhaling, lift your upper body, sit up, and in a continuous motion, bend forward to place your palms on the floor beyond your feet. This is niralamba paschimatanasana (*see figure 11-55*).

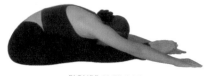

FIGURE 11-55 ◆◆◆

Stay in this position for three breaths. As you are inhaling, raise your trunk and roll back to return to the lying-down position. While doing so, you may round your back after reaching the seated position, and lower your back slowly. Starting from your tailbone stretch one vertebra after the other until the back of your head and the backs of your hands touch the floor to reach the plough pose (*see figure 11-56*).

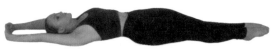

FIGURE 11-56 ◆◆◆

You may do this cycle, paschimatana and halasana, three times, and then inhaling roll back to the lying-down position. You can see that this combination is helpful to give a dynamic stretch to your pelvis and help achieve a good pelvic tilt. During the forward movement, your arms and your torso get involved to stretch your low back, and on the reverse movement your lower extremities help to achieve similar results.

Exhaling, raise your legs and your body and land your feet on your palms for the plough pose. Clasp your big toes with your fingers (*see figure 11-57*).

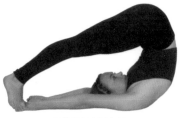

FIGURE 11-57 ◆◆◆

Stay in this position for three breaths. Then, as you exhale, slowly lower your waist and stretch your spine, so that your bodyweight is slowly shifted to your back from your neck. In this position, which is the upward-looking stretch pose (*urdhwa-mukha paschimatanasana*), you will be able to lift your head and touch your knee with your forehead (*see figure 11-58*).

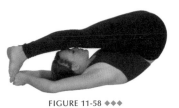

FIGURE 11-58 ◆◆◆

Exhale, hold your breath and gently rock your body back and forth a couple of times; transferring your weight alternately from the back of your neck to your back and again to your neck—all the time holding your toes with your hands.

Exhale and hold your breath; bend your knees slightly and roll to the posterior stretch pose, all the while holding your toes with you hands (*see figure 11-59*).

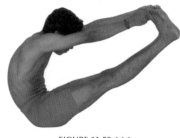

FIGURE 11-59 ◆◆◆

It is a good idea to use a soft mat or blanket to support your ankles and heels when landing as you complete the movement (*see figure 11-60*).

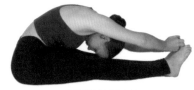

FIGURE 11-60 ◆◆◆

Stay in paschimatanasana (posterior stretch pose) for three breaths.

Next, exhale; hold your breath while still in plough pose holding your toes. Bend your knee slightly and roll back, still holding your toes. As you complete the roll back movement, stretch your knees nicely to reach plough pose. All the while you will be holding your toes. Stay in this position for a breath and repeat the movements three times. Then from the plough position, roll your body back to the lying-down position (*see figure 11-61*).

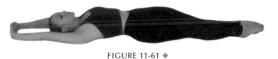

FIGURE 11-61 ◆

You may repeat the sequence three to six times.

Roll back to the plough pose on exhalation (*see figure 11-62*).

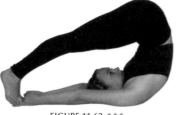

FIGURE 11-62 ◆◆◆

Now support your back. During the following inhalation, raise your trunk. Bend your knees, arch your spine, and lower your legs. Slowly land on your feet as you continue to arch your spine (*see figure 11-63*).

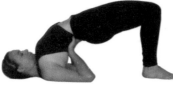

FIGURE 11-63 ◆◆◆

Inhaling stretch your legs for uttana-mayurasana (*see figure 11-64*).

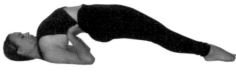

FIGURE 11-64 ◆◆◆

Stay in this position for a breath.

Now exhaling, bend your knees and draw your legs closer to your body (*see figure 11-65*).

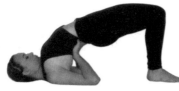

FIGURE 11-65 ◆◆

During the following exhalation, roll your body back to the plough position (*see figure 11-66*).

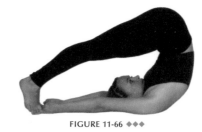

FIGURE 11-66 ◆◆◆

Stay. This cycle can be repeated three to six times. You can practice the three movements in one cycle—from figures 11-53 to 11-60. Then finally roll down to the lying-down position and rest.

PUMPING AND JUMPING (UTPLUTI)

Lifting one's body and jumping while supporting oneself on one's hands form a set of sequences quite popular these days. We will examine some of them. These emanate from the downward-facing-dog (DFD) pose.

From DFD (*see figure 11-67*), exhale, hold your breath and jump through your hands (*see figures 11-68 and 11-69*) and stay balanced with your legs stretched (*see figure 11-70*).

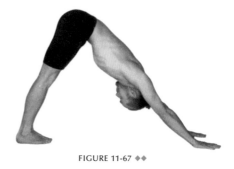

FIGURE 11-67 ◆◆

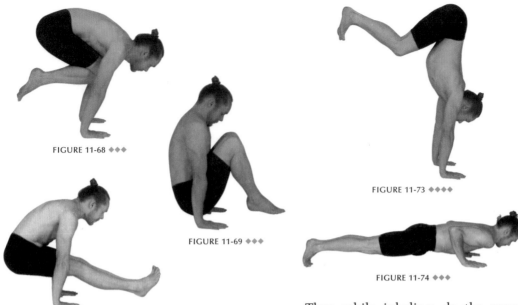

FIGURE 11-68 ◆◆◆

FIGURE 11-69 ◆◆◆

FIGURE 11-73 ◆◆◆◆

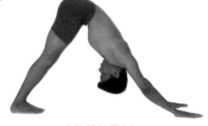

FIGURE 11-74 ◆◆◆

FIGURE 11-70 ◆◆◆

Inhaling lower your body to the floor for staff pose (*see figure 11-71*).

Then while inhaling, do the upward-facing-dog pose. On the next exhalation, return to the downward-facing-dog position.

From DFD, (*see figure 11-75*), exhale, hold your breath, and jump through the space between your hands but keeping your knees bent.

Balance with your knees bent (*see figure 11-76*).

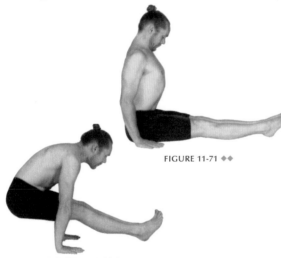

FIGURE 11-71 ◆◆

FIGURE 11-72 ◆◆◆

FIGURE 11-75 ◆◆

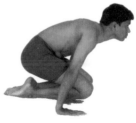

FIGURE 11-76 ◆◆◆

Stay in this position for three breaths. To return, inhale, hold your breath, and lift your body (*see figure 11-72*).

Jump back (*see figure 11-73*) to chaturanga-dandasana (*see figure 11-74*).

Stay in this position for a breath. Now inhaling, you lower yourself to the floor for vajrasana (see figure 11-77).

Stay in this position for three breaths, keeping your hands on your thighs and keeping your back erect in vajrasana (see figure 11-78).

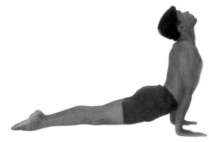

FIGURE 11-81 ◆◆◆

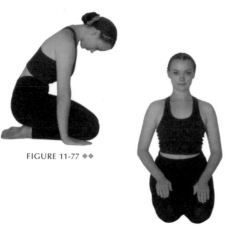

FIGURE 11-77 ◆◆

FIGURE 11-78 ◆◆

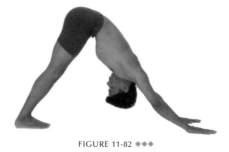

FIGURE 11-82 ◆◆◆

In DFD (see figure 11-83), exhale, and keeping your right knee bent, jump through your hands and balance in tiryang-mukha utpluti position (see figure 11-84).

Inhale, hold your breath, lift yourself (see figure 11-79) and jump back to chaturanga-dandasana (see figure 11-80), the UFD (inhaling) (see figure 11-81), and DFD (exhaling), and DFD (exhaling) (see figure 11-82).

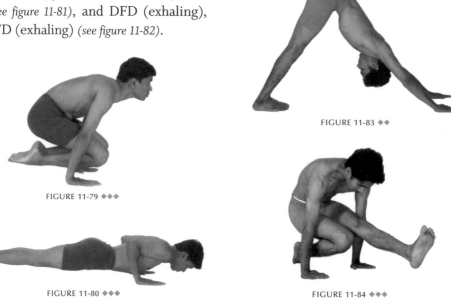

FIGURE 11-79 ◆◆◆

FIGURE 11-83 ◆◆

FIGURE 11-80 ◆◆◆

FIGURE 11-84 ◆◆◆

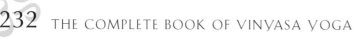

Inhale hold your breath and slowly lower yourself to the tiryang-mukha asana sthiti.

Again while in DFD (*see figure 11-85*), exhale, and keeping your left knee slightly bent and pressing down through your palms, jump through your hands to utpluti in tiryang-mukha sthiti (*see figure 11-86*).

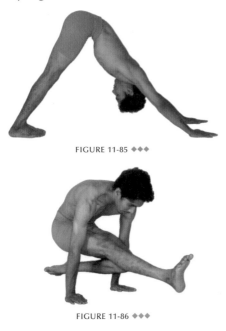

FIGURE 11-85 ◆◆◆

FIGURE 11-86 ◆◆◆

Inhale; hold your breath, and slowly position yourself in tiryang-mukha sthiti.

Start the sequence from the DFD position. Exhaling, grab your right leg with your right hand and tuck your right foot on the left thigh beside your groin, in the half-lotus position (*see figure 11-87*).

Lower your right hand, and place your palm on the floor in line with your other hand. Stay in this position for a breath. Exhale. Holding your breath, bend your left knee slightly. Pressing through your palms, gently hop forward through the space between your hands and balance yourself (*see figure 11-88*).

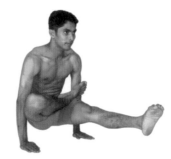

FIGURE 11-88 ◆◆◆◆

Slowly lower your body to the half-lotus seated pose. Inhale, hold your breath, lift your body, and balance on your hands. Exhale, hold your breath, and jump back to the starting position.

You may repeat the movement on the other side. First the starting position (*see figure 11-89*).

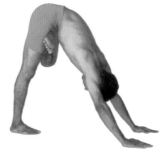

FIGURE 11-89 ◆◆

In this, your left leg is in the half-lotus position. When you jump through your

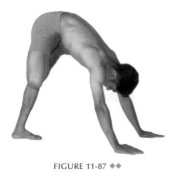

FIGURE 11-87 ◆◆

hands as explained in the previous vinyasas, you will be in the lifted-half-lotus position *(see figure 11-90)*.

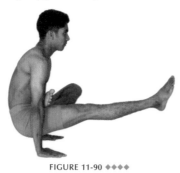

FIGURE 11-90 ◆◆◆◆

This sequence will start from adho-mukha swanasana, with one leg in ekapada sirsasana *(see figure 11-91)*.

Exhale and hold your breath. Bend your left knee slightly and gently hop and land between your palms, pressing them against the floor. Keep your left leg straight. You are now in durvasasana *(see figure 11-92)*.

After three breaths, hop back to the starting position. Inhaling lower your right leg to get to the downward-facing-dog pose. You may repeat the same movements with your left leg in ekapada sirsasana sthiti, to reach durva asasana *(see figure 11-93)*.

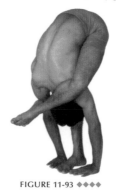

FIGURE 11-93 ◆◆◆◆

From DFD *(see figure 11-94)*, exhale, hold your breath, jump around your hands, and entwine your arms and cross your legs at your ankles *(see figure 11-95)*.

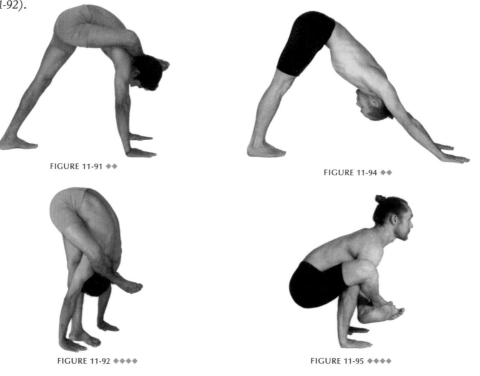

FIGURE 11-91 ◆◆

FIGURE 11-94 ◆◆

FIGURE 11-92 ◆◆◆◆

FIGURE 11-95 ◆◆◆◆

Stay balanced for three breaths.

Another vinyasa: Stay in DFD position *(see figure 11-96)*.

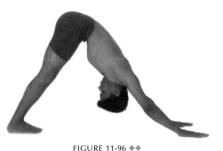

FIGURE 11-96 ◆◆

Jump and entwine your legs, but keep your legs stretched forward *(see figure 11-97)*.

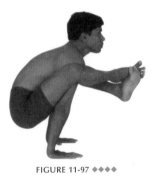

FIGURE 11-97 ◆◆◆◆

Inhale hold your breath, lean forward, and jump back to chaturanga-dandasana, UFD, (inhaling), and DFD (exhaling). This is a vinyasa of bhuja peedasana, or the shoulder-pressure pose.

From DFD, *(see figure 11-98)* again exhale, hold your breath, and hop gently and place your knees abutting your shoulders.

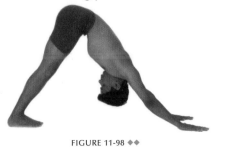

FIGURE 11-98 ◆◆

Your knees should be kept bent *(see figure 11-99)*.

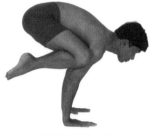

FIGURE 11-99 ◆◆◆◆

Stay in this position for three breaths. Inhaling, jump back to chaturanga-dandasana, do UFD (inhaling), and then do DFD (exhaling). This is another vinyasa of Bhuja peedasana.

From the previous asana position, stretch your legs up and back a little bit, and lift your head and open your chest as you are inhaling *(see figure 11-100)*.

Stay in this position for three breaths. While exhaling return to bhuja peedasana, and then inhaling jump back to chaturanga-dandasana, then UFD (inhaling), and then DFD (exhaling).

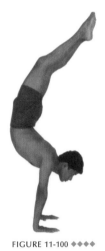

FIGURE 11-100 ◆◆◆◆

Let us consider some more postures balancing on your hands. While in the DFD pose, exhaling turn your palms inward. Then bend your knees while exhaling, and keep your knees on the floor. Place your

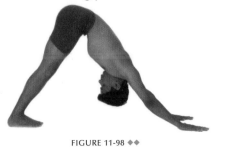

FIGURE 11-101 ◆◆◆◆

lower abdomen against your elbows, and balancing on your hands lift your body (see figure 11-101).

Stay in this position for six breaths with long exhalations. Retrace the steps of the sequence to return to DFD. This is mayur-asana, or the peacock pose.

The same asana can be done with your thumb bent for better support (see figure 11-102).

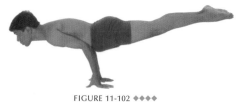

FIGURE 11-102 ◆◆◆◆

Now from DFD, while exhaling, gently jump, bending your knees and placing your knees on your right shoulder. Stay in this position for a breath. Inhaling, stretch your legs to the right side with your right shoulder supporting your legs (see figure 11-103).

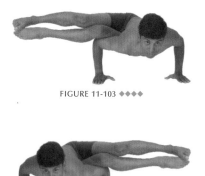

FIGURE 11-103 ◆◆◆◆

FIGURE 11-104 ◆◆◆◆

This is Astavakrasana, named after a physically handicapped (but mentally very tough) sage with a crooked body. Stay in

this position for three breaths. Exhale, bend your knees, and on the next inhalation jump back to chaturanga-dandasana, then UFD (inhaling), and then DFD (exhaling).

This may be repeated on the other side, following the same procedure (see figure 11-104).

While in DFD, exhaling, bring your right leg up and place it behind your left shoulder in the ekapada sirsasana position (see figure 11-105).

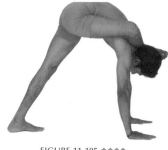

FIGURE 11-105 ◆◆◆◆

Now exhale, hold your breath, and jump through your hands, anchoring your hands and balancing your body (see figure 11-106).

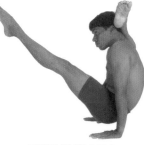

FIGURE 11-106 ◆◆◆◆

This is chakora asana.

The same procedure may be done on the left side as well (see figure 11-107), with chakora asana (see figure 11-108).

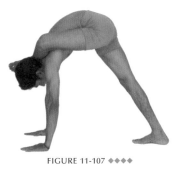

FIGURE 11-107 ◆◆◆◆

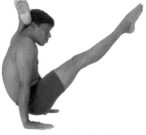

FIGURE 11-108 ◆◆◆◆

SALUTATIONS TO DIRECTIONS
(DING-NAMASKARA)

All yoga students are familiar with the surya namskara, or sun salutations. Here we will see a lesser-known namaskara sequence dedicated to the guardian angels of the various directions, called *ding-namaskara*. Like surya namaskara, it is done with mantras; the mantras are taken from the ancient Vedas.

First, start from sam-sthiti with your hands folded in anjali and facing east, because the Veda mantra starts with salutation to the eastern direction. Inhaling slowly raise both arms over-

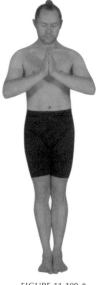

FIGURE 11-109 ◆

head, and keep your palms together in the anjali gesture *(see figure 11-109)*.

Then as you are exhaling, slowly bend forward halfway to ardha-uttanasana (half-forward-stretch pose) toward the eastern direction *(see figure 11-110)*.

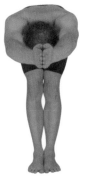

FIGURE 11-110 ◆◆

Now as you are holding your breath out, mentally chant the mantra (or the translation of it). Or, you may listen to a recording of the mantra. Or, stay in the posture holding your breath for five seconds and proceed to the next vinyasa.

OM! Namh prachyai diseyascha deva-ta yetasyam prativasanti yetabhyasch namah!

(Om. I bow to the east and the guardian angels that permeate it.)

Now as you are inhaling, get back to samasthiti, and as you breathe out turn to south. Inhale and during the following exhalation, bend forward to half-forward-stretch position (*see figure 11-111*).

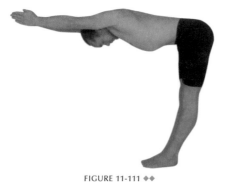

FIGURE 11-111 ◆◆

Hold your breath and chant the following mantra:

OM! Namo dakshinayai diseyascha devata yetasyam prativasanti yetabhyasch namah!

(Om. I bow to the south and the guardian angels that permeate it.)

Inhaling, please return to samathiti and as you breathe out, turn 90 degrees to face west (*see figure 11-112*).

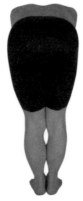

FIGURE 11-112 ◆◆

Inhale and on the following exhalation, bend forward to half-forward-stretch position. While you hold your breath, you may do any one of the options available. The mantra is:

OM! Namh prateechyai diseyascha devata yetasyam prativasanti yetabhyasch namah!

(Om. I bow to the west and the guardian angels that permeate it.)

Inhaling please return to samathiti, and as you breathe out turn 90 degrees to face north. Inhale, and on the following exhalation, bend forward to the half-forward-stretch position (*see figure 11-113*).

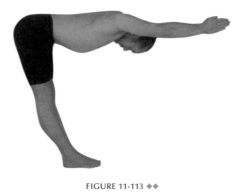

FIGURE 11-113 ◆◆

While you hold your breath, you may do any one of the options available. If you want to use the manta it is:

OM! Nama udeechyai diseyascha devata yetasyam prativasanti yetabhyasch namah!

(Om. I bow to the north and the guardian angels that permeate it.)

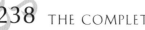

Now inhale and return to samasthiti; exhaling, turn 90 degrees to the east. Now inhaling, raise your head (and look up if you wish), or just raise your arms with your palms in the anjali position *(see figure 11-114)*.

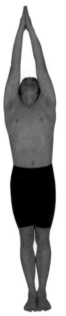

FIGURE 11-114 ◆

As you hold your breath, you may use the following mantra:

OM! Nama urdhwayai diseyascha devata yetasyam prativasanti yetabhyasch namah!

(Om. I bow to the upward direction and the guardian angels that permeate it.)

Facing still east, inhale once again and as you are exhaling, bend down and forward to uttanasana, but keep your palms in the anjali gesture and place your hands on the floor *(see figure 11-115)*, and say the following mantra if you wish. The side view is shown in figure 11-116.

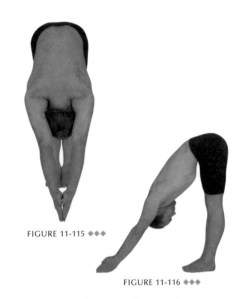

FIGURE 11-115 ◆◆◆

FIGURE 11-116 ◆◆◆

OM! Namo adharayai diseyascha devata yetasyam prativasanti yetabhyasch namah!

(Om. I bow to the downward direction and the guardian angels that permeate it.)

Return to samasthiti. Again as you breathe out, bend forward to the half-forward-stretch position, but keep your arms spread out at about 45 degrees *(see figure 11-117)*.

The side view is shown in figure 11-118.

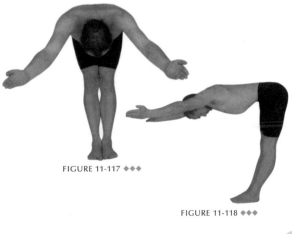

FIGURE 11-117 ◆◆◆

FIGURE 11-118 ◆◆◆

The relevant mantra is:

OM! Namo avantharayai diseyascha devata yetasyam prativasanti yetabhyasch namah!

(Om. I bow to the intermediate direction and the guardian angels that permeate it.)

You may slowly inhale and return to samasthti *(see figure 11-119)*.

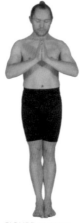

FIGURE 11-119 ◆

This concludes the salutations to the directions subroutine.

FLYING BIRD POSE SEQUENCE (KHAGASANA)

The next sequence, a fun sequence, is the bird (flying) pose.

Stand in tadasana *(see figure 11-120)*.

Keep your chin down and do a few ujjayi breaths. Lift your arms overhead during a slow, smooth inhalation *(see figure 11-121)*.

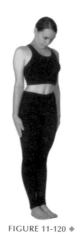

FIGURE 11-120 ◆

While exhaling, bend forward to ardha uttanasana *(see figure 11-122)*.

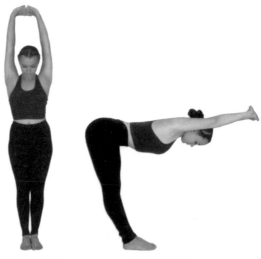

FIGURE 11-121 ◆   FIGURE 11-122 ◆◆

Stay in this position for one or two breaths.

During the next inhalation, slowly bring your arms laterally to shoulder level. This is a variation of ardha-uttnasana, or the half-forward-stretch pose. It is also known as khagasana, or the bird posture, because it resembles a bird flying with its wings opened *(see figure 11-123)*.

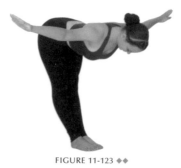

FIGURE 11-123 ◆◆

Stay in this position for three long inhalations and exhalations. Then exhale slowly and hold your breath. Bend your knees slightly and jump (or hop) forward (see figure 11-124) by about a foot and land gently on your toes, then on your feet, and squat on your haunches all in one smooth movement (see figure 11-125).

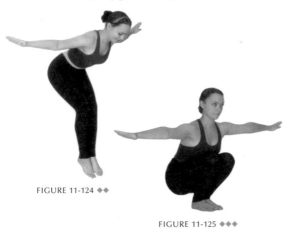

FIGURE 11-124 ◆◆

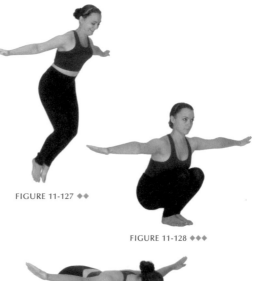

FIGURE 11-127 ◆◆

FIGURE 11-125 ◆◆◆

FIGURE 11-128 ◆◆◆

This is a variation of khagasana, because it resembles a bird landing. Stay in this position for a few breaths.

Now from the khagasana vinyasa position, inhale, rise, straighten your knees, and get back to the ardha-utkatasana/khagasana position (see figure 11-126).

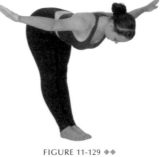

FIGURE 11-129 ◆◆

Stay in this position for a few breaths. Inhaling, get back to flying bird posture position (see figure 11-129).

Stay in this position for a breath.

You may repeat the cycle a few times.

While in the half-forward khagasana position, stretch your arms overhead (see figure 11-130).

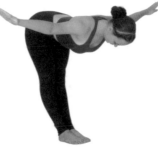

FIGURE 11-126 ◆◆

Then exhale, hold your breath, and gently jump (or hop) (see figure 11-127) back by about a foot, keeping your "wings" spread. Land gently on you toes (on the balls of your feet); in one motion place your feet on the floor and sit on your haunches (see figure 11-128).

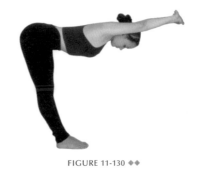

FIGURE 11-130 ◆◆

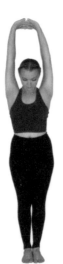

Exhale once again, and on the next inhalation raise your upper body and return to tadasana (see figure 11-131).

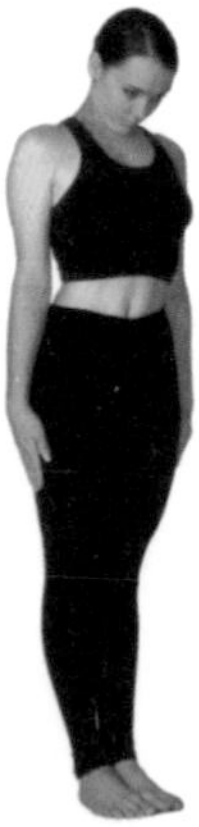

Exhaling, lower your arms to samsthiti (see figure 11-132).

Children love this sequence. And I know several adults who love this even more.

FIGURE 11-131 ◆

FIGURE 11-132 ◆

DOWNWARD-FACING-DOG/UPWARD-FACING-DOG/PLOUGH SEQUENCE

We are very familiar with the "dog-faces" poses with chaturanga-dandasana, which form a popular sequence of exercises. Here we consider a more involved sequence, with the downward- and upward-facing-dog poses and the plough.

Start the sequence from samasthiti (see figure 11-133).

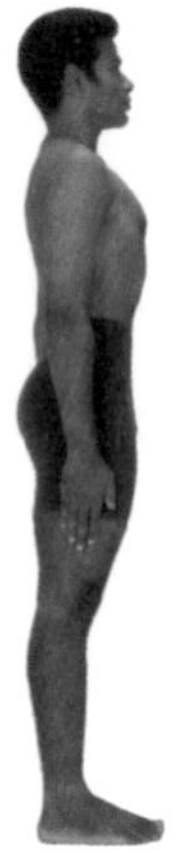

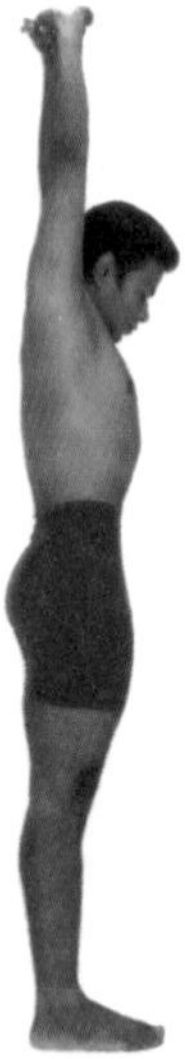

FIGURE 11-134 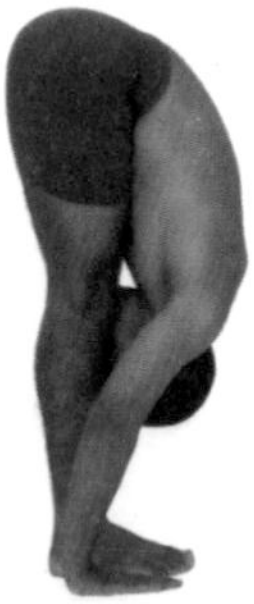 ◆   FIGURE 11-135 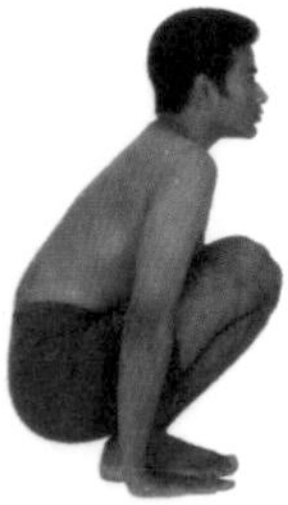 ◆◆◆   FIGURE 11-136 ◆◆◆

Inhaling, raise both arms overhead and interlock your fingers (see figure 11-134).

After a few ujjayi breaths, while exhaling, bend forward to uttanasana (see figure 11-135).

Inhale, and during exhalation, squat on your haunches in utkatasana (see figure 11-136).

Exhale, hold your breath, and lift your body (utkatasana utpluti), as you press through your palms (see figure 11-137).

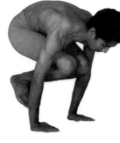

FIGURE 11-137 ◆◆◆

Inhale, hold your breath, and jump back to chaturanga-dandasana (see figure 11-138).

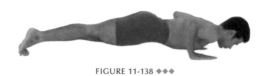

FIGURE 11-133 ◆

FIGURE 11-138 ◆◆◆

Stay in this position for a few breaths and make sure that your breathing is smooth and even. Exhaling, lift your waist. Flex the dorsas of your feet to assume the downward-facing-dog pose (*see figure 11-139*).

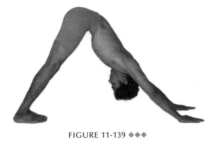

FIGURE 11-139 ◆◆◆

Stay in this position for a few breaths. Inhaling, stretch out your ankles, and lower your legs as you straighten your back. Continuing your inhalation, nicely arch your spine, bring your pelvis down as low as possible and look up. Stay in this position for three breaths in this pose, the upward-facing-dog pose (urdhwa-mukha swanasana). (*See figure 11-140*).

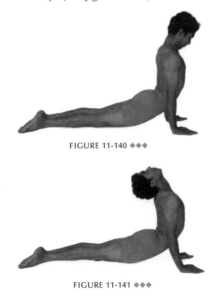

FIGURE 11-140 ◆◆◆

FIGURE 11-141 ◆◆◆

Keep your chin locked, and stay in this position for three long, smooth ujjayi breaths. Now inhaling, lift your heart a little more and gently toss your head back (*see figure 11-141*).

Now as you very deeply exhale, pressing down through your palms, round your back, and try to maintain a firm chin lock. Continuing your exhalation, stretch out your ankles to place your toes and the dorsum of your feet on the floor. Lower your trunk, round your back as much as you can, and bring your head into the space between your two palms (*see figure 11-142*).

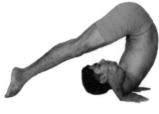

FIGURE 11-142 ◆◆◆◆

Gently place the back of your head and neck on the floor in the space between your palms, which are pressing against the floor (*see figure 11-143*).

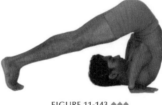

FIGURE 11-143 ◆◆◆

Now you are in plough posture. Stay in this position for three breaths.

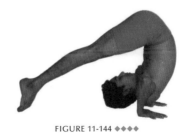

FIGURE 11-144 ◆◆◆◆

Now as you slowly inhale, pressing down through your palms, lift your body off the floor, keeping the chin lock intact (*see figure 11-144*).

Straighten your back, and pull your waist up as you flex the dorsa of your feet to plant your feet on the floor. You are now in the downward-facing-dog pose (*see figure 11-145*).

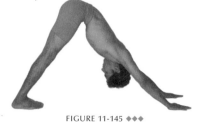

FIGURE 11-145 ◆◆◆

During the next inhalation, as explained earlier, arch your spine to assume the upward-facing-dog pose (*see figure 11-146*).

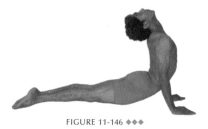

FIGURE 11-146 ◆◆◆

You may continue to do the cycle of the three poses a few times. Finally, rest in the downward-facing-dog pose for a few breaths, drawing in your rectum and your lower abdomen, while maintaining the chin lock (*see figure 11-147*).

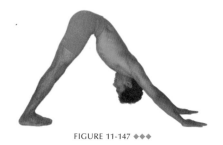

FIGURE 11-147 ◆◆◆

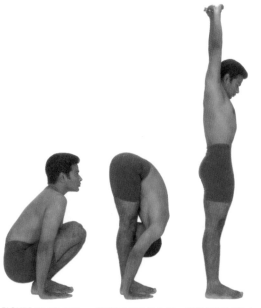

FIGURE 11-148 ◆◆◆   FIGURE 11-149 ◆◆◆   FIGURE 11-150 ◆

Exhale, hold your breath, and jump gently to land between your palms in utkatasana (*see figure 11-148*).

On the next inhalation, stretch your knees for uttanasana (*see figure 11-149*).

While you are inhaling, return to tadasana (*see figure 11-150*).

This sequence is a very powerful cycle, strengthening the arms and giving maximum flexion to the spine as well. The torso and the lower extremities also get an excellent work out. The sequence could be very tiring, so take a rest at the end of every cycle or even every vinyasa if need be. Persons with a delicate or stiff neck should not attempt the plough from the upward-facing-dog position.

UTTANASANA-UTKATASANA

A compact minisequence, which we will see now, has been found to be very useful for getting back into shape by many yoga students.

Start the sequence from samasthiti *(see figure 11-151)*.

Inhaling, raise your arms overhead and interlock your fingers *(see figure 11-152)*.

Exhaling, bend down to uttanasana *(see figure 11-153)*.

Stay in this position for a breath and then while exhaling, squat on your haunches in utkatasana *(see figure 11-154)*.

Stay in this position for a breath, and while inhaling straighten your knees,

while pressing down through your palms, and place your face on your knees. You are back in uttanasana *(see figure 11-155)*.

Repeat the movements in figures 11-153 through 11-155, with the appropriate breathing, three to six times.

If your capacity for holding your breath out (bahya kumbhaka) is good—say, about twenty seconds at a time—then you may try to do this cycle several times while holding your breath. Inhaling return to samasthiti, and stay in this position for a few breath to return to normal breathing. You may do the sequence again more times. Well, it is said that one can burn calories very fast by performing this sequence. The key is however, relaxed external breath holding.

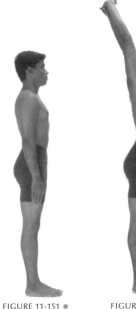

FIGURE 11-151 ◆

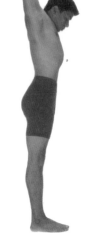

FIGURE 11-152 ◆

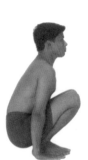

FIGURE 11-153 ◆◆◆

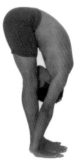

FIGURE 11-154 ◆◆◆

FIGURE 11-155 ◆◆◆

THE
WINDING DOWN
PROCEDURE

URING THE HUNDREDS of lessons I had with my teacher, all the asana sessions, which lasted for an hour, always ended with some pranayama practice.

Whenever I teach asanas, I devote the last 25 to 30 percent of the time to pranayama and some form of *pratyahara* (the fifth anga, or limb, of ashtanga yoga), ending with some meditative prayer. Here is a suggested winding down procedure.

First choose a comfortable seated pose. It would be good to take a yogic pose—the following are some that I recommend.

YOGIC POSTURES FOR YOGIC BREATHING EXERCISES

◆ **PADMASANA** or lotus pose
(*see figure 12-1*)

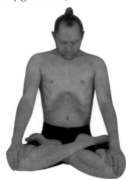

FIGURE 12-1 ◆◆◆

◆ **SIDDHASANA** (*see figure 12-2*)

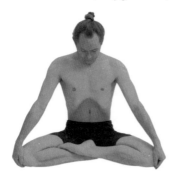

FIGURE 12-2 ◆◆◆

◆ **GOMUKHASANA** (*see figure 12-3*)

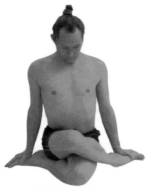

FIGURE 12-3 ◆◆◆

◆ **VAJRASANA** (*see figure 12-4*)

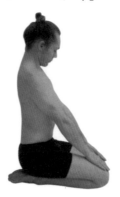

FIGURE 12-4 ◆◆◆

◆ **VIRASANA** (*see figure 12-5*)

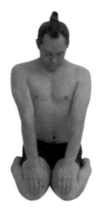

FIGURE 12-5 ◆◆◆

The steps needed to reach these postures have been described in detail in earlier chapters.

KAPALABHATI

In a yogic posture, you may start from *kapalabhati*, or bellows-like breathing. In this procedure, keeping your back straight and chin down, you vigorously blow out air repeatedly for a specified number of times. More about kapalabhati and its numerous therapeutic benefits are discussed in my book *Yoga for the Three Stages of Life*. For a start you may do this twelve times, wait and breathe normally for about thirty seconds, repeat it another two times. You may gradually become able to do this up to 108 times, and adepts do much more—even twice that many. However, one has to be careful in this practice. Contraindications may include acute sinusitis, hernia, pregnancy, and heavy menstruation.

While you are doing kapalabhati, you may change the position of your hands (hasta vinyasa) to increase the efficacy of the procedure. The three hand positions are

- Palms on your knees as shown in figure 12-6.

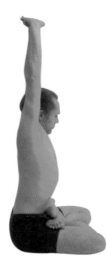

FIGURE 12-7 ◆◆◆

- Arms overhead (you may raise your arms as you are inhaling). (*See figure 12-7*).

  Here your rib cage is moved up, providing more freedom for the abdominal contents to move up and down and hence be massaged better.

- Palms on your shoulder blades with your hands crossed (*see figure 12-8*).

  Here your rib cage is kept up because your arms and your shoulders are locked. Both the air expelled and the movement in the abdominal and pelvic region are enhanced in this position. And kapalabhati is a very invigorating procedure.

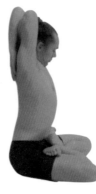

FIGURE 12-8 ◆◆◆

You may do kapalabhati 36 times in each of the three positions to make it a total of 108. It would take about a minute or a little longer to do the procedure. Then keep your eyes closed and watch your breath for about thirty seconds without interfering with your breathing. Your breath may appear suspended for a few moments and slowly your breathing will resume. This is kapalabhati.

SIMPLE PRANAYAMA

A procedure that you may try is ujjayi, or throat breathing. You have used it right through asana vinyasa practice. In pranayama there are four factors:

- Exhalation (*rechaka*)
- Inhalation (*puraka*)
- Holding your breath after inhalation (*ontara kumbhaka*)
- Holding your breath out after exhalation (bahya kumbhaka)

All these are deliberate practices with total focus on your breathing. Pranayama consists of mastery over all these aspects.

If you want to start the practice of pranayama, it will be better to proceed step by step. We have to master all the aspects of pranayama individually and then proceed to do pranayama proper. The vinyasa krama of learning pranayama will be to first practice exhalation. Only when the exhalation is complete and under control, you will be able to purka, or inhalation, well. Patanjali in his treatise gives this order: bahya (breathing out), *abhyantara* (breathing in), and *stambha vritti* (restraint of breath). So, let us start with exhalation.

Exhalation

If exhalation can be improved, the rest can also improve. The first step after doing kapalabhati is to breathe out slowly (ujjayi exhalation) as long and as smoothly as possible. Sometimes it may be useful to make use of sound (not music) or basically mouth a single note while exhaling. You can breathe out making the sound of a bee, a humming sound, which is known as *bhra-* mari. Another useful approach will be to chant "OM" with a throaty sound. OM can be split into A, U, and then Om. First chant "Aaaaaaaaaaaa" as long as possible, making use of the first musical note, "sa," which corresponds to "doe" in the Western system. Chant "Aaaa." Then on the next musical note, "ri," corresponding to the note "ro," chant "Uuuuuuuuuuuuuu" (as in "mood") smoothly and as long as you can. Then chant "OoooooooooooM" (as in "yoke"), breaking open your throat, and on the note "ga," corresponding to Western note "me." While chanting "OM," ensure that you mouth is wide open and no part of your mouth, tongue, teeth, or lips get in the way. According to the ancients, it should merely break open your throat (*kantham bhitwa*). Sometimes we tend to chant "OM" as it sounds in "worm," which should be avoided. Do not try to bring in "effects" such as the sound of a gong, by modulating your voice. Chant the sequence three to six times, and chant "OM" another six times. This will slowly improve the length and quality of your exhalation, which has to be long and smooth. According to many texts, the exhalation should be continuous and uniform like the flow of oil (or honey). Then practice long exhalation the ujjayi way, dispensing with the sound "prop."

Inhalation

Once you are able to empty your lungs well, the "filling" of your lungs, or puraka, becomes much easier and more fruitful. After a complete exhalation, wait for a moment and inhale by the ujjayi method, smoothly and uniformly. The texts give the example of drinking water through a small tube like the stem of a blue lily (*nila utphala nala*). While inhaling, keep your chest muscles relaxed. Gradually, you will feel a healthy, pleasant stretch inside your chest with the whole chest opening out in all directions. After inhalation is complete, hold your breath for a moment consciously, and then slowly exhale. Now the inhalation practice will be coupled with the exhalation practice. Practice several times with total attention on the movement of your breath.

Holding Your Breath After Inhalation

According to patanjali, the next parameter in pranayama will be the holding of your breath after inhalation (*sthamba vritti*). Now, you will start with long exhalation, wait for a moment, inhale as smoothly and as long as possible and then hold your breath for a short period, say three seconds to start with. Repeat this cycle several times for a few days, by which time you will have a good control of all the three aspects of breathing we have so far discussed.

Holding Your Breath Out After Exhalation

This is given as the last aspect of pranayama by Patanjali, who allocates it a separate sutra as *caturta*, or fourth. You may exhale smoothly, then inhale, then hold your breath, then exhale, and hold your breath out for say five seconds for start. This is breath holding after exhalation, also known as *bahya kumbhaka*. This is a very important aspect of pranayama, because it is during this external breath holding that you can effectively and usefully employ the bandhas, the anal lock and the pelvic/abdominal lock.

Having got used to having good control over each aspect of yogic breathing, you are in a position to do pranayama per se. We will

still stick to ujjayi. First do kapalabhati 108 times as detailed earlier. Then make a definite commitment to do a specific number of rounds of pranayama. You must decide beforehand the number of rounds you will do. Often, people start pranayama without any definite plan. One day they may do a few and suddenly end their practice and walk away. Or sometimes if they feel good, they keep on doing it without number. The *Hathayoga Pradipika* clearly says that the yoga practitioner should decide on the type of pranayama (say ujjayi) beforehand, the duration of each aspect of pranayama (say 5, 10, 10, 15 seconds), and the number of times (say 3, 10, or 80).

THE LOCKS (BANDHAS)

During the external holding of your breath (bahya kumbhaka), you may attempt to do anal and abdominal locks. These bandhas are ideally introduced during the practice of pranayama. The complete exhalation facilitates the movement of the pelvic floor and the diaphragm so that the pelvic, abdominal, and thoracic organs can be accessed and gently massaged.

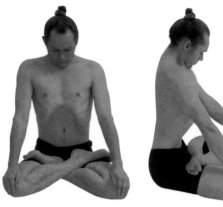

FIGURE 12-9 ◆◆◆   FIGURE 12-10 ◆◆◆

The figures shown give the status of the abdomen while doing the bandhas after exhalation. The three bandhas in the lotus pose are shown here.

Holding of the three bandhas in lotus pose is shown in figure 12-9. The side view is shown in figure 12-10.

The three bandhas in parvatasana, or the hill pose, is shown in figure 12-11.

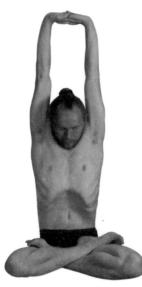

FIGURE 12-11 ◆◆◆

They are shown in the bhadrasana, or auspicious pose, in figure 12-12. The side view is shown in figure 12-13.

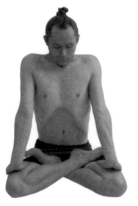
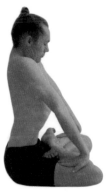

FIGURE 12-12 ◆◆◆   FIGURE 12-13 ◆◆◆

They are shown in gomukhasana, or the cow-head pose in figure 12-14.

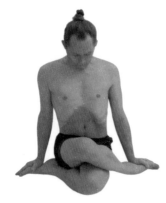

FIGURE 12-14 ◆◆◆

They are shown in vajrasana, or the thunderbolt pose, in figure 12-15. The side view is shown in figure 12-16.

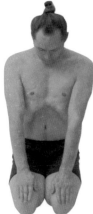

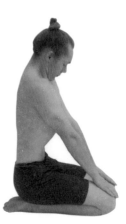

FIGURE 12-15 ◆◆◆   FIGURE 12-16 ◆◆◆

They are shown in virasana, the hero pose, in figure 12-17. The side view is shown in figure 12-18.

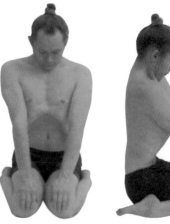 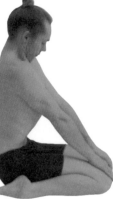

FIGURE 12-17 ◆◆◆   FIGURE 12-18 ◆◆◆

They are shown in siddhasana, the accomplished pose, in figure 12-19.

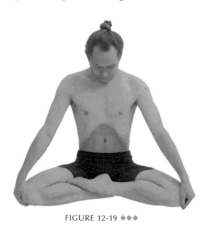

FIGURE 12-19 ◆◆◆

It is good to practice pranayama with the bandhas, or locks, to get the full benefit of vinyasa yoga practice. Following are some closeup views of the bandhas, illustrating standing, crouching, and resting one's hands on one's thighs.

Uddiyana bandha is shown in figures 12-20 and 12-21.

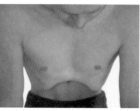

FIGURE 12-20 ◆◆◆

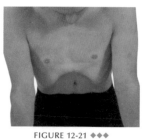

FIGURE 12-21 ◆◆◆

A fuller view is shown in figure 12-22. A straight view is shown in figure 12-23.

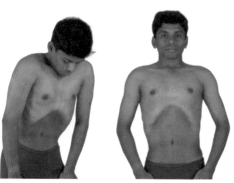

FIGURE 12-22 ◆◆◆   FIGURE 12-23 ◆◆◆

Remaining in this position, you can also do the *nauli kriya*. It is a process by which you are able to isolate and tighten the rectus abdominus, and push back all other muscles and organs backward toward your spine and upwards toward your diaphragm.

Central (*madhya*) nauli is shown in figures 12-24 and 12-25.

The full view is shown in figures 12-26 and 12-27.

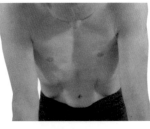

FIGURE 12-24 ◆◆◆◆

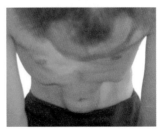

FIGURE 12-25 ◆◆◆◆

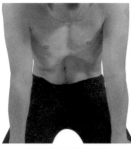

FIGURE 12-28 ◆◆◆◆

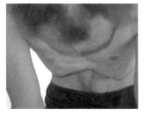

FIGURE 12-29 ◆◆◆◆

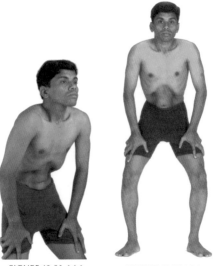

FIGURE 12-26 ◆◆◆   FIGURE 12-27 ◆◆◆

Nauli on the right side (dakshina) is shown in figure 12-28.

Nauli on the left side (vama) is shown in figure 12-29.

We have seen the abdominal exercises that are possible during breath holding after exhalation. These bandhas, kriyas like nauli, and kapalabhati have a tonic effect on the internal organs. Mere asana practice does not give the full, intended benefits of yoga. Yoga is considered a *sarvanga sadhana,* or a science whose practice is beneficial to all parts of the body, including the internal organs. So vinyasa yoga practice will include not only asana vinyasa practice but also a good measure of concentrated pranayama and the use of locks after exhalation.

PRATYAHARA—SEALING THE SENSES (SHANMUKHI MUDRA)

The next step is to closely follow your breath without any distractions from the senses. Closing off all the senses in the face by a special procedure called pratyahara accomplishes this. Here, a particular mudra or "sealing" of sense organs is used to achieve the result. It is known as shanmukhi mudra, or sealing of the six portals (two eyes, two ears, the nose, and the mouth). It is also termed *yoni mudra*, or sealing the "breeding place." This is done after completing pranayama practice. Close your ears with your thumbs; close the tops of your eyelids, above your eyeballs with your index fingers; and close your lids with your middle fingers, kept below your eyeballs. Then close (partially) your nostrils with your ring fingers. Place your little fingers just by either side of your mouth. Keep your elbows stretched out laterally at the level of your shoulders. Keep your back straight, keep your head straight, and closely watch your breath. If your mind wanders, gently coax your mind back to your breath. The position of shanmukhi mudra can be done in any of the main sitting yogic poses after pranayama. The recommended poses are lotus, vajrasana, siddhasana, and virasana. Shanmukhi mudra in vajrasana is shown in figure 12-30.

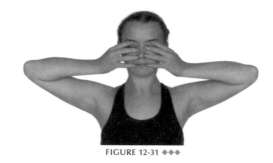

FIGURE 12-31 ◆◆◆

the nostrils. Ring fingers and the little fingers are kept over and below the closed mouth. This procedure also is shanmukhi mudra, a version while seated in lotus pose shown in figure 12-32. A close-up is shown in figure 12-33.

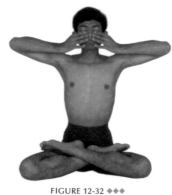

FIGURE 12-32 ◆◆◆

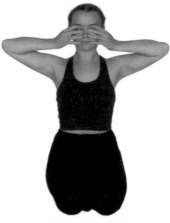

FIGURE 12-30 ◆◆◆

A closeup of the hand and fingers positions is shown in figure 12-31.

Some of the old texts suggest a slightly different position of the fingers. The index finger is kept below the eyeball closing the eyelid. The middle fingers partially close

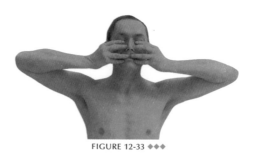

FIGURE 12-33 ◆◆◆

You may stay in shanmukhi mudra for a long time. I suggest at least five minutes. At the end of it, you may review the quality of your observation of your breath. How often did your mind wander? What was the span of attention? The purpose is to reduce the number of distractions every time you practice and also increase the time during which your attention remains on your breath. Slowly and surely both these parameters will improve. You will stay with the breath longer (*ekagra*) and the frequency of your becoming distracted (*vikshepa*) will lessen. You may be able to monitor your own practice of "concentration" quite easily.

After some days or weeks of practice, while in shanmukhi mudra slowly and deliberately direct or focus your attention (with some help from your teacher) on different centers of your body, one at a time. One point of attention is the middle of your eyebrows, which you should look at inwardly, visualizing a bright luminous object like the rising sun. Another object of concentration could be your mantra, which you can repeat while in shanmukhi mudra. Actually this position of your hands helps you to keep your back erect and also your neck straight. An erect back and straight neck are mentioned in the great *Bhagavat Gita* as useful preconditions for *dhyana*, or meditation.

Doing asanas, following strictly the disciplines of *yama* (restraint) and *niyamais* (self-control), is a necessary condition for yoga practice. Classical ashtanga yoga itself can be considered a vinyasa krama. Yama and viyama are the first two vinyasas. Following these, practice of asana by the vinyasa krama method will ensure that there is a perfection of the body position. It will ensure that your body is so well conditioned that you will completely forget the existence of your body when you go to the next vinyasa, which is pranayama. You see, your body will not be another source of distraction. Pranayama helps to remove the dross in the body and the mind. Asana removes the *rajo guna* (energy) and pranayama reduces laziness and the *tamo guna* (mental darkness). Only then does the mind become *satwic* (enlightened and sharp) so that it can refreshingly concentrate on any subtle object it has to contemplate. You could also see that when people practice dhayna, or meditation—except for a blessed few—most have minds that are continually and habitually distracted by unrelated thoughts (*rajas*), or that just fall asleep. So, asana practice and pranayama practice have a definite role to play in the scheme of things in traditional yoga. Then shanmukhi mudra helps to restrain the naturally outgoing senses so they are at rest. We make use of this quality time in shanmukhi mudra to start the internal practice (*antaranga sadhana*).

The repeated attempts to focus on breath or any other object such as a mantra or a yogic spot inside your body will be the next *anga*, or step in ashtanga (vinyasa) yoga. As your mind repeatedly wanders, gently bring it back to the subtle object you are focusing on. Over a period of time, the distracting tendencies will lessen and the focusing tendencies will increase as a result of dharana practice. This will result in the mind being completely focused on the object during the entire duration of your internal practice. It may one day lead you to be with the object you are meditating on, even forgetting yourself completely, which is called *samadhi*, or the final vinyasa of ashtanga yoga.

Many people are happy with asana practice. But even the creator of hatha yoga, Svatmarama, says that his hatha yoga should be considered as a stepping stone to the sublime raja yoga, or yoga of light or enlightenment. So, the internal practices could be the logical next step in the yogi's spiritual progress. Mantra chants, meditation on mantras or sublime thoughts, study and contemplation on spiritual thoughts as contained in texts like the *Yoga Sutras* will be the next step.

One can never get bored with yoga. It is so versatile, so complete. It deals with how to help your body, how to help your mind find happiness and transform itself, to know and understand what "is" and so to know what should be called the Self. The whole philosophy and practice of yoga is developed for the good of each and every individual—so that he or she can find the Self individually, and thereby divine the undercurrent of happiness in all life.

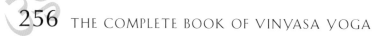

GLOSSARY

ADHO-MUKHA: downward-facing

AKARNA: to the ear

AKUNCHA: contraction or bend

ANA: breath

ANGA: step (or limb)

ANJALI: hands held together as for prayer

ANJALI MUDRA: the gesture of anjali

ANJANEYA: the monkey-god

ANNA KOSA: stomach

ANTARA: internal

ANTARA KUMBHAKA: holding your breath after inhalation

ANTARANGA SADHANA: internal practice (of the mind)

ANULOMA: with the grain, refers to movement or breathing

APANA: pelvis or lower abdomen

APANA VAYU: the neurological force operating on the lower abdomen

APANASANA: pelvic floor poses

ARDHA: half

ASANA: a yogic pose

ASANA SIDDHI: perfection in a yogic pose

ASANA STHITI: the basic or "home" position of an asana

ASHTAVAKRA: the name of a sage with a crooked body

BAHYA: external

BANDHA: lock

BHADRA: peaceful or auspicious

BHAGIRATA: name of a king

BHAIRAVA: an aspect of Shiva

BHANGI: position

BHARADWAJA: name of a Vedic sage

BHERUNDA: name of a yogi

BHRAMARI: making a humming sound (like a wasp) while exhaling

BHUJA: arm

BHUJANGA: cobra

BIJAKSHARA MANTRA: a one-syllable basic mantra

BINDU KOSA: prostate

BRAHMANA KRIYA: expansion, inhalation

CHAKORA: moonbeam bird

CHAKRA: wheel

CHATURA: four

DAKSHINA: right

DANDA SAMARPANA: lying prostrate like a stick.

DANDA: staff or stick

DHANUS: bow

DHYANA: meditation

DURVASA: name of a sage
DWI: two

EKA: one
EKAGRA: one-pointedness of the mind
EKAPADA: one-legged or one-footed

GARBHA KOSA: uterus
GARBHA PINDA: fetus
GARUDA: eagle
GODHA: iguana
GOMUKHA: cow-head
GURUMUKHA: direct from the preceptor

HALA: plough
HANUMAN: a monkey-god, son of Anjaneya
HASTA: hand or arm
HASTASANA: forward stretch of the arms
HRIDAYA KOSA: heart

JALANDHARA BANDHA: the chin lock
JANU: knee
JATARA: belly
JIHVA BANDHA: the tongue lock
JIVANA PRAYATNA: literally, effort of life;
   breathing

KANTHAM BHITWA: opening your throat
   when chanting
KAPALA: skull
KAPALABHATI: bellow-like breathing
KAPOTA: pigeon
KARNAPIDA: blocked ears
KASHYAPA: name of a sage
KAYAKLESA: positions and activities that
   are painful and injurious
KHAGA: bird
KONA: angle
KOSAS: sacs
KRAUNCA: heron

KUKKUTA: rooster
KUMBHAKA: breath holding
KURMA: turtle

LAGHU: simple
LANGHANA KRIYA: literally, activity of
   reduction; exhalation
LAUKIKA MANTRA: chanting the name of a
   deity as part of a non-vedic mantra
LAYA: to merge
LOLA: swing

MADHYA: central
MAHA MUDRA: the great seal
MAHABANDHA: the great lock
MAKARA: crocodile
MALA KOSA: the large intestines
MALA: garland
MANDALA: circular ambulation
MANDUKA: frog
MARICHI: name of a sage
MATSYENDRA: name of a yogi, or kingfish
MAYURA: peacock
MUDRA: seal
MUDRA: seals; also, pleasant gestures
MULA BANDHA: rectal lock
MUTRA KOSA: bladder

NAMASKARA: salutation, greeting
NARA: man
NATARAJA: dancing Shiva
NAULI KRIYA: process of isolating and
   tightening the rectus abdominus, and
   push back all other muscles and organs
   backward toward the spine and upward
   toward the diaphragm
NAVA: boat
NIDRA: sleep
NIRALAMBA: without support
NIYAMAS: self control

NYASAS: association of a particular part of the body with specific deities, mantras, or gestures

PADA: foot or leg
PADA HASTA: hand(s)-to-feet
PADANGUSHTA: big toe
PADMA: lotus
PARIVRITTI: crossed, or with a twist
PARSVA: side
PARSVA VAYU: hemiplegia
PARYANKA: couch
PASA: noose
PASCHIMATANA: back stretch
PAVANAMUKTASANA: wind-release pose
PINCAMAYURA: peacock with stretched-feathers
PLAVANA: jump through
PRAKRITI: nature
PRANASTHANA: the "Place of Breath
PRANASTHANA: the place of breath(pl delete this line, repeated)
PRANAYAMA: yogic breathing
PRASA: assemblage
PRASARANA: sweeping movement of the arms
PRASARITA: spread
PRATIKRIYA: counterpose
PRATYAHARA: the fifth anga of Ashtanga yoga
PRISHTA: back
PRISHTANJALI: back salute
PURAKA: inhalation
PURNA: complete

RAJAKAPOTA: king pigeon
RAJAS: unrelated thoughts; the aspect of energy in nature; one of the three constituents of prakriti
RAJO GUNA: characteristic of activity

RAKTA SANCHARA: blood circulation
RECAKA BALA: the efficacy of exhalation
RECHAKA: exhalation
RICHIKA: name of a sage

SADHANAS: practice for achievement
SAHITA: aided
SALABA: locust
SALAMBA: with support
SAMA: equal or same
SAMADHANA: mental peace
SAMADHI: forgetting oneself completely, but being in the object of meditation while meditating
SAMANTRAKA-SURYANAMASKARA: the sun salutation with mantras
SAMAPATTI: total mental concentration
SAMASTHITI: a state of balance
SARVANGA: all-parts
SARVANGA SADHANA: a science or practice that is beneficial to all parts of the body
SATWIC: the characteristc of light/order; one of three constituents of prakriti
SAVA: corpse
SETHUBANDA: bridge
SHANMUKHI MUDRA: closing of all six ports (or sensory organs)
SIDDHA: accomplished
SIMHA: lion pose
SIRSA: head
SKANDA: a son of Shiva
SRUTI: pitch
STHAMBA VRITTI: holding your breath after inhalation
SUKHA: comfort; literally, agreeable mental space
SUPTA: supine
SWANA: dog
SWASA KOSA: lungs

TADA: straight tree

TADASANA-SAMASTHITI: a state of balance (an even distribution of weight while standing)

TAILA DHARAAVAT: like the flow of oil

TAMO GUNA: characteristic of darkness/heaviness; one of the three constituents of prakriti

TAPA: austerity

TAPASVINS: sages doing penance

TATAKA MUDRA: pond gesture

TIRYANG-MUKHA: backward-facing

TOLANGULASANA: balance pose (tolangin: scales)

TRI: three

TRIKONA: triangle

TRIVIKRAMA: the conqueror of three worlds

UDDIYANA BANDHA: abdominal lock

UJJAYI: slow throat breathing

UPAVISHTA: seated, with legs spread

URDHWA: upward

USHTRA: camel

UTKATA: squat

UTPLUTI: lifting or pumping up

UTTANA: upright

UTTANASANA: forward bend

UTTITA: extended

VAJRA: thunderbolt

VAMA: left

VASETH: to stay put; to remain

VASISHTA: name of a Vedic sage

VATAYANA: horse

VIKSHEPA: distraction

VIMANA: aircraft, or chariot of the gods

VINYASA: variation

VIPARITA: inverted, or upside-down

VIRA: hero

VIRABHADRA: warrior

VRIKSHA: tree

VRISCHIKA: scorpion

VYAYAMA: exercise

YAMA: restraint

YATI: caesura

YOGASANA: yogi posture

YONI MUDRA: sealing "the breeding place"

YUKTI: union

INDEX
OF POSES AND SEQUENCES

THE FIRST FULL, photo-illustrated description of each pose is given here, supplemented where applicable with the location of photos giving another perspective of that same pose, or pages containing variations of the pose.

In all cases, the page numbers of descriptive text are followed by italicized page numbers of its corresponding photographs.